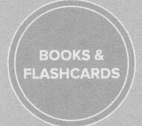
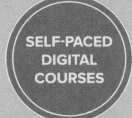
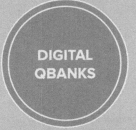
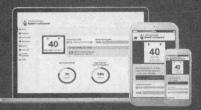

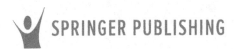

PEDIATRIC NURSING CERTIFICATION EXPRESS REVIEW

PEDIATRIC NURSING CERTIFICATION EXPRESS REVIEW

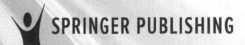

Springer Publishing Company, LLC
11 West 42nd Street, New York, NY 10036
www.springerpub.com

Acquisitions Editor: Elizabeth Nieginski
Compositor: diacriTech

ISBN: 978-0-8261-5853-6
ebook ISBN: 978-0-8261-5854-3
DOI: 10.1891/9780826158543

Printed by BnT

The author and the publisher of this Work have made every effort to use sources believed to be reliable to provide information that is accurate and compatible with the standards generally accepted at the time of publication. The author and publisher shall not be liable for any special, consequential, or exemplary damages resulting, in whole or in part, from the readers' use of, or reliance on, the information contained in this book. The publisher has no responsibility for the persistence or accuracy of URLs for external or third-party Internet websites referred to in this publication and does not guarantee that any content on such websites is, or will remain, accurate or appropriate.

Library of Congress Control Number: 2022904417

Contact sales@springerpub.com to receive discount rates on bulk purchases.

Publisher's Note: **New and used products purchased from third-party sellers are not guaranteed for quality, authenticity, or access to any included digital components.**

Printed in the United States of America.

CONTENTS

PREFACE

If you have purchased this *Express Review*, you are likely well into your exam prep journey to certification. This book was designed to be a high-speed review—a last-minute gut check before your exam day. We created this review, which is a quick summary of the key topics you'll encounter on the exam, to supplement your certification preparation studies. We encourage you to use it in conjunction with other study aids to ensure you are as prepared as possible for the exam.

This book follows the most recent exam content outlines from the PNCB and ANCC, and uses a succinct, bulleted format to highlight what you need to know. The aim of this book is to help you solidify your retention of information in the month or so leading up to your exam. It is written by certified pediatric nurses who are familiar with the exam and the content you need to know. Special features appear throughout the book to call out important information, including:

- **Complications:** Problems that can arise with certain disease states or procedures
- **Nursing Pearls:** Additional patient care insights and strategies for knowledge retention
- **Alerts:** Need-to-know details on how to handle emergency situations or when to transfer care
- **Pop Quizzes:** Critical-thinking questions to test your ability to synthesize what you learned (answers in appendix)
- **List of Abbreviations:** A useful appendix to help guide you through the alphabet soup of clinical terms

We know life is busy. Being able to prepare for your exam efficiently and effectively is paramount, which is why we created this *Express Review*. You have come to the right place as you continue on your path of professional growth and development. The stakes are high, and we want to help you succeed. Best of luck to you on your certification journey. You've got this!

PASS GUARANTEE

If you use this resource to prepare for your exam and you do not pass, you may return it for a refund of your full purchase price. To receive a refund, you must return your product along with a copy of your original receipt and exam score report. Product must be returned and received within 180 days of the original purchase date. Excludes tax, shipping, and handling. One offer per person and address. Refunds will be issued within 8 weeks from acceptance and approval. This offer is valid for U.S. residents only. Void where prohibited. To begin the process, please contact customer service at CS@springerpub.com.

GENERAL EXAMINATION INFORMATION

OVERVIEW

- Congratulations on taking one step closer to becoming a certified pediatric nurse. Included in this chapter is information about the examination for certification as a pediatric nurse through both the PNCB and the ANCC. While the blueprints for both exams differ, this book is organized by organ system, focusing on assessment and diagnosis, health promotion, planning, implementation, management of care, and evaluation, and serves as a review for both exams.

PNCB CERTIFICATION

- The PNCB's CPN® program has met the accreditation standards of the National Commission for Certifying Agencies.
- The eligibility and requirements for certification as a CPN through the PNCB are posted on its website at www.pncb.org.
- Due to information and scheduling processes updating periodically, the best source of information about eligibility, application process, fees, scheduling, test site information, and other details about the exam can be viewed in the *Steps to CPN Certification* page at www.pncb.org/cpn-certification-st eps.

About the Examination

- The exam is based on U.S. standards of practice.
- The exam is 3 hours long and contains 175 multiple-choice questions, including 150 scored and 25 unscored items.
- The three content areas of the exam are Assessment, Health Promotion, and Management.
- The PNCB provides a test blueprint on their website with percentages and resources to help the nurse prepare.
- The nurse has a 90-day window to take the examination after applying.
- Nurses should self-schedule through Prometric, a licensed testing center with multiple locations.

Eligibility

- The nurse must have a current RN license in the United States, Canada, American Samoa, Guam, Northern Mariana Islands, or the U.S. Virgin Islands. The license must be unencumbered, valid, and unrestricted.
- The nurse must also report a minimum of either of the following:
  - 1,800 hours as an RN with pediatric clinical experience within the past 2 years
  - 5 years of pediatric RN experience and 3,000 pediatric nursing hours within the last 5 years, provided that at least 1,000 hours are within the past 2 years

How to Apply

- Applications to take the certification exam are accepted online through the PNCB website after making an account.
- See the PNCB website for No Pass, No Pay eligibility.
- Members of the Society of Pediatric Nurses receive a discount on the initial exam fee.
- A special accommodations form may be submitted if requesting special accommodations under ADA.

How to Recertify

- Once certified as a CPN, recertification through PNCB is required annually between November 1 and January 31 each year.
- The fee to recertify is between $65 and $85, depending on the date of recertification. See www.pncb. org/cpn-recertification for current pricing.
- The nurse must maintain a current, active, unencumbered license to recertify.
- To recertify, 15 hours of documented completed activity is required. Examples of accepted activity hours include contact hours, clinical practice, professional practice learning, or academic credit.

How to Contact PNCB

Website: www.pncb.org/contact-us
Phone: 301-330-2921
Toll-free number: 1-888-641-2767
Fax: 301-330-1504
Pediatric Nursing Certification Board
9605 Medical Center Drive, Suite 250
Rockville, MD 20850

ANCC CERTIFICATION

- The ANCC's Pediatric Nursing (PED-BC™) board certification exam is a competency-based exam that provides an assessment of clinical knowledge and skills of pediatric nurses.
- The ANCC Pediatric Nurse board certification is valid for 5 years and is accredited by the Accreditation Board for Specialty Nursing Certification.
- You can review the website, www.nursingworld.org/our-certifications/pediatric-nurse/, which provides information about eligibility, the application process, fees, scheduling, testing site information, and other pertinent information. This information changes from time to time; therefore, the ANCC website is the most reliable resource for these details.

About the Examination

- This computer-based examination contains 150 questions, including 125 scored and 25 unscored items.
- ANCC provides a test blueprint with an explanation of examination content on their website.
- The nurse has a 90-day window to take the examination after applying.
- Testing can be done at a Prometric Testing Center or via live remote proctoring.
- For details and procedural steps to request accommodations for testing, review the instructions in the testing handbook.

Eligibility

- The nurse must have a current, active RN license in the United States. Visit the ANCC website for eligibility for candidates outside of the United States.
- The nurse must have completed 2 years of full-time practice as an RN.
- The nurse must have recorded a minimum of 2,000 hours of clinical practice in pediatric nursing within the last 3 years.
- The nurse must have completed 30 hours of continuing education in pediatric nursing within the last 3 years.

How to Apply
- Applications to take the certification exam are accepted online.
- Members of the American Nurses Association receive a discounted testing price.

How to Recertify
- Once certified, recertification through ANCC is required every 5 years. A renewal application must be submitted and can be submitted up to 1 year prior to renewal.
- A renewal fee is required. See www.nursingworld.org/our-certifications/pediatric-nurse/ for current pricing.
- The nurse must maintain a current, active, unencumbered license to recertify.
- To recertify, completion of at least 75 continuing education hours is required in the pediatric nursing specialty, plus an eligible activity in at least one of the following categories:
  - Academic credits
  - Presentations
  - Evidence-based practice, quality improvement project, publication, or research
  - Preceptor hours
  - Professional service
  - Practice hours
  - Assessment

How to Contact ANCC
Website: www.nursingworld.org/our-certifications/
Email: aprnvalidation@ana.org
Toll-free number: 1-800-284-2378
ANCC Certification Registration
8515 Georgia Ave, Suite 400
Silver Spring, MD 20910

RESOURCES

Pediatric Nursing Certification Board. (2021, November). *PNCB exam candidate handbook.* https://www.pncb.org/sites/default/files/resources/PNCB_Exam_Candidate_Handbook.pdf

Pediatric Nursing Certification Board. (n.d.[a]). *CPN recertification.* https://www.pncb.org/cpn-recertification

Pediatric Nursing Certification Board. (n.d.[b]). *Recertification: A guide for maintaining your credential.* https://www.pncb.org/sites/default/files/resources/CPN_Recert_Guide.pdf

Pediatric Nursing Certification Board. (n.d.[c]). *Steps to CPN certification.* https://www.pncb.org/cpn-certification-steps

2

GROWTH AND DEVELOPMENT

DEVELOPMENTAL STAGES

DEVELOPMENTAL STAGES

Overview

- *Growth* is an increase in size and weight.
  - Linear growth reflects skeletal growth.
  - Weight correlates with nutritional status and fluid balance.
  - Head circumference is associated with brain growth.
- *Development* is a process of continuous change and advancement.
- Development includes:
  - Expanding abilities and skills through social maturation
  - Increasingly complex thoughts and behaviors
- Patterns of growth and development include:
  - Cephalocaudal: growth from head to toe
  - Proximodistal: growth from near to far or from midline trunk to distal tips of extremities
  - Differentiation: development from general to specific or from simple to more complex functions
- *Chronologic age* is months or years since birth.
- *Mental age* is the level of cognitive function.
- *Corrected age*, or *adjusted age*, is the chronologic age reduced by the number of weeks born prematurely.
  - *Prematurity* is birth before 40 weeks gestation.
  - Corrected gestational age is used to evaluate milestones for infants born prematurely until they are 2 years old.
- Developmental age periods and stages include:
  - Infancy
  - Toddler
  - Preschooler
  - School-age
  - Adolescence

 POP QUIZ 2.1

An infant was born 6 months ago at 28 weeks gestation. What is the infant's corrected age?

Infancy

- *Infancy* encompasses birth to 12 months.
- Within this period, birth to 28 days is considered the *neonatal period*.
- Infancy is characterized by rapid motor, cognitive, and social development.
- The infant is completely dependent on family.

Physical Assessment
- The expected vital signs are:
  - Temperature: 97.7 °F to 98.6 °F (36.5 °C–37 °C), recommended axillary or rectal routes
  - Heart rate: 100 to 180 beats/min

(continued)

Physical Assessment (continued)
- Respiratory rate: 30 to 57 breaths/min
- Blood pressure: 72 to 104 mmHg/37 to 56 mmHg
- Birth weight:
  - Up to 10% of birth weight is expected to be lost by 4 days old, but this weight should be regained by 2 weeks old.
  - Birth weight should double by 6 months and triple by 12 months.
- Growth:
  - Birth length increases by 50% by 12 months.
  - Length increases by about 1 in. per month for the first 6 months of infancy.
  - Weight increases by about 1.5 lb. per month for the first 5 months of infancy.
- Posterior fontanel closes by 2 months.
- Pulses are expected to be +2 and equal bilaterally.
  - Assess upper extremity pulses at the radial and brachial arteries.
  - Evaluate lower extremity pulses at the dorsalis pedis, posterior tibial, and femoral arteries.
  - Start assessment at the most distal pulse and work toward the heart if the more distal pulse is not +2.
- Teeth start to erupt between 6 and 10 months; six to eight teeth are present by 1 year. Indications of teething include drooling, biting on fingers and toys, and irritability.
- Several primitive reflexes are expected during infancy (Table 2.1).

Table 2.1 Primitive Reflexes

Reflex	Age	Elicit By	Expected Infant Response
Stepping	Birth to 4 weeks	Holding infants upright with their feet touching a flat surface	Infant responds by making stepping movements.
Palmar grasp	Birth to 4 months	Placing an object in the infant's palm	Infant responds by grasping the object.
Rooting	Birth to 4 months	Touching infant's cheek	Infant responds by turning head toward the touch and making sucking movements.
Sucking	Birth to 4 months	Touching the roof of the mouth	Infant responds by making sucking movements with mouth.
Tonic neck	Birth to 4 months	Turning the infant's head to one side	Infant responds by extending the arm and leg on that side and flexing the arm and leg on the opposite side.
Moro (startle reflex)	Birth to 6 months	Startling infants or causing a sudden change in their balance	Infant responds by abducting their arms out to the side and then drawing their arms inward toward body.
Plantar grasp	Birth to 8 months	Touching the soles of the infant's feet	Infant responds by turning their toes downward.
Babinski	Birth to 1 year	Stroking the outer edge of an infant's foot upward from heel to toes	Infant responds by their toes fanning upward and out.

Source: Data from Hockenberry, M., Wilson, D., & Rodgers, C. (2017). *Wong's essentials of pediatric nursing.* Elsevier.

Health Promotion

- Car seat safety
  - Avoid airbag injury and other injuries, such as SCWOARA, by using a rear-facing car seat that is placed in the back seat.
  - Ensure the shoulder harness is at or below the level of the infant's shoulders.
  - Only use a federally approved car seat and check the expiration date.
  - Do not leave infant alone in vehicle.
- Dental health
  - Avoiding milk or juice bottles while infants are falling asleep can markedly decrease dental caries.
  - Prevent propping bottle during feedings to avoid aspiration of formula, middle ear infections, and pooling of formula or juice that can lead to dental caries.
- Infant bonding
  - Breastfeeding is an essential element of maternal–infant bonding.
  - Cuddling and holding infants will help them feel secure and promote trust.
  - Kangaroo care, or skin-to-skin contact, encourages touch for parents with infants and has benefits for premature and full-term infants, including:
    - ○ Decreased crying, increased sleep time, and increased weight gain for infants
    - ○ Improved breathing patterns, oxygenation levels, and stabilized heart rate for infants
    - ○ Increased bonding and confidence caring for infant by family members
    - ○ Increased milk supply for mothers and improved breastfeeding sessions
  - Reading, singing, and mimicking baby's sounds helps to promote communication.
- Nutrition
  - Breastfeeding (human milk) is the optimal option for infant nutrition.
    - ○ Human milk is biologically active and benefits the infant in several ways.
      - Antimicrobial agents help decrease the risk of acute illness, such as upper respiratory infections and ear infections.
      - GI-developing factors stimulate growth, motility, and maturation of the intestines.
      - The immune system is stronger in breastfed infants, and breast milk provides immunomodulatory factors that help prevent NEC, a common diagnosis in the NICU.
      - Breastfed infants have less illness overall, fewer hospitalizations, and a lower rate of SIDS.
    - ○ Breast milk fat contents include lipids, triglycerides, and cholesterol that are necessary for optimal growth.
    - ○ Encourage exclusive breastfeeding for the first 6 months with continuation until 1 year or longer as able or desired. WHO recommends breastfeeding until 2 years old.
    - ○ Through skin-to-skin contact, breastfeeding can enhance neurodevelopment.
    - ○ Give all breastfed infants a vitamin D supplement.
  - Iron-fortified formula is the only recommended alternative to breast milk.
    - ○ Formulas are available in ready-to-feed, concentrated liquid, and powder.
    - ○ The difference in formulas is primarily the source of protein.
      - Amino acid
      - Soy
      - Whey
    - ○ Advise family that nondairy or plant-based alternatives such as soy milk are not recommended for infants.
    - ○ Do not give cow's milk to children under 1 year old because cow's milk does not provide enough iron and has too much protein, sodium, and potassium.
    - ○ Fruit juice is not recommended for children under 1 year of age.
    - ○ Introduce iron-fortified cereals for infants over 6 months old.
  - Solid foods
    - ○ Solid foods can be introduced at 6 months of age.
    - ○ Developmental signs that infants are ready for solid foods are that they can sit without support, have good head control, and they open their mouth when food is offered.

 ALERT!

Many foods can be a choking risk to infants. Avoid feeding infants nuts, peanuts, grapes, and raw carrots. Cut food into small pieces.

(continued)

Health Promotion (continued)

- ○ New foods should be introduced one at a time over a period of 5 to 7 days to monitor and watch for allergies or intolerances.
- ○ Offer and expose infants to a wide variety of healthy foods and textures over time.
- Teach family to never give honey to infants due to the risk of botulism.
  - ○ *Clostridium botulinum* spores cause botulism poisoning. Spores can be ingested from environmental dust or soil and raw honey.
  - ○ Clinical characteristics of botulism include weakness, feeding difficulties, hypotonia, and a weak cry. The infection can be life threatening and may require a prolonged hospital stay.
  - ○ Diagnosis of botulism includes stool toxin detection.
  - ○ Treatment of botulism includes botulism immunoglobin known as BIG-IV or BabyBIG and should be implemented as the treatment plan as early as possible.
- Safe sleep
  - Infants at age 4 to 12 months should get 12 to 16 hours of sleep per day. Infants at age 12 months old should be sleeping through the night and also take one to two naps per day.
  - It is acceptable to share the bedroom with the infant but avoid co-sleeping.
  - Offer pacifier during naps and bedtime.
  - Place infants on their backs to sleep using a firm sleep surface with tightly fitted sheets to prevent SIDS. (See Chapter 16 for more information about SIDS.)
  - Remove pillows, extra blankets, crib bumpers, and stuffed animals from cribs.
- Safety
  - Avoid screen time for infants.
  - Avoid secondhand smoke.
  - Never shake a baby. Their neck muscles cannot yet support their heads, and shaking can cause brain damage or abusive head trauma also known as Shaken Baby Syndrome.
  - Prevent choking by cutting food into small pieces when infants start to eat solids.
  - Prevent choking by not allowing infants to play with small toys, objects, or other choking hazards.
  - To protect skin from sun, keep infant in shade or add protective clothing such as hats. Sunscreen should be applied if at least 6 months old.
- Treat teething pain with a combination of pharmacologic and nonpharmacologic methods.
  - Consider a dose of acetaminophen if irritability interrupts sleeping and feeding.
  - Offer frozen teething rings when the infant is awake and playing.

Nursing Interventions

- Create a warm, quiet environment and comfort infants with swaddles and soft voices.
- Distract infants during procedures with rattles or brightly colored toys. Child life specialists can be consulted and utilized during procedures.
- Educate family on health promotion topics and expected growth trends. New or first-time parents may need more guidance.
- Educate family about medications and other substances that may cross into the breast milk. Breastfeeding mothers should check with their physicians prior to taking any supplements or medications.
- Evaluate family's understanding of health promotion topics, car seat safety, nutrition, safe sleeping, and other safety measures.
- Interact with infants using age-appropriate play, which includes rattles, teething toys, reading books out loud, and mirrors.
- Notify provider of any abnormal vital signs, abnormal reflexes, or physical assessment findings, such as cleft palate, jaundice, murmur, hip clicks, or any other suspected congenital anomalies.
- Promote daily tummy time and position changes in hospitalized patients to prevent plagiocephaly.
  - *Plagiocephaly* is a flat spot on back or side of head.
  - Some infants with plagiocephaly need to wear a helmet to help mold the head shape.
- Use containment and maintain warmth when performing physical assessments.
  - Observe the infant and perform inspection first to not disturb infant.

- Auscultate lungs, heart, and abdomen while the infant is quiet and calm.
- Provide a warm and nonstimulating environment for assessment.
- Undress only necessary body area for assessment to maintain warmth and prevent heat loss.
- Test reflexes last.

ALERT!

When performing pediatric physical assessments and procedures, leave the most invasive procedures for last. For example, when taking vital signs, observe and count respirations first and take an axillary temperature last.

Toddler

- The toddler age group is from 1 to 3 years old.
- Toddlers learn by exploring their environment and continue to have rapid physical, motor, and language development.

Physical Assessment

- Expected vital signs:
  - Temperature: 97.8 °F to 98.9 °F (36.6 °C–37.2 °C)
  - Heart rate: 80 to 140 beats/min
  - Respiratory rate: 22 to 46 breaths/min
  - Blood pressure: 86 to 106 mmHg/42 to 63 mmHg

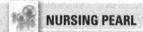

NURSING PEARL

To estimate how tall the child will be as an adult, double the child's height at age 2 years.

- Physical findings:
  - Anterior fontanel closes by 18 months.
  - Gait will have a bowlegged appearance.
  - Growth for toddlers:
    - Weight increases by about 4 to 6 lb. per year.
    - Height increases by about 3 in. per year.
  - Head circumference and chest circumference are equal by 2 years old.
- Language development is usually as follows:
  - 1 year old: using one-word sentences
  - 2 years old: using two-to-three-word sentences
  - 3 years old: combining three to four words to create simple sentences
- Toilet training can begin when the child expresses physical, mental, and psychological readiness:
  - Has voluntary control and ability to stay dry at least 2 hours, or wakes from a nap dry
  - Recognizes the urge to urinate or defecate and is able to communicate needs

Health Promotion

- Educate family on the benefits of creating routines for toddlers for mealtimes and bedtimes.
- Play and therapeutic play can be used to help children cope with fears and express feelings. Child life specialists can assist with play and distraction.
- Play provides distraction.
- Play helps child feel more comfortable in their environment.
- Play can help relieve separation anxiety.
- Environmental safety
  - Cover electrical outlets to prevent burns.
  - Keep small objects such as candy, coins, batteries, or magnets out of reach to avoid the risk of aspiration or choking.
  - Place candles, pot handles, electrical cords, and lighters out of reach to prevent burns.
  - Place safety gates at top and bottom of stairs to prevent falls.
  - Secure cabinets that contain chemicals, cleaners, or medications with safety locks.

(continued)

Health Promotion (continued)

- Supervise children when they are near bathtubs, pools, and bodies of water to prevent accidental drowning.
- Nutrition
  - Avoid using food for reward or punishment:
    - Early development of healthy eating habits can have a positive influence on overall health and decreases chronic diseases such as obesity, cardiovascular disease, and diabetes.
    - Using food, especially unhealthy snacks, for rewards can cause the toddler to overeat for nonnutritional reasons.
  - Limit fruit juice to 4 oz per day and avoid sugary nonnutritive drinks such as sports drinks and soda.
  - Offer toddlers between the ages of 1 to 2 years vitamin D supplemented whole milk rather than reduced fat alternatives.
    - Milk provides protein, calcium, and vitamins A and D.
    - The recommended consumption is two 8 oz cups per day.
    - Children over 2 years old may have low-fat milk.
  - Remember that toddlers are generally picky eaters.
    - Offer a variety of healthy foods and allow them to select.
    - Provide frequent opportunities to try new foods, but do not force or pressure toddlers to eat new foods.
    - Recognize that it may take 8 to 10 times to accept a new food.
  - Schedule meal and snack times.
    - Have child sit in highchair or booster seat.
    - Serve food in small portions and cut food into small pieces.
    - To prevent choking, encourage toddler to sit and chew food thoroughly.
- Safety and health
  - Assist with and encourage brushing teeth and flossing. Toddlers should start having regular dental check-ups.
  - Screen time is not recommended for children younger than 18 months old.
  - Sunscreen should be applied when outside to protect skin.
  - Toddlers sleep 11 to 12 hours per day on average, including one nap. It is important to maintain a regular bedtime schedule and routine.
- Vehicle safety
  - Do not leave toddler alone in a vehicle.
  - Use appropriate car seat for child's age, weight, and height.
    - Keep toddlers in rear-facing car seats until age 3 or until they meet the maximum weight and height requirements.
    - Transition to a forward-facing car seat when children outgrow their rear-facing car seat.

POP QUIZ 2.2

Parents bring their 18-month-old boy in for a well-baby visit, state they think he is getting big for his car seat, and ask if they can stop using it soon. What is the most appropriate response?

Nursing Interventions

Nursing interventions are similar for toddlers and preschoolers. See Preschooler section for specific nursing interventions.

Preschooler

- The preschooler age group is from 3 to 6 years old.
- During the preschool age, the rate of physical growth and language development slows and stabilizes.

Physical Assessment

- Expected vital signs:
  - Temperature: 97.8 °F to 98.9 °F (36.6 °C–37.2 °C)

- Heart rate: 65 to 120 beats/min
- Respiratory rate: 20 to 29 breaths/min
- Blood pressure: 89 to 112 mmHg/46 to 72 mmHg
- Growth for preschoolers:
  - Weight increases by about 4.5 to 6.5 lb. per year.
  - Height increases by about 2.4 to 3.5 in. per year.
- Language development is usually as follows:
  - Children ages 4 to 5 years old combine four to five words to create sentences.
  - Language is a preschooler's primary method of communication.
- Most often, all deciduous teeth have erupted by preschool age.

Health Promotion

- Encourage preschoolers' development through age-appropriate play, which includes playing with balls, puzzles, painting, and playing dress-up.
- Play and therapeutic play can be used to help children cope with fears and express feelings. Child life specialists can assist with developmental play, coping, and distraction.
  - Play provides distraction.
  - Play helps a child feel more comfortable in their environment.
  - Play can help relieve separation anxiety.
- Environmental safety
  - Cover electrical outlets to prevent burns.
  - Keep small objects such as candy, coins, batteries, or magnets out of reach to avoid the risk of aspiration or choking.
  - Place candles, pot handles, electrical cords, and lighters out of reach to prevent burns.
  - Secure cabinets that contain chemicals, cleaners, or medications with safety locks.
  - Supervise children when they are near bathtubs, pools, and bodies of water to prevent accidental drowning.
- Nutrition
  - Avoid using food for reward or punishment.
  - Avoid sugary nonnutritive drinks such as sports drinks and soda.
  - Preschoolers are recommended to have five servings of fruits and vegetables per day.
  - Schedule meal and snack times.
- Safety and health
  - Assist with and encourage brushing teeth and flossing. Preschoolers should continue to have regular dental check-ups.
  - Preschoolers should have 2 hours or less of screen time per day.
  - Sunscreen should be applied when outside to protect skin.
- Vehicle safety
  - Do not leave preschoolers alone in a vehicle.
  - Encourage wearing helmets when riding tricycles or scooters to prevent head trauma.
  - Teach preschool-aged children to look both ways before crossing the street.
  - Use appropriate car seat for child's age, weight, and height. Use a forward-facing car seat with harness until at least age 5 or until they reach the maximum weight and height requirements. Then, they can move into a booster seat in the back seat.

Nursing Interventions

The following are nursing interventions for toddlers and preschoolers.

- Allow children to touch equipment when it is safe and appropriate to do so to help become comfortable with new equipment.
- Avoid using figures of speech because the child may interpret what is said literally. For example, during the process of a hospital admission, if a child hears that they are "being taken to the floor" they may interpret this literally and think they will be taken out of bed and placed on the floor of the room, rather than what was intended, which is moving them to a room on a specialized floor or unit.
- Distract toddlers during procedures by reading a book or blowing bubbles.

(continued)

Nursing Interventions (continued)
- Encourage children to sit on a family member's lap during procedures, exams, and physical assessments.
- Give the child choices during assessment, such as which arm to look at first.
- Interact with toddlers using age-appropriate play, which includes blocks, push-pull toys, and finger painting. Interact with preschoolers using age-appropriate play, which includes playing with balls, puzzles, painting, and playing dress-up.
- Length should be assessed using recumbent position using a length board until children are 2 years old or until they are able to stand alone, then height can be measured using a stadiometer.
- Monitor for signs of regression, especially during hospitalizations or stressful situations.
- Notify provider of any missed milestones or abnormal vital sign values.
- Use direct and concrete language when communicating with toddler and preschooler.
  - Tell them how or what they will feel; do not lie to children by telling them something will not hurt when it will.
  - Temper tantrums are common for toddlers. Use consistent and age-appropriate expectations to help promote independence and prevent their frustrations.

School Age
- The school-age period of development includes children 6 to 12 years old.
- During these years, children attend a school environment or begin a more formal education. This is a period of gradual growth, both physically and emotionally.
- School age children progressively become more complex in their ability to communicate and create social relationships.

Physical Assessment
- Expected vital signs for school age children include:
  - Temperature:
    - 7 years old: 98.2 °F (36.8 °C)
    - 9 years old: 98 °F (36.7 °C)
    - 11 years old: 98 °F (36.7 °C)
  - Heart rate: 70 to 110 beats/min
  - Respiratory rate: 16 to 24 breaths/min
  - Blood pressure:
    - 6 to 9 years old: 97 to 115 mmHg/57 to 76 mmHg
    - 10 to 12 years old: 102 to 120 mmHg/61 to 80 mmHg
- Caloric needs are less for school age children than preschool age and adolescent age groups.
- Gait becomes steady.
- Growth slows down.
  - Weight increases by about 4.4 to 6.6 lb. per year.
  - Height increases by about 2 in. per year.
- First permanent teeth erupt around 6 years old.
  - By age 13, most permanent teeth will be in place.
  - First molars erupt at 6 to 7 years old.
  - Second molars erupt at 11 to 12 years old.
- On average, puberty begins at age 10 for females and age 12 for males.

Health Promotion
- Dental care
  - Fluoride supplements may be recommended by pediatrician or dentist if the level of fluoride in local tap water is not enough to prevent cavities.
  - Remind school age children to brush their teeth after meals, snacks, and at bedtime, and to floss daily.
  - School age children should continue to have regular dental check-ups.

- Environmental safety
  - Advise children and family to use sunscreen when outside to protect skin.
  - Educate family about car safety.
    - ○ Remember to use an approved car restraint system, or booster seat, until children reach 4 ft. 9 in. and are big enough to use a seat belt properly.
    - ○ Until age 13, children should sit in the back seat, and they should always be wearing a seat belt.
  - Teach children cooking safety precautions to prevent burns and fires.
- Nutrition
  - Discuss risk factors for eating disorders and provide resources if appropriate.
  - Encourage children to eat nutritious snacks rather than sugary snacks and to avoid frequently eating fast food.
  - Emphasize that skipping meals should be avoided.
  - Focus on teaching positive aspects of healthy choices, not just the effects of unhealthy eating.
- Physical activity
  - Encourage 1 hour or more of physical activity per day.
    - ○ Many children in this age group play organized team sports.
    - ○ Physical activity in school age children is linked to improved cognition and a decrease in depression symptoms.
  - Remind family that children should wear proper safety equipment and helmets when doing activities.
  - Set limits on amount of screen time allowed per day and set parental controls to restrict viewing inappropriate content.
  - Stress that children need to be supervised when swimming or around bodies of water.
- Psychosocial issues
  - Encourage peer relationships and participation in group activities or team sports.
  - Promote positive body image.
  - Teach school-age children about substance misuse.
  - Teach children about available resources related to bullying.

Nursing Interventions

- Demonstrate and explain nursing equipment before using it. School age children are interested in the functionality of equipment, how it works, and why and how it is being used.
- Distract children with small talk or counting down until end of the procedure.
- During hospitalizations, establish a daily routine including procedures, medications, meals, activities, therapies, television time, and bedtimes. Play and therapeutic play can be used to help children cope with fears and express feelings related to hospitalization and procedures.
- Educate and answer questions about puberty and body changes.
- Incorporate health screenings into the plan of care.
  - Hearing screenings should be conducted at school entry and at ages 6, 8, and 10 years old.
  - Many schools also offer vision screenings.
  - Family should be educated on following up with any necessary specialists, such as audiologists, ophthalmologists, and optometrists, for any necessary interventions or further assessments.
- Initiate scoliosis screening for school-age children by examining for lateral curvature of the spine.
- Notify provider of concerns for scoliosis, substance abuse, mental health issues, or eating disorders or abnormal vital sign values.
- Relate to school-age children using age-appropriate activities which include board games, jump rope, riding bicycles, crafts, and organized sports.

Adolescence

- Adolescence is the period between childhood and adulthood.
- Adolescent children have rapid physical, cognitive, social, and emotional growth.
- The developmental period spans from ages 12 to 20.

Physical Assessment

- Expected vital signs for this age group include:
  - Temperature: 97.8 °F (36.6 °C)
  - Heart rate: 60 to 100 beats/min
  - Respiratory rate: 12 to 22 breaths/min
  - Blood pressure:
    - ○ 12 to 15 years old: 110 to 131 mmHg/64 to 83 mmHg
    - ○ 16 years old: 108 to 145 mmHg/63 to 94 mmHg
- Growth stops during adolescence.
  - Females stop growing about 2 to 2.5 years after the onset of menarche.
  - Males usually stop growing between 18 to 20 years old.
- Puberty is the beginning of physical change and the development of secondary sex characteristics.
  - Tanner staging or sexual maturity rating describes the sequence of secondary sex characteristics of adolescents through puberty (Figures 2.1 and 2.2).
  - Female sexual maturation occurs in order of:
    - ○ Breast development
    - ○ Pubic hair growth
    - ○ Axillary hair growth
    - ○ Menstruation
  - Male sexual maturation occurs in order of:
    - ○ Testicular enlargement
    - ○ Pubic hair growth
    - ○ Penile enlargement
    - ○ Axillary hair growth

Stage I

Stage II

Stage III

Stage IV

Stage V

Stage I

Stage II

Stage III

Stage IV

Stage V

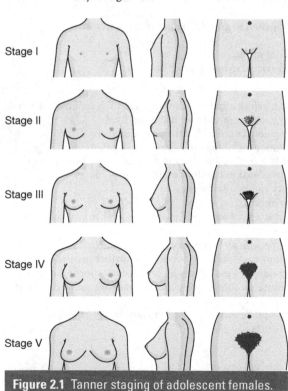

Figure 2.1 Tanner staging of adolescent females.

Source: From Ruggiero, K., & Ruggiero, M. (2020). *Fast facts handbook for pediatric primary care: A guide for nurse practitioners and physician assistants.* Springer Publishing Company.

Figure 2.2 Tanner staging of adolescent males.

Source: From Ruggiero, K., & Ruggiero, M. (2020). *Fast facts handbook for pediatric primary care: A guide for nurse practitioners and physician assistants.* Springer Publishing Company.

- ○ Facial hair growth
- ○ Vocal changes
- Wisdom teeth, or third molars, may start to emerge at 17 years old.

Health Promotion
- Environmental safety
  - Avoid tanning beds and wear sunscreen to prevent sunburns.
  - Keep guns and medications in a locked cabinet to prevent self-harm.
- Nutrition
  - Encourage healthy food choices for meals and snacks.
  - Monitor for signs of overeating, restrictive eating, and excessive exercise (see Eating Disorders in Chapter 15).
  - Provide support for patients seeking treatment or therapy for eating disorders.
- Physical activity
  - Educate on how to prevent sports-related injuries, such as wearing protective equipment properly, proper stretching and warm ups, and avoiding over-training.
  - Encourage at least 60 minutes of physical activity per day. Physical activity should be moderate to vigorous and include aerobic activity, muscle-strengthening activity, and bone-strengthening activity.
  - Provide education on stress and competition for adolescents that play on sports teams.
- Psychosocial issues
  - Demonstrate a nonjudgmental attitude to enhance the likelihood of adolescent asking questions regarding psychosocial issues.
  - Discuss online safety and cyber bullying.
  - Present accurate information on sexual health and preventing and screening for STIs.
  - Provide information on reproductive health, pregnancy, and effective contraception methods.
  - Offer support for bullying, depression, and suicidal thoughts.
  - Screen female patients for signs of pregnancy.
  - Teach risks and dangers of substance use and abuse. Discuss substance use and abuse including e-cigarettes.
- Vehicle safety
  - Educate on not getting into a car with an impaired driver.
  - Encourage seat belt use.
  - Discuss dangers of cell phone use and substance use while driving.
  - Support attendance of driver's education courses.

Nursing Interventions
- Assess for risk-taking behaviors such as substance abuse, self-harm, and sexual activity.
- During hospitalizations, modify nursing care to support the adolescent.
  - Encourage group activities and socialization if stable enough.
  - Provide flexible routines and activities.
  - Encourage adolescents to take an active role in their care.
- Educate adolescents by providing age-appropriate verbal and written explanations of procedures and diagnoses.
- Notify provider of concerns for substance abuse, mental health issues, or eating disorders.
- Remember that age-appropriate activities include sports, nonviolent video games, reading, social interaction, and social media.
- Respect the need for privacy and independence.

ERIKSON'S PSYCHOSOCIAL STAGES OF DEVELOPMENT

Overview
- Erikson's psychosocial stages of development is a theory developed to explain psychosocial and personality development.

Overview *(continued)*

- Each stage is based on a conflict between a favorable or positive component and an unfavorable or negative component.
- The stages are aligned with the developmental age periods.

Stages

- Trust versus mistrust (birth to 1 year old)
  - Infants develop trust through their family providing stability, consistency, loving care, and meeting their basic needs. Family can promote healthy development through trust by responding when an infant cries and providing consistent affection, attention, comfort, and basic needs such as feeding.
  - Mistrust develops when trust-promoting experiences are inconsistent, unreliable, or inadequate.
  - The infant's temperament is developed and displayed through trust or mistrust.
  - Successful completion of this stage results in hope.
- Autonomy versus shame and doubt (1–3 years old)
  - Children develop autonomy through controlling themselves and their environment.
    - Autonomy is developed by family supporting and encouraging independence and providing ritualism.
    - Toddlers want to display their newly acquired motor and mental skills by doing things independently.
  - Feelings of shame and doubt develop when children are made to feel self-conscious, when others shame them, or when skills are done for them.
  - Family should avoid reacting negatively or punishing children for mistakes.
  - Positive resolution of this stage results in positive self-esteem and willpower.
- Initiative versus guilt (3–6 years old)
  - Children take initiative and pursue activities and play that give them satisfaction.
  - During this stage, children develop a conscience.
  - Feelings of guilt surface if their actions do not align with expectations of family.
  - To develop initiative, offer explanations, encourage imagination, and allow initiation of activities.
  - Family should encourage children to make good choices and encourage using their imagination during play.
  - Positive resolution of this stage results in a sense of purpose.
- Industry versus inferiority (6–12 years old)
  - Children engage in tasks and activities that can show achievement.
    - They start to have an interest in hobbies.
    - They learn to compete, cooperate, and form social relationships with others and seek approval from peers.
  - Promote healthy development by supporting and encouraging independence while providing guidance and supervision.
  - Support the development of self-esteem by setting reasonable expectations and giving praise for accomplishments.
  - An inferiority complex develops if children do not feel confident in their abilities or if they believe that too much is expected of them.
- Identity versus role confusion (12–18 years old)
  - Adolescents search for purpose and self-identity; they develop a sense of their role in society and think about their future and career.
  - During this stage, adolescents value peers' opinions and place value in how others perceive them.
  - Family can encourage adolescents to identify their own values and passions to help identify their own identity.
  - Successful resolution of this stage results in fidelity.

POP QUIZ 2.3

An infant's parent provides care by feeding on a reliable schedule and providing comfort every time the infant cries. Which of Erikson's psychosocial stages is the parent nurturing the infant to develop?

PIAGET'S THEORY OF COGNITIVE DEVELOPMENT

Overview

- Piaget's theory of cognitive development is a theory developed to understand the way children think and how they develop intellectually.
- The theory presents children's cognitive development as a continuous process through four stages, and each stage builds on the development from the previous stage.

Stages

- Sensorimotor (birth to 2 years old)
  - Children progress developmentally from having primitive reflexes to having repetitive and imitative behaviors.
  - Curiosity and experimentation drive cognitive development; infants experience learning through sensation and movement.
  - During this period, infants begin to use language to express wants and needs.
  - Object permanence develops (knowing that an object exists even though it is not visible to them).
  - Separation anxiety may develop at this stage.
- Preoperational (2–7 years old)
  - Children's thinking is concrete during the preoperational stage.
  - Cognitive development is reflective of their use of imitation, symbolic play, drawing, and how they start to use verbal associations.
  - Development at this stage reflects reasoning becoming intuitive.
  - Three key elements of this stage are:
    - *Animism*: giving lifelike qualities to describe inanimate objects
    - *Egocentrism*: the inability to see things from another perspective and only able to see things from their own point of view
    - *Magical thinking*: believing that their thoughts can cause events to occur
- Concrete operational (7–11 years old)
  - Children can consider points of view other than their own, and they can categorize objects.
  - Development at this stage reflects reasoning becoming inductive.
  - During this stage, thinking becomes logical and less self-centered.
  - The key developmental accomplishment of this stage is conservation, which is the ability to realize that physical factors remain the same even when the outward appearance changes.
- Formal operational (11–15 years old)
  - During this stage, adolescents' thinking is abstract.
  - They are able to draw logical conclusions and make hypotheses.
  - They are also able to understand cause and effect.

GROWTH CHARTS

Overview

- Growth charts use a series of percentile curves to demonstrate the distribution of weight, length/height, and head circumference in the pediatric population. They track and compare body measurements at a point in time against children of the same age.
- Growth patterns help assess the overall health of a child.
- Serial measurements must be assessed to determine a growth pattern.
  - Abnormal growth patterns may indicate:
    - Low socioeconomic levels or lack of education about nutrition.
    - Nutritional disorders or failure to thrive.
    - Underlying diseases such as cystic fibrosis, inflammatory bowel disease, genetic conditions, or hormone deficiencies

(continued)

Overview *(continued)*

- Specialists are frequently involved in the management of children with an abnormal growth pattern. Common specialists include:
  - Dieticians
  - Endocrinologists
  - Gastroenterologists
- There are two types of growth charts: WHO growth charts and CDC growth charts. Refer to the CDC's growth charts web page for examples of both types of growth charts.

WHO Growth Charts

- Charts include weight, length, and weight for length sections.
- The WHO growth charts are the standard of how infants should grow under optimal conditions.
- The WHO growth charts use the second and the 98th percentiles as outer ranges to indicate abnormal growth.
- They reflect growth patterns of infants who are breastfed for at least 4 months and are still breastfeeding at 1 year.
- Use for all infants and children from birth to 2 years, whether breastfeeding or not, and calculate length using a recumbent position.

CDC Growth Charts

- Charts include sections for weight, height, and BMI for age.
- CDC growth charts are references of typical growth patterns of children in the United States. They are not based on ideal growth patterns.
- CDC growth chart uses fifth and 95th percentiles as outer ranges to indicate abnormal growth.
  - Between fifth and 95th percentiles is considered normal range.
  - Between 85th and 95th percentiles is considered in the overweight category.
  - Below the fifth percentile is considered in the underweight category.
- Obtain a series of accurate measurements when transitioning from WHO growth charts to CDC growth charts.
- Use for patients between the ages of 2 and 20 years old.
- Use standing height for stature measurement.

MILESTONES

Overview

- Children and infants grow and develop rapidly over the first few years of life.
- *Milestones* are behaviors and skills that are met as the infant or child learns to move, play, speak, and act.
- Milestones are based on:
  - *Fine motor skills*, which are the coordination of small muscle movement in the hands, wrists, and fingers
  - *Gross motor skills*, which are coordination of large muscle movements in the arms, legs, and torso
  - *Cognitive development*, which includes skills used for thinking, learning, language development, and sensory processing

COMPLICATIONS

If a child is missing milestones, it could be an indicator of a developmental delay. Providers should be notified of these concerns in order to facilitate screening for general development delays and autism. Early intervention specialists, occupational therapists, and physical therapists are often involved to help with motor, speech, or cognitive impairments.

Infant

- 1 month
  - Demonstrates head lag
  - Strong reflex movements
- 2 months
  - Begins to smile
  - Lifts head when prone
  - Turns head toward sounds
- 3 months
  - Recognizes familiar faces
  - Lifts head and shoulders when prone
  - Smiles socially
  - Tracks objects with eyes
  - Vocalizes with cooing
- 4 months
  - Able to roll from front to back
  - Begins to babble
  - Separation anxiety may begin
  - Vocalizes a laugh
- 6 months
  - Able to hold a bottle
  - Begins to imitate sounds
  - Holds head upright unsupported
  - Rakes objects with hands
  - Rolls from back to front
  - Sits with support
- 7 months
  - Plays peek-a-boo
  - Sits leaning forward on both hands
- 8 months
  - Sits without support
  - Transfers objects from hand to hand
- 9 months
  - Creeps on hands and knees
  - Develops pincer grasp
  - Pulls to standing position
  - Understands the word "no"
- 12 months
  - Can say "mama" and "dada"
  - Uses one-word sentences to communicate
  - Walks with hands held

Toddler

- 15 months
  - Builds a two-block tower
  - Can use a cup
  - Creeps up stairs
  - Walks independently
- 18 months
  - Able to run
  - Builds a three- or four-block tower
- 2 years

(continued)

Toddler *(continued)*

- Combines two-to-three-word sentences to communicate
- Runs and jumps
- Walks up and down stairs

ALERT!

Children should be screened for general development using standardized tools at 9, 18, and 30 months.

Preschooler

- 3 years
  - Able to dress themselves
  - Combines three to four words to form complex sentences
  - Learns to pedal a tricycle
  - Stands on one foot
- 4 years
  - Able to skip and hop
  - Can throw ball overhead and can catch ball
  - Communicates using four-to-five-word sentences
- 5 years
  - Able to draw a person
  - Handedness is established
  - Knows the days of the week
  - Skips on alternate feet

School Age

- 6 to 8 years
  - Able to tie their shoes
  - Wants independence from caregivers
  - Wants to be liked and accepted by friends and peers
- 9 to 11 years
  - Able to see the point of view of others
  - Gains a sense of responsibility
  - Has increased attention span
  - Starts to form stronger, complex peer friendships

Adolescents

- 12 to 14 years
  - Has ability for complex thought
  - Shows concern about body image, looks, and clothing
  - Shows interest and is influenced by peers
- 15 to 17 years
  - Able to give reasons for their choices
  - Develops work habits
  - Expresses concern for the future

POP QUIZ 2.4

The nurse is admitting a new patient who just turned 4 years old. When taking the child's history and completing a physical assessment, what developmental milestones should the nurse expect the child to have met?

FAMILY DYNAMICS AND ENVIRONMENTAL INFLUENCES

Overview

- Assessing the family dynamic and the child's environment can help to promote family-centered nursing care. It includes respecting, collaborating with, and including patients and their families in care decisions and treatment plans.
- Family dynamics, social influences, home life, and children's environments can impact their overall health, growth, and development.
- Part of the nurse's role is to perform family and household assessments. This is done to evaluate how these influences impact families and to educate families on the best ways to promote safety, proper development, and healthy lifestyle choices.

 COMPLICATIONS

A patient may appear to be noncompliant or have worsening symptoms, but it could be due to lack of education or barriers to care. Nurses need to assess environmental influences to be able to intervene and assist the family and patient in receiving the correct resources or care.

Nursing Interventions

- Assess the family dynamic (see Diversity in Chapter 17).
  - Evaluate whether there is a primary caregiver for the patient.
  - Evaluate whether there is a support system for both the patient and any other caregivers.
  - Evaluate whether siblings are involved and if they are affected or need to be supported.
- Assess for family coping mechanisms (see Diversity in Chapter 17).
  - Educate on positive coping mechanisms.
  - Evaluate family stress and how the family has coped with or reacted to past illnesses and hospitalizations.
  - If family could benefit from support with coping, refer to social worker or psychologist.
- Assess the family and patient readiness to learn (see Therapeutic Communication in Chapter 17).
  - Evaluate family's education levels.
  - Evaluate whether there are any known learning disabilities or language barriers.
  - Evaluate learning preferences for family and patients.
  - Evaluate family's acceptance of illness, condition, or treatment.
  - Evaluate family's understanding of discharge teaching.
- Assess for any barriers to care.
  - Evaluate barriers to attending follow-up appointments, such as transportation issues, child care issues for siblings, or scheduling issues.
  - Evaluate for financial concerns and refer to social work or case management for insurance or supply issues.
  - Evaluate patient and family compliance to treatment plan and educate or discuss alternatives if noncompliant.

IMMUNIZATIONS

Overview

- Immunizations are administered routinely starting in infancy and throughout childhood to prevent infectious diseases and their complications. An important aspect of health promotion is discussing childhood immunizations with family during routine visits.
- Immunizations have helped to eliminate and decrease the spread of infectious diseases in communities around the world.

 ALERT!

Vaccines that use live, attenuated viruses, such as MMR, rotavirus, varicella, and influenza nasal spray, are contraindicated in immunocompromised patients.

(continued)

Overview (continued)

- Recommendations for routine immunizations (Table 2.2) are based on age. There is a recommended catch-up schedule for children not completely immunized as infants.
- Anticipated side effects include pain, redness, and swelling at injection site and mild fever. Live vaccine side effects can mimic the disease process.

Nursing Interventions

- Administer multiple vaccines together as recommended.
- Administer IM injections in the vastus lateralis muscle in infants and young children. *Vastus lateralis muscle* is the anterolateral aspect of the middle or upper thigh.
- Administer IM injections in the deltoid muscle for children 3 years old and older.
  - *Deltoid site* is the densest part of deltoid muscle, 1 to 2 in. below the acromion process. It may be used when adequate muscle mass is developed, usually at 3 years old.
- Choose the correct needle size for age, route, and site.
- Do not immunize patients with current severe febrile illness, a history of a life-threatening reaction to a previous dose, or a severe allergy to a component of the immunization.
- Do not routinely premedicate with antipyretics.
- Follow CDC immunization schedule based on age.
- Follow CDC catch-up schedule for patients with missed immunization doses.
- Obtain informed consent from parents or guardians prior to administration.
- Provide and review VIS with patients and family prior to administration.
- Document lot numbers and site of administration in the medical record.

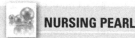 **NURSING PEARL**

Serum titers are done to check for immunity or the presence of antibodies from previous infection or disease or to confirm a previous vaccination. Titers are often drawn if a child does not have complete vaccination records or if they have recently immigrated and need evidence of immunization for school enrollment.

Table 2.2 Routine Immunization Schedule

Indications	Doses/Age	Recommendations, Contraindications, and Precautions
Hepatitis B		
• Immunization protects against hepatitis B. • *Hepatitis B* is a liver disease that leads to serious lifelong illness.	• *Three doses* • Birth • 1–2 months • 6–18 months	• None
DTaP		
• Immunization protects against diphtheria, tetanus, and pertussis. • Diphtheria leads to difficulty breathing, heart failure, and death. • Tetanus can cause muscle stiffening (i.e., lockjaw). • Pertussis can cause severe coughing and difficulty breathing.	• *Five doses* • 2 months • 4 months • 6 months • 15–18 months • 4–6 years	• DTaP for children less than 7 years old • Contraindicated with a history of coma, decreased level of consciousness, or prolonged seizures within 7 days of a previous dose • Contraindicated with history of Guillain-Barré syndrome

Table 2.2 Routine Immunization Schedule *(continued)*

Indications	Doses/Age	Recommendations, Contraindications, and Precautions
HiB		
• Immunization protects against *Haemophilus influenza* type B (Hib). • Hib can cause bacterial meningitis.	• *Three to four doses (*depending on manufacturer type)* • 2 months • 4 months • 6 months* • 12–15 months	• None
Pneumococcal (PCV13)		
• Immunization protects against pneumococcal disease. • Pneumococcal disease is the most common cause of pneumonia.	• *Four doses* • 2 months • 4 months • 6 months • 12–15 months	• None
Rotavirus		
• Immunization protects against rotavirus. • Rotavirus can cause severe diarrhea leading to dehydration.	• *Two doses* • 2 months • 4 months	• Live vaccine • Administered orally • Contraindicated in infants with history of intussusception and SCID • Series starts before 15 weeks of age • Contraindicated in immunocompromised infants
Inactivated polio virus		
• Immunization protects against poliomyelitis. • Polio infects the spinal cord and can cause paralysis.	• *Four doses* • 2 months • 4 months • 6–18 months • 4–6 years	• None
MMR		
• Immunization protects against measles, mumps, and rubella. • Measles can cause fever, cough, red watery eyes, rash, seizures. • Mumps can cause fever, headache, muscle aches, and may lead to deafness or swelling of the brain and spinal cord. • Rubella can cause fever, rash, and arthritis.	• *Two doses* • 12–15 months • 4–6 years	• Live vaccine • No administration within 4 weeks of other vaccines • Contraindicated in immunocompromised patients • Cautious use in patients with a history of bleeding disorders or seizures

(continued)

Table 2.2 Routine Immunization Schedule *(continued)*

Indications	Doses/Age	Recommendations, Contraindications, and Precautions
Varicella		
• Immunization protects against varicella (chickenpox). • Varicella can cause itchy rash, fever, skin infections, and swelling of the brain.	• *Two doses* • 12–15 months • 4–6 years	• Live vaccine • No administration within 4 weeks of other vaccines • Contraindicated in immunocompromised patients • Cautious use in patients with a history of bleeding disorders or seizures
Hepatitis A		
• Immunization protects against hepatitis A. • Hepatitis A is transmitted from person to person via fecal-oral route and can cause diarrhea, nausea, and vomiting.	• *One dose* • 12–18 months	• None
Tdap		
• Immunization protects against tetanus, diphtheria, and pertussis.	• *One dose* • 11–12 years	• Recommended for children 7 years and older • A booster dose every 10 years throughout life to provide continued protection • Contraindicated with a history of allergic reaction with previous dose (or dose of DTaP), or severe, life-threatening allergies, history of coma, decreased level of consciousness, or prolonged seizures within 7 days of a previous dose • Contraindicated with history of Guillain-Barré syndrome and history of severe pain and swelling after previous dose of any vaccine that protects against tetanus or diphtheria
HPV		
• Immunization protects against HPV. • HPV can cause cervical, vaginal, penile, and anal cancers.	• *One dose* • 11–12 years	• May be administered beginning at age 9
Meningococcal ACWY		
• Immunization protects against meningococcal disease. • Meningococcal disease can cause meningitis.	• *Two doses* • 11–12 years • 16 years	• Recommended for people with HIV, history of splenectomy, and college freshmen living in residence halls

Table 2.2 Routine Immunization Schedule *(continued)*

Indications	Doses/Age	Recommendations, Contraindications, and Precautions
Influenza		
• Immunization protects against viral influenza. • Flu typically spreads each year between October and May and can cause complications, especially in infants and young children.	• *Annual* • 6 months+	• Possible recommendation of two doses per year for children 6 months through 8 years • Live, attenuated flu vaccine as a nasal spray available for children age 2 and older • Follows live vaccine contraindications • Contraindicated with history of Guillain-Barré syndrome within 6 weeks of previous influenza dose
Palivizumab		
• Immunization prevents serious lower respiratory tract disease caused by RSV in high-risk infants.	• *1–5 doses, monthly during first year and second year of life* • Premature infants born before 29 weeks gestation and administered in the first year of life during RSV season, or older infants in high-risk categories	• Recommended for infants born before 29 weeks, or those born before 32 weeks with chronic lung disease and an oxygen requirement for at least 28 days, or congenital heart disease receiving medication to control congestive heart failure or with pulmonary hypertension • Contraindicated to continue monthly dosing if infant is diagnosed with RSV

Any immunization may be contraindicated for a patient who is severely immunocompromised or allergic to any of the components of the vaccine. Discuss individual cases with the provider.

Nursing Interventions *(continued)*

- Reduce discomfort during administration.
  - Apply topical anesthetic prior.
  - Give oral sucrose to infants.
  - Let toddlers and preschoolers sit with and be comforted by family.
  - Provide distraction.

Patient and Family Education

- Inform family of expected side effects such as injection site pain, redness and swelling at injection site, and mild fever, and provide a list of adverse reactions to report.
- Delay live vaccines for up to 11 months after receiving an antibody-containing product, such as blood products or IVIG.
- Discuss catch-up schedule with family for patients behind on immunizations.
- Encourage family to stay up to date on their child's immunizations (Table 2.2).

 ALERT!

In October of 2021, the U.S. FDA authorized the Pfizer-BioNTech COVID-19 vaccine for children ages 5 to 11. This authorization followed the August 2021 emergency use authorization for children ages 12 to 15. Nurses can support vaccine adverse event reporting to the Vaccine Adverse Event Reporting System. Reporting is required for severe adverse effects, cases of the multisystem inflammatory syndrome in children, or cases of COVID-19 hospitalization or death. Nurses can remind families that inquire about the COVID-19 vaccine to ensure they are up to date on all standard vaccines. Nurses can also recommend catch-up schedules for any families who have fallen behind on recommended vaccines. For more information, consult the FDA or CDC.

Patient and Family Education *(continued)*

- Lack of immunizations, especially in a community or close geographical area, can cause outbreaks of disease.
- Manage vaccine fever side effect by giving a cool bath or nonaspirin pain reliever.
- Treat injection site soreness and swelling using a cool, damp cloth.
- Offer immunizations if patients have mild illness or the common cold.

ALERT!

Vaccine adverse effects to report include anaphylaxis, difficulty breathing, dizziness, hoarseness, hives, lethargy, pallor, rash, tachycardia, and wheezing.

POP QUIZ 2.5

What should the nurse tell a parent to expect as side effects of her child's 4-month immunizations and how to manage them at home?

RESOURCES

AAP. (2014). Updated guidance for palivizumab prophylaxis among infants and young children at increased risk of hospitalization for respiratory syncytial virus infection. *Pediatrics, 134*(2), 415–420. https://pediatrics.aappublic ations.org/content/134/2/415.full

AAP. (2016). SIDS and other sleep-related infant deaths: Updated 2016 recommendations for a safe infant sleeping environment. *Pediatrics, 138*(5), e20162938. https://pediatrics.aappublications.org/content/138/5/e20162938

American Heart Association. (2016). *Pediatric advanced life support provider manual.* American Heart Association.

Centers for Disease Control and Prevention. (2010). *Growth charts.* U.S. Department of Health and Human Services, Centers for Disease Control and Prevention. https://www.cdc.gov/growthcharts/index.htm

Centers for Disease Control and Prevention. (2013). *Use and interpretation of the WHO and CDC growth charts for children from birth to 20 years in the United States.* U.S. Department of Health and Human Services, Centers for Disease Control and Prevention. https://www.cdc.gov/nccdphp/dnpa/growthcharts/resources/growthchart.pdf

Centers for Disease Control and Prevention. (2015). *Growth chart training.* U.S. Department of Health and Human Services, Centers for Disease Control and Prevention. https://www.cdc.gov/nccdphp/dnpao/growthcharts/who/using/transitioning.htm

Centers for Disease Control and Prevention. (2020a). *Current VISs.* U.S. Department of Health and Human Services, Centers for Disease Control and Prevention. https://www.cdc.gov/vaccines/hcp/vis/current-vis.html

Centers for Disease Control and Prevention. (2020b). *Keep child passengers safe.* U.S. Department of Health and Human Services, Centers for Disease Control and Prevention. https://www.cdc.gov/injury/features/child-passe nger-safety/index.html

Centers for Disease Control and Prevention. (2021a). *Children's oral health.* U.S. Department of Health and Human Services, Centers for Disease Control and Prevention. https://www.cdc.gov/oralhealth/basics/childrens-oral-he alth/index.html#:~:text=Fluoride%20varnish%20can%20prevent%20about,the%20primary%20(baby)%20teeth. &text=Children%20living%20in%20communities%20with,whose%20water%20is%20not%20fluoridated.&text= Similarly%2C%20children%20who%20brush%20daily,toothpaste%20will%20have%20fewer%20cavities

Centers for Disease Control and Prevention. (2021b). *Immunization schedules.* U.S. Department of Health and Human Services, Centers for Disease Control and Prevention. https://www.cdc.gov/vaccines/schedules/hcp/imz /child-adolescent.html

Centers for Disease Control and Prevention. (2021c). *Immunization schedules.* U.S. Department of Health and Human Services, Centers for Disease Control and Prevention. https://www.cdc.gov/vaccines/schedules/hcp/imz /catchup.html

Hockenberry, M., Wilson, D., & Rodgers, C. (2017). *Wong's essentials of pediatric nursing.* Elsevier.

Leonard, J. (2020). Spinal cord injury without radiographic abnormality. *UpToDate.* https://www.uptodate.com/cont ents/spinal-cord-injury-without-radiographic-abnormality-sciwora-in-children

McLeod, S. (2018a). Erik Erikson's stages of psychosocial development. *Simply Psychology.* https://www.simplypsych ology.org/Erik-Erikson.html

McLeod, S. (2018b). Jean Piaget's theory of cognitive development. *Simply Psychology.* https://www.simplypsychology .org/piaget.html

Pegram, P. S., & Stone, S. M. (2020). Botulism. *UpToDate*. https://www.uptodate.com/contents/botulism?search=inf
ant%20botulism&source=search_result&selectedTitle=1~18&usage_type=default&display_rank=1#H25

Ruggiero, K., & Ruggiero, M. (2020). *Fast facts handbook for pediatric primary care: A guide for nurse practitioners
and physician assistants*. Springer Publishing Company.

U.S. Food and Drug Administration. (2021a). *FDA approves first COVID-19 vaccine*. U.S. Department of Health and
Human Services, U.S. Food and Drug Administration. https://www.fda.gov/news-events/press-announcements/
fda-approves-first-covid-19-vaccine

U.S. Food and Drug Administration. (2021b). *FDA authorizes Pfizer-BioNTech COVID-19 vaccine for emergency
use in children 5 through 11 years of age*. U.S. Department of Health and Human Services, U.S. Food and Drug
Administration. https://www.fda.gov/news-events/press-announcements/fda-authorizes-pfizer-biontech-covid
-19-vaccine-emergency-use-children-5-through-11-years-age

Vaccine Adverse Event Reporting System. (n.d.). *Frequently asked questions*. U.S. Department of Health and Human
Services, Vaccine Adverse Event Reporting System. https://vaers.hhs.gov/faq.html

World Health Organization. (2020, May 22). *At least 80 million children under one at risk of diseases such as
diphtheria, measles and polio as COVID-19 disrupts routine vaccination efforts, warn Gavi, WHO and UNICEF*.
https://www.who.int/news/item/22-05-2020-at-least-80-million-children-under-one-at-risk-of-diseases-such-as
-diphtheria-measles-and-polio-as-covid-19-disrupts-routine-vaccination-efforts-warn-gavi-who-and-unicef

3

MEDICATION ADMINISTRATION, OVER-THE-COUNTER ANALGESICS, AND COMPLEMENTARY THERAPIES

MEDICATION ADMINISTRATION

Overview

- Pediatric medication dosing is based on age, body weight (in kilograms), and body surface area.
- Routes of medications include oral, optic, otic, nasal, enteral, parenteral, and rectal.

Routes of Administration

Oral Route

- Avoid adding medication to bottle to ensure child receives full medication dose even if they do not finish bottle. Instead, use a syringe and place small amounts in the sides of the mouth.
- For children, determine ability to swallow tablets and pills prior to administration.
- Mix medications in small amounts of sweet tasting foods, such as applesauce.
- Offer a drink of water or juice after administering medication.
- Preparations include liquids, chewable tablets, and capsulated pills or tablets.

COMPLICATIONS

Medication administration errors and adverse effects of medications can be prevented by performing the six rights of medication checks prior to administration and evaluating the patient's response to the medication. (See Nursing Interventions.) The right dose is an important check for pediatric patients due to dosing based on weight.

NURSING PEARL

When giving infants oral medications, gently stroking their cheek can help to open their mouth.

Enteral Route

- Enteral is the preferred route of administration for patients who receive nutrition via NG, ND, GT, or JT.
    - Confirm placement and patency of tube prior to medication administration.
    - Do not add medication to formula bags.
    - Flush tubing with water before and after each medication administration.
- Preparations include liquids, elixirs, and crushed or dissolvable pills mixed with water.

Parenteral Route

- Choose the correct needle size based on age, site, and type of injection: IM or IV.
- IM injection sites

(continued)

Parenteral Route (continued)

- Include vastus lateralis muscle and deltoid muscle.
  - Insert needle at a 90-degree angle.
- Peripheral venous access devices or peripheral IV access
  - Use for short-term and intermittent medications.
  - Assess for infiltration and phlebitis.
  - Transparent dressings should be used to view the insertion site.
- Subcutaneous sites: outer upper arm, anterolateral thighs, abdomen, upper hip
  - Determine appropriate site for age of patient and medication.
  - Insert needle at a 45-degree angle.
- Central venous access devices
  - Central venous access devices include peripherally inserted central catheters, tunneled catheters, and implanted ports (see Vascular Access Devices in Chapter 6).
  - Prevent central line-associated bloodstream infections with routine dressing changes using chlorhexidine.
  - Remember to change dressing when visibly soiled, wet, or no longer intact.

POP QUIZ 3.1

A parent asks why the nurse is not adding the medication to the bottle of formula since the infant does not like the taste of the medication. What is the correct response?

Nursing Interventions

- Ask for and verify two patient identifiers to confirm patient prior to administration.
- Assess for any allergies.
- Assess the six rights of medication administration:
  - Right documentation
  - Right dose
  - Right drug
  - Right patient
  - Right route
  - Right time
  - Recently, additional rights have been added to include the right assessment, right indication, right evaluation, patients' right to education, and the patients' right to refusal.
- Be aware of high-alert or high-risk medications and check with another nurse.
- Calculate the safe dose for each medication.
- Consult provider and pharmacist prior to crushing a medication.
- Do not crush enteric-coated or sustained-release tablets or capsules.
- Educate patient on medication use, side effects, and dosing.
- Evaluate patient for response to medication.
- Notify the provider if any dose is subtherapeutic or toxic.

Patient and Family Education

- Always use the measuring device packaged with medication to ensure the correct amount.
- Avoid using kitchen teaspoons, tablespoons, or paper cups to measure doses.
- In case of emergencies, have poison control center phone number available.
- Lock the safety cap on bottles and containers of medications.
- Store medications in a safe place out of reach of children.

POP QUIZ 3.2

What actions should the nurse take prior to administering an enteral medication through an NG tube to ensure safe nursing practice?

OVER-THE-COUNTER ANALGESICS

Overview

- Use of over-the-counter medications and analgesics is common. Common use increases the potential for unintentional overdoses and poisonings.
- Common over-the-counter medications include acetaminophen, aspirin, and ibuprofen (Table A.2).
- Acetaminophen
  - Safe dosing or therapeutic dosing is 10 to 15 mg/kg every 4 hours, or a maximum of 90 mg/kg per day.
  - Subtherapeutic is dosing less than 10 mg/kg/ dose.
  - Toxic dosing is greater than 15 mg/kg/dose or more than 90 mg/kg per day.
- Aspirin
  - Aspirin is sometimes used for anti-inflammatory and antiplatelet effects and is commonly used to treat Kawasaki disease; it should be administered to children only under the guidance of the provider.
  - Aspirin is contraindicated for use in children and adolescents with acute viral illnesses such as the chicken pox or flu due to association with Reye's syndrome.
  - *Reye's syndrome* is rapidly progressing encephalopathy with hepatic involvement.
    - Early signs include nausea, vomiting, and changes in behavior.
    - Later symptoms include confusion, seizures, and loss of consciousness.
- Ibuprofen
  - Ibuprofen is commonly used as an analgesic and antipyretic.
  - Dosing for 6 months old to less than 12 years is 10 mg/kg/dose with maximum of 400 mg/dose every 4 to 6 hours as needed.
  - Dosing for children 12 to 17 years is 400 mg every 4 to 6 hours as needed.

> **COMPLICATIONS**
>
> Acetaminophen is the most common accidental drug poisoning in children, which can lead to hepatotoxicity, organ or renal failure, and possibly death. Other symptoms of acetaminophen poisoning include confusion, jaundice, nausea, pallor, pancreatitis, sweating, upper right abdominal pain, and vomiting.

Nursing Interventions

- Ask about over-the-counter usage to prevent interactions and overdoses.
- Calculate doses prior to administration.
- Monitor GI status and liver function after acetaminophen overdose.

Patient and Family Education

- Do not administer ibuprofen to infants under 6 months old.
- Do not give children aspirin unless under the instruction of the provider.
- Ensure safe storage of medications and keep them out of the reach of children.
- Read all over-the-counter product labels carefully.

PROCEDURAL SEDATION

Overview

- *Procedural sedation* is defined by the International Committee for the Advancement of Procedural Sedation as "the administration of one or more pharmacologic agents to facilitate a diagnostic or therapeutic procedure while targeting a state during which airway patency, spontaneous respiration, protective airway reflexes, and hemodynamic stability are preserved, while alleviating anxiety and pain."

(continued)

Overview *(continued)*

- Procedural sedation includes administering medications that cause sedation or dissociation, with or without analgesics.
  - Sedation refers to the ability of the patient to lie very still.
  - Analgesia is pain relief.
  - Dissociation is the product of mind–body separation.
- Many different health providers in a variety of settings practice procedural sedation, including:
  - Dentists
  - Emergency room providers
  - Physician/surgeons in outpatient clinics
  - Inpatient hospital units for procedures, and diagnostic tests
    - CT or MRI
    - PICC placement, fracture reduction, chest tube insertion, dressing changes
- The goal of procedural sedation is for the patient to tolerate a procedure and prevent pain, anxiety, and movement. The desired depth of sedation is dependent on the procedure to be performed, the anticipated degree of pain, the experience and credentials of the provider, and patient factors.
- The three levels of sedation-analgesia are:
  - Minimal sedation:
    - Anxiolysis
    - Causes altered cognitive function
    - Respiratory and cardiovascular function typically not altered
  - Moderate sedation/analgesia:
    - Depresses consciousness
    - Includes using both sedatives and analgesics
  - Deep sedation
    - Responds to painful stimuli
    - Requires careful monitoring as there is a risk of altered respiratory function
  - General anesthesia
    - Used to induce general anesthesia
    - Respiratory and cardiovascular function possibly altered
- Medications commonly used are ketamine and propofol. Monitoring requirements include:
  - Adequacy of ventilation
  - Frequent vital signs according to facility policy
    - Typically, every 5 minutes during procedure
    - Post procedure, every 15 minutes until patient returns to baseline
  - End-tidal CO_2 monitoring
  - Patient responsiveness

ALERT!

- Precaution should be used with special needs patients and patients who have the following:
  - Airway abnormalities
  - Allergies to sedation and/or pain medications
  - History of respiratory obstruction
  - History of sleep apnea

COMPLICATIONS

Complications of procedural sedation include:
- Airway obstruction
- Cardiac arrest
- Hypotension/hypertension
- Respiratory depression
- Tachycardia

Nursing Interventions

- Advise the patient and family regarding what to expect and answer all questions.
- Encourage family support and child life involvement, if available.
- Ensure appropriate fasting status prior to sedation, giving the patient appropriate NPO times for solids and clear liquids.
- Gather the appropriate equipment, including:
  - Airway equipment

- Intravenous access (see Chapter 6)
- Medications
- Monitoring equipment
  - Cardiac/respiratory monitor
  - Blood pressure cuff
  - End-tidal CO_2 ($EtCO_2$)
  - Pulse-oximeter
- O_2 administration supplies
- Reversal drugs, if needed
- Suction
- Make a preprocedural phone call to the patient's family and give instructions for the procedure (if they are at home).
- Monitor and document vital signs continuously during the procedure and observe for changes that indicate transition between levels of sedation. Monitor patient after the procedure during recovery until the patient meets the criteria for discharge.
- Provide appropriate distraction if the patient is awake during the procedure. Utilize child life therapists to assist with this process.

Patient and Family Education

Discharge instructions should contain the following:
- Diet should begin with clear liquids and then proceed with solids, as tolerated.
- If nausea/vomiting occurs, wait at least 30 minutes before trying clear liquids again. This is normal. If nausea/vomiting continues, and the patient is unable to keep anything down, they should call the physician's office.
- Some medications cause some patients to have flushed faces for 24 hours after the procedure. This is not a cause for worry or concern.
- More tiredness than usual is common for the rest of the day.

COMPLEMENTARY AND ALTERNATIVE THERAPIES

Overview

- Complementary medicine is used in addition to standard or conventional treatments, and alternative therapies are used in place of standard or conventional treatments.
- Possible indications for complementary and alternative medicine include:
  - Anxiety
  - Chronic conditions
  - Common colds
  - Gastrointestinal problems
  - End-of-life care
  - Insomnia
  - Musculoskeletal issues
  - Nausea
  - Pain
  - Stress
- There are multiple classifications of complementary therapies used by children and adolescents.
  - Traditional Chinese therapies
  - Energy therapy
  - Chiropractic or manipulative therapy
  - Mind–body therapy
  - Natural products

 ALERT!

Supplements and herbal therapies may interact with conventional medications. For example, St. John's wort interacts with antidepressants to cause serotonin syndrome and may interact with cyclosporine levels leading to transplant rejection.

Common Types of Complementary Medicine

Traditional Chinese Medicine

- Acupuncture uses fine needles to release endorphins by stimulating pressure points and is used to treat the following conditions:
  - Chronic pain
  - Headaches
  - Nausea
- For children, alternatives to using acupuncture are acupressure and magnetic acupressure.
  - *Acupressure* is a form of massage using hands and fingers, rather than needles, on pressure points. It still encourages the flow of qi, or energy, through the body and has been used to help with pain, nausea, and constipation.
  - *Magnetic acupressure* uses magnets, rather than needles, on pressure points or on body parts, such as the ears.
  - Many herbal supplements are used in traditional Chinese medicine for a variety of chronic conditions.

Energy Therapy

- Healing via therapeutic touch involves healing through intention and invisible energy from the healer.
- Reiki is an example of energy therapy.

Manipulative Therapy

- Chiropractic treatments align the spine to promote health and heal acute illnesses.
- Children and adolescents use chiropractic therapy to relieve headaches and to improve immune system responses.
- Massage focuses on stimulating muscles and connective tissues and is commonly used in infants to help with relaxation, sleep, gas, cramps, and colic.

Mind–Body Therapy

- *Biofeedback* uses a device to measure and give audio, visual, or kinesthetic feedback about the body's physiologic response, such as temperature or heart rate. It helps the child to learn how to control a body function and is often used in pain management and ADHD.
- *Guided imagery* involves immersive meditation to promote relaxation. It has been used for palliation of cancer treatment side effects and for managing stress and pain. Use with caution in children with a history of abuse to avoid unintended PTSD.
- *Meditation* enhances awareness of emotional, cognitive, and sensory feelings and involves a specific focus of attention. It is used to decrease blood pressure, reduce negative behaviors or actions, and improve coping.
- *Yoga* uses breathing, body postures, and meditation to connect the mind and body. It is beneficial for stress management, pain management, and to improve emotional behaviors.

Natural Products

- Echinacea is commonly used for management and prevention of infections.
- Ginger is used as an aid to reduce nausea during chemotherapy.
- Melatonin treats circadian rhythm disorders and may enhance sleep.
- *Probiotics* are live microorganisms, or good bacteria, ingested to replenish and balance gastrointestinal flora. Probiotics are used to manage irritable bowel syndrome, diarrhea, eczema, and the common cold.

Nursing Interventions

- Advocate to include patient preferences for complementary treatment in the plan of care.
- Ask about natural product usage when taking patient history or completing medication reconciliation.

- Check for interactions between supplements, vitamins, and herbs with prescribed medications.
- Ensure safety and efficacy prior to administering any complementary medicine products.
- Remain objective and nonjudgmental about patient practices related to their culture or complementary alternative medicine use.

Patient and Family Education

- Educate family on potential adverse effects or misleading marketing.
- Encourage family to research risks and benefits of complementary medicine prior to use.
- Notify the provider of any complementary or alternative medicine use.

 POP QUIZ 3.3

What questions should the nurse include in the subjective history of an adolescent patient regarding OTC medication and supplement use to help avoid any medication interactions and unintentional overdoses?

RESOURCES

Beardsley, E. (2018, December 6). *Nursing grand rounds: Procedural sedation.* Seattle Children's Hospital. www.seattlechildrens.org/globalassets/documents/healthcare-professionals/nursing-grand-rounds/ngr-procedural-sedation-dec2018.pdf

Burchum, J., & Rosenthal, L. (2019). *Lehne's pharmacology for nursing care* (10th ed.). Elsevier.

Centers for Disease Control and Prevention. (2020a). *Protect your children: Store & use medicines safely.* U.S. Department of Health and Human Services, Centers for Disease Control and Prevention. https://www.cdc.gov/patientsafety/features/safe-medicine-children.html

Centers for Disease Control and Prevention. (2020b). *Recommended intervals between administration of antibody-containing products and measles or varicella-containing vaccine* [Fact Sheet]. U.S. Department of Health and Human Services, Centers for Disease Control and Prevention. https://www.cdc.gov/vaccines/pubs/pinkbook/downloads/appendices/a/mmr_ig.pdf

Cravero, J. P., & Roback, M. G. (2021). Procedural sedation in children outside of the operating room. *UpToDate.* https://www.uptodate.com/contents/procedural-sedation-in-children-outside-of-the-operating-room

Green, S. M., Irwin, M. G., Mason, K. P., & International Committee for the Advancement of Procedural Sedation (2021). Procedural sedation: providing the missing definition. *Anaesthesia, 76*(5), 598–601. https://doi.org/10.1111/anae.15213

Hockenberry, M., Wilson, D., & Rodgers, C. (2017). *Wong's essentials of pediatric nursing.* Elsevier.

Kemper, K. (2019). Complementary and alternative medicine in pediatrics. *UpToDate.* https://www.uptodate.com/contents/complementary-and-alternative-medicine-in-pediatrics?search=chiropractic&source=search_result&selectedTitle=3~45&usage_type=default&display_rank=3#H13

Lexicomp. (2021a). Acetaminophen: Pediatric drug information [Drug Information]. *UpToDate.* https://www.uptodate.com/contents/acetaminophen-paracetamol-pediatric-drug-information?search=acetaminophen&source=panel_search_result&selectedTitle=2~148&usage_type=panel&kp_tab=drug_pediatric&display_rank=1#F129282

Lexicomp. (2021b). Aspirin: Pediatric drug information [Drug Information]. *UpToDate.* https://www.uptodate.com/contents/aspirin-pediatric-drug-information?search=aspirin&source=panel_search_result&selectedTitle=2~148&usage_type=panel&kp_tab=drug_pediatric&display_rank=1

Lexicomp. (2021c). Ibuprofen: Pediatric drug information [Drug Information]. *UpToDate.* https://www.uptodate.com/contents/ibuprofen-pediatric-drug-information?search=ibuprofen&source=panel_search_result&selectedTitle=2~148&usage_type=panel&kp_tab=drug_pediatric&display_rank=1

Ventola, C. L. (2010). Current issues regarding complementary and alternative medicine in the United States. *Pharmacy & Therapeutics, 35*(8), 461–468. https://www.ncbi.nlm.nih.gov/pmc/articles/PMC2935644/#:~:text=Dietary%20Supplements%20Are%20the%20Most%20Frequently%20Used%20CAM%20Therapy&text=Echinacea%20and%20fish%2C%20omega%2D3,Figures%206%20and%20%E2%80%8B7).&text=Other%20popular%20therapies%20included%20deep,%2C%20massage%20therapy%2C%20and%20yoga

NEUROLOGIC SYSTEM

ASSESSMENT AND MANAGEMENT

Body Temperature Regulation

- Body temperature can be affected by environmental factors, but it is regulated by the hypothalamus, so injury or surgery near the hypothalamus can affect thermoregulation.
- Body temperature is most commonly measured and monitored via axillary temperature in newborns and infants. Older children's temperatures can be measured via axillary, oral, temporal, and tympanic temperatures. The most accurate measurement of temperature is a rectal temperature.
- Maintaining thermoregulation is essential for newborns and infants, and extreme changes in temperature should be avoided.
- Newborns have a decreased ability to maintain thermoregulation.
  - Newborns cannot shiver; metabolism and oxygen requirement increase when a newborn is too cold.
  - To maintain warmth immediately after birth, newborns should be warmed by drying with a warm blanket, and then placed and assessed in an open bed with a radiant warmer or an isolette.
- Infants require close monitoring of their body temperature.
  - A cold infant is 97.7 °F (36.5 °C) or less.
  - Infants can lose heat very quickly, four times faster than adults.
  - Just a 1 degree drop in temperature causes the baby's oxygen use to increase by 10%.
- Inability to maintain body temperature can lead to cold stress, and cold stress can lead to hypoxia, acidosis, and hypoglycemia.
- Symptoms of cold stress include:
  - Heart arrhythmias
  - Hypoglycemia
  - Lethargy
  - Poor feeding
  - Red, cold skin
  - Weak cry

NURSING PEARL

Educate families on how to properly obtain the temperature of the infant. The teach back method is a way to confirm understanding of learning. The nurse will explain and demonstrate taking the infant's temperature, and then the family will complete a return demonstration of taking the baby's temperature.

ALERT!

If the infant is less than 3 months old and has a rectal temperature greater than 100.4 °F (38 °C), this is an emergency and needs to be assessed by a provider urgently. Fever could be a sign of infection. Since infants have immature immune systems and are more susceptible to infection, they are at much higher risk for bacterial and viral infections.

ALERT!

The body surface of an infant is three times greater than an adult. Infants lose body heat four times quicker than adults.

Fall Risk

- Children are at high risk of falling. Factors include:
  - Curiosity
  - Immature motor skills
  - Inadequate supervision
  - Lack of judgment
  - Male gender
- Children from families with lower income or income below the federal poverty level may have a higher risk of falls due to the possibility of:
  - Family stress
  - Hazardous environments
  - Healthcare inequities
  - Maternal/paternal youth or families with less than a high school education
  - Overcrowding
  - Single parenting
  - Untreated mental illness
- Falls at home or in the community can often be prevented.
  - Always supervise infants and children. Direct supervision is the best prevention.
    - Do not leave infants unattended on a surface where they could fall.
    - Do not leave small children unattended.
    - Keep side rails up on cribs.
    - Use baby monitors when possible.
  - Do not use walkers.
  - Install safety rails on beds for toddlers.
  - Move furniture away from windows.
    - Ensure windows do not open more than 4 inches.
    - Secure cords for window blinds.
  - Place child-resistant gates at the top and bottom of stairs.
  - Use safety straps with high chairs and shopping carts.
  - Use helmets and kneepads when participating in sports and riding tricycles and bikes.
  - Utilize playgrounds with shock-absorbing surfaces like wood chips, mulch, rubber, or sand.
- Hospital risks and safety precautions:
  - Risks include:
    - Admitting diagnosis
    - Age
    - Cognitive/physical impairment
    - Degree of sedation
    - Degree of supervision
    - Developmental stage
    - Fall history
  - Safety precautions:
    - Accompany patients when walking.
    - Assess and document a fall risk assessment for each patient, according to policy. Place sign on door or bracelet on patient for awareness if they are a fall risk.
    - Avoid leaving young children unattended; employ hospital staff or volunteers to sit with children when their family or caregiver is unavailable.
    - Educate family and the patient about fall prevention and safety.
    - Ensure patients wear nonskid socks when out of bed.
    - Keep the environment free of extra equipment and other potential hazards.
    - Keep side rails up and beds and wheelchairs locked.
    - Place hospital beds in lowest possible position.
    - Place personal items in close reach.

 NURSING PEARL

Talk with caregivers about their home and community and nearby environmental conditions. Offer suggestions on how they could provide a safer environment, if necessary. There are online tools available that help caregivers provide the safest possible environment; nurses should assist with printed handouts or direct to online resources. Provide community resources, if needed.

Pain Assessment

- Pain assessment in children is based on the cognitive and developmental level of each patient.
- If present, families can be a resource for assessing a child's pain. Family input is invaluable for the child with any developmental delays.
- Use the most appropriate pain scale based on age and cognitive function to make a more accurate assessment. There are numerous pain scales available in pediatrics. These pain scales are available in different languages and use different ethnic pictures.
- The most common pediatric pain scales used are:
  - N–PASS
    - Used for premature infants
    - Based on:
      - Physiologic parameters such as heart rate, respiratory rate, and blood pressure
      - Behavioral responses such as crying, facial expressions, muscle tone, and sleep patterns
  - CRIES
    - Used for infants from 38 weeks gestation to 6 months old
    - Assessment based on observations and objective measurements
    - Assesses crying, oxygenation, vital signs, facial expressions, and sleeplessness
  - FLACC
    - Used for patients ages birth to 3 years old
    - Behavioral scale based on five observable characteristics: facial expression, leg movement, activity, cry, and inconsolability
    - Revised FLACC scale available for children over 3 with cognitive impairment
  - FACES
    - Used for patients ages 3 and older
    - Self-reporting scale in which the child chooses the face that most closely represents their pain
  - Numeric
    - Used for patients 6 and older who are able to self-report pain
    - Self-reporting scale in which the child rates pain on a scale from 0 to 10
  - Oucher
    - Used for patients 3 to 12 years old
    - Self-report photograph scale for pain intensity
    - Uses picture and numbers
    - Pictures from 0 to 10 progressively showing more distress with higher numbers

Pain Management

- Choose an appropriate pain management modality after completing an initial assessment of the child's illness or disorder.
- Common *pharmacologic* therapy includes:
  - Acetaminophen (Table A.2) can be used for mild pain or used with narcotics to help moderate and severe pain.
  - Nonsteroidal anti-inflammatory drugs such as ibuprofen (Table A.2) and ketorolac can be used for mild to moderate pain.
  - Opioids, such as morphine, hydromorphone, oxycodone, and hydrocodone can be used for moderate and severe pain such as after surgery, for children experiencing sickle-cell crisis, and cancer patients.
  - Fentanyl is used during and after surgery and for procedural sedation.
  - Side effects of opioids include:
    - Confusion
    - Constipation

 ALERT!

Codeine should be avoided in the pediatric population. In 2015, the American Academy of Pediatrics advised that codeine no longer be given to children under 18 due to serious side effects including serious breathing problems and death.

(continued)

Pain Management *(continued)*

- ○ Excessive sleepiness
- ○ Itching
- ○ Nausea
- ○ Slow breathing or respiratory depression
- Common *nonpharmacologic* therapies include:
  - Distraction, hypnosis, imagery, and psychotherapy
  - Massage, heat/cold therapy, and acupuncture
  - Nonnutritive sucking for infants
  - Relaxation, biofeedback, art, and play therapy
  - Oral 24% sucrose solution (per facility policy):
    - ○ Infants may use during painful procedures.
    - ○ Sucrose provides taste stimulation to the cellular membrane receptors in the brain, in which the endogenous opioid system is located.
    - ○ Sucrose solution can be placed directly in the mouth in drops, and then infants can be given pacifier for nonnutritive sucking.
    - ○ Note: sucrose is contraindicated in infants with sucrose or fructose intolerance and glucose malabsorption.

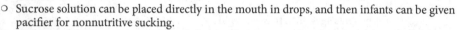

NURSING PEARL

When sending a patient home with pain medication, verify any drug allergies and make sure medications are compatible. Ask if the child can swallow pills or needs a liquid. Explain how often the medication can be taken and if it should be given with food. Check family's understanding by asking them to repeat instructions and demonstrate administration. Send written instructions home with family.

ATTENTION DEFICIT HYPERACTIVITY DISORDER

Overview

- *ADHD* is a common neurobehavioral disorder.
- There are three presentations of ADHD:
  - Inattention
  - Hyperactive/impulsive
  - Combined
- About 9.4% of children have been diagnosed with ADHD.
  - The cause of ADHD is not definitively known, but a combination of organic, genetic, and environmental factors is thought to be involved. An imbalance of dopamine, norepinephrine, and serotonin is a factor. Common risk factors include:
    - ○ Exposure to toxins, alcohol, cocaine, and nicotine in utero
    - ○ Family association between parents, children, and siblings: over 50% chance of children having ADHD when parents have ADHD
    - ○ History of traumatic brain injury
- It is common to have coexisting conditions with ADHD, including:
  - Anxiety disorder
  - Conduct disorder
  - Depressive disorder
  - Oppositional defiant disorder
  - Reading disability

COMPLICATIONS

Some complications of ADHD include:
- Accidents/injuries
- Excess weight
- Poor self-esteem
- Risky behavior
- Sleep problems
- Substance abuse
- Trouble interacting with others

Signs and Symptoms

- Hyperactivity and impulsivity
  - Always active
  - Difficulty remaining still or seated
  - Fidgety
  - Impatient
  - Overly talkative
  - Restless
  - Unable to play quietly
- Inattention
  - Difficulty maintaining focus and attention
  - Difficult tasks avoided
  - Easily distracted
  - Forgetful, loses things
  - Lacks ability to complete assignments
  - Poor listening skills
  - Struggles to follow through on homework and chores
- Impaired social skills and difficult family and peer relationships
- Sleep impairment
- Underachievement in school

NURSING PEARL

Sleep disturbances that are common in children with ADHD include bedtime resistance, awakening at night, trouble waking in the morning, daytime sleepiness, and sleep-related breathing problems.

Diagnosis

Labs
There are no labs specific to diagnose ADHD.

Diagnostic Testing
- To rule out other causes for the child's behavior, a physical examination, including vision, hearing, and neurologic evaluation is done. Psychologic tests are then performed.
- There are several tools to help screen for symptoms of ADHD and aid in diagnosis:
  - The National Institute for Children's Health Quality Vanderbilt Assessment Scale
  - ADHD Rating Scale-5 for Children and Adolescents
  - Swanson, Nolan and Pelham scale
  - Conners Comprehensive Behavior Rating Scales

Treatment

- Behavioral therapy and/or medications, depending on the child's age and severity of symptoms
  - Behavioral therapy is recommended for children under 6 years old.
  - Both behavioral therapy and medication is recommended for children 6 years and older.
- Stimulant medications:
  - Dexmethylphenidate, methylphenidate, amphetamine, atomoxetine, and extended-release guanfacine (see Table 4.3*)
    - ○ Stimulants work by increasing dopamine and norepinephrine in the brain.
    - ○ The medication should be titrated to the best response in the patient.
    - ○ The stimulants are available in short-acting, intermediate-acting, and long-acting preparations.
- Nonstimulant medication: atomoxetine: causes fewer side effects (see Table 4.3)
- Treatment involving family and teachers for success

---

* Table 4.3 is located at the end of this chapter.

Nursing Interventions

- Engage with patient and family using an open communication style.
- Provide family with informational written materials that are easy to understand.
- Provide support and celebrate successes.
- Send and retrieve screening and assessment tools to family and teachers to aid in initial diagnosis and follow-up status.

Patient and Family Education

- Administer medications as instructed.
- Family may contact the provider's office between office visits with questions or concerns.
- Family should learn about the chronic condition and importance of following treatment plan and ask any questions they may have.
- Family should remember self-care, especially when feeling overwhelmed.
- Support groups are available where they can express feelings and receive help from other families experiencing the same things.

AUTISM SPECTRUM DISORDER

Overview

- *Autism spectrum disorder* is a series of complex neurodevelopmental disorders that range from mild to severe and are characterized by difficulties in social communication and restrictive or repetitive behavior.
- Children are usually diagnosed when they are toddlers, and the disorders are more common in boys.
- The exact cause of autism spectrum disorder is unknown, but it is thought to be a combination of genetic and environmental factors.

COMPLICATIONS

Feeding issues are common in children with autism spectrum disorders and stem from hypersensitivities and the need for routine and sameness. This can include aversions to tastes and textures and can lead to restricted eating patterns.

Signs and Symptoms

- Abnormal, or avoidance of, eye contact
- Atypical response to certain sights, smells, or textures
- Communication impairment
- Constipation
- Decreased response to name
- Intolerance to change
- Limited social interaction
- Repetitive behaviors

Diagnosis

Labs
There are no labs specific to diagnose autism spectrum disorder.

Diagnostic Testing
Autism spectrum disorder screening.

Treatment

- Applied behavior analysis therapy
- Occupational therapy
- Positive reinforcement
- Speech therapy

Nursing Interventions

- Assess for self-injury behaviors such as head banging, arm biting, and skin scratching.
- Communicate and create individualized plan of care. Help to create a schedule or structured routine if desired.
- Early identification and early intervention are the keys for improving outcomes. Notify provider of any concerns related to social and neurocognitive development.
- Evaluate and adapt to preferences for auditory and visual stimulation. Assess if a private room or certain lighting would help during hospitalization.
- Goals of management include:
  - Encouraging effective communication
  - Improving play skills
  - Increasing social functioning
  - Promoting independent functioning
  - Reducing nonfunctional or negative behaviors.
- Refer to specialist if there are concerns about social interaction, communication, or atypical behaviors.
- Support family in development of individualized education program with child's school.

Patient and Family Education

- Develop and keep a structured routine to help prevent negative behaviors.
- Consider use of assistive technology, a tool that is especially helpful for children who are nonverbal to help improve or assist with communication abilities.
- Contact the local school about early intervention or special education eligibility.
- Promote independence by incorporating applied behavioral analysis therapy techniques at home.
- Reiterate and clarify myths that there is no link between vaccines and autism.

POP QUIZ 4.1

The nurse notices that a toddler admitted for constipation does not respond to his name. What other signs would the nurse assess for before referring to a developmental evaluation for autism spectrum disorder?

CEREBRAL PALSY

Overview

- *CP* is a group of conditions involving permanent motor dysfunctions that affect muscle tone, posture, and movement.
- The conditions are nonprogressive, but symptoms and functional abilities evolve as the nervous system matures.
- Diagnosis is usually made when the patient is 12 to 24 months of age.
- There are four types of CP, but spastic and dyskinetic are the most common types.
  - Spastic
    - Most common type and characterized by the affected portion of the body
    - Spastic diplegia/diparesis: only legs are affected
    - Spastic hemiplegia/hemiparesis: one side only, arms usually more affected than legs
    - Spastic quadriplegia/quadriparesis: affects all four limbs, trunk, and face
  - Dyskinetic
    - Involuntary, uncoordinated movement
    - Body in constant motion
    - Muscle tone can change from hypertonic to hypotonic daily

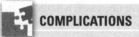

COMPLICATIONS

Complications include muscle spasticity and contractures that may affect movement and cause pain.

(continued)

Overview (continued)

- Ataxic
  - Awkward, wide gait
  - Not usually diagnosed until patient is walking
- Mixed: more than one type
- Causes of CP:
  - Brain damage
  - Maternal infection
  - Maternal nutritional deficiencies
  - Kernicterus: condition caused by Rh incompatibility
  - Prematurity
  - Prenatal lack of oxygen supply
- Neurodevelopmental disabilities associated with CP:
  - Chronic pain
  - Drooling
  - Epilepsy
  - Feeding difficulties, failure to grow properly
  - GI disorders
  - Orthopedic abnormalities
  - Osteopenia
  - Pulmonary diseases
  - Urinary disorders
  - Sleep disorders
  - Speech, hearing impairment
  - Vision problems

Signs and Symptoms

- Abnormal muscle tone (hypertonic/hypotonic)
- Asymmetrical crawling
- Developmental delays the first year
- Difficult to hold infant due to stiffness
- Excessive docility, irritability
- Failure to meet milestones
- Failure to thrive
- Hand preference before age of 1
- Increased or decreased reflexes
- Poor sleep
- Spasticity

Diagnosis

Labs
There are no labs specific to diagnose CP.

Diagnostic Testing
- Clinically through serial examination, prenatal history, and possible imaging to determine cause
- Testing for underlying cause or for clinical/historical concerns:
  - Genetic testing
  - EEG
  - MRI
  - Thrombophilia testing

Treatment

- Goal of treatment: maximize function and independence and reduce effect of disability
- Multidisciplinary team manage physical, psychological, social, and educational needs
- Treatment options:
  - Medications (see Table 4.3)
    - Baclofen
    - Benzodiazepines
    - OnabotulinumtoxinA
  - Orthotics
  - Orthopedic surgical interventions
    - Lengthening or releasing muscles/tendons
    - Osteotomy
    - Hip surgery to correct subluxation, dysplasia
    - Spinal fusion to correct scoliosis
  - Physical and occupational therapy

Nursing Interventions

- Advocate and encourage physical therapy, age-appropriate activities, and socialization.
- Assess and monitor pain levels.
- Assist with ROM exercises and promote mobility.
- Assure family that the goal is for the patient to achieve maximal function and independence.
- Provide emotional support as family accepts this lifelong process.
- Provide resources for support groups and reputable online information.
- Teach family that CP can be treated, but there is no cure.

Patient and Family Education

- Attend appointments to monitor medications and patient status.
- Family to take time for themselves, if possible. (Utilize community day or respite care.)
- Learn about medications and side effects.
- Learn how to apply and use orthotics and other aids correctly.

HEAD INJURY

Overview

- Head injury is very common in infants and children due to having large heads in contrast to their body size and neck muscles that are not fully developed.
- Most head injuries do not end in serious TBI.
- A minor injury in infants can cause intracranial injury, skull fracture, or concussion.
- Head injuries can vary by severity and are characterized by mild, moderate, and severe.
  - Mild head injuries include:
    - A cut (shallow) in the scalp
    - Confusion, headache, problems with balance or concentration
    - Raised or swollen bump or bruise
  - Moderate to severe head injuries require immediate medical attention and may include any of the above plus:
    - Coma
    - Difficulty walking
    - Loss of consciousness

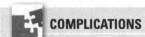 **COMPLICATIONS**

Long-term complications of head injury can include permanent brain damage, cerebral palsy, chronic seizure disorder, paralysis, blindness (shaken baby syndrome), motor problems, developmental delays, and learning disabilities.

(continued)

Overview *(continued)*

- ○ Loss of short-term memory
- ○ Repeated nausea and vomiting
- ○ Seizures
- ○ Severe headache that does not go away
- Severe head injuries: focal
- Head injuries can also vary by type:
  - Blunt trauma to the head can cause bruising to the brain tissue.
  - A contusion causes bleeding and swelling inside of the brain around the area where the head was struck or sometimes on the opposite side of the brain where the head was struck.
  - *Penetrating brain injury* is when something enters or penetrates the brain such as a bullet or sharp object.
  - Shaken baby syndrome
    - ○ Usually a result of abuse, rigorous shaking, or striking an infant against a hard surface causes major head trauma, brain swelling, skull fractures, bleeding into the brain, and retinal hemorrhages.
    - ○ Depending on the severity of the injury, death or permanent disability may occur.
  - Intraparenchymal brain hemorrhage
    - ○ Tears in the brain tissue or vasculature, which causes bleeding
  - Diffuse axonal injury
    - ○ Tissue shearing of the gray and white matter
    - ○ Usually as a result of an acceleration/deceleration injury
  - Epidural hematoma (Figure 4.1)
    - ○ Bleeding above the dura mater of the brain and below the skull
    - ○ Usually caused by an arterial bleed; neurologic status decompensates quickly
  - Subdural hematoma (Figure 4.1)
    - ○ Bleeding below the dura mater but above the brain
    - ○ Usually caused by a venous bleed; neurologic status decompensates a little slower than epidural bleeds.
  - Subarachnoid hemorrhage (Figure 4.1)
    - ○ Tearing of small vessels in the pia mater
    - ○ Can be acute or chronic
      - *Acute*: within a short time of the injury
      - *Chronic*: slow forming (usually occurs in the elderly)

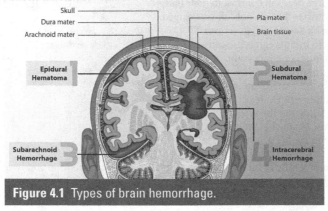

Figure 4.1 Types of brain hemorrhage.

Source: MyUpchar.

Signs and Symptoms

- Altered mental status
- Drainage of CSF from the ear or the nose
- Headache
- Hemotympanum (blood in the space behind the tympanic membrane)
- Lethargy
- Loss of consciousness
- Nausea/vomiting
- Periorbital ecchymosis (raccoon's eyes)
- Posterior auricular ecchymosis (Battle sign)
- Scalp hematoma (especially significant in infants)
- Seizure
- Slow response, repetitive questioning

 ALERT!

An isolated scalp hematoma, along with the mechanism of injury, are important indicators of potential TBI in infants. Also, seizure indicates a high risk for TBI. If abuse is suspected, report to the appropriate authorities.

Diagnosis

Labs

- There are no labs specific to diagnose a head injury. However, the following may be helpful when determining severity and treatment:
  - Arterial blood gases
  - CBC
  - CMP
  - Urinalysis
  - PT, PTT, INR
  - Type and screen

 ALERT!

When monitoring GCS, trends are more important than single scores.

Diagnostic Testing

- Head CT
- MRI
- X-ray for severe TBI with multiple injuries:
  - Cervical spine
  - AP chest
  - AP pelvis
- GCS used in measuring impaired consciousness and coma
- Pediatric scale for patients 2 years old and younger (Table 4.1)
- Interpretation of table:
  - Possible scores range from 3 to 15
  - Score 13 and over:
    - Mild brain injury
  - Score 9 to 12:
    - Moderate brain injury
  - Score 8 and below:
    - Severe brain injury

Treatment

- Will be determined by the type and severity of injury
- Mild head injury:
  - May be treated with mental rest for one to two days following the injury
  - Symptoms treated
  - Usually resolves in 3 to 4 weeks

(continued)

Table 4.1 GCS for Pediatrics

Sign	Pediatric GCS	GCS	Score
Eye opening	Spontaneous	Spontaneous	4
	To sound	To command	3
	To pain	To pain	2
	None	None	1
Verbal response	Age-appropriate vocalization, smile, or orientation to sound; interacts (coos and babbles) and follows objects	Oriented	5
	Cries, irritable	Confused, disoriented	4
	Cries to pain	Inappropriate words	3
	Moans to pain	Incomprehensible sound	2
	None	None	1
Motor response	Spontaneous movements (obeys verbal command)	Obeys commands	6
	Withdraws to touch (localizes pain)	Localizes pain	5
	Withdraws to pain	Withdraws	4
	Abnormal flexion to pain (decorticate posture)	Abnormal flexion to pain (decorticate posture)	3
	Abnormal extension (decerebrate posture)	Abnormal extension to pain (decerebrate posture)	2
	None	None	1
Total			15

Source: Data from Brazelton, T., & Gosain, A. (2020). Classification of trauma in children. *UpToDate.* https://www.uptodate.com/contents/classification-of-trauma-in-children?search=pediatric%20glasgow%20coma%20scale&source=search_result&selectedTitle=1~125&usage_type=default&display_rank=1

Treatment *(continued)*

- Severe head injury:
  - Nonsurgical
    - Frequent neurologic exams (usually every hour for 24 hours in the PICU)
    - Monitor for increasing ICP from brain swelling
    - Prevent hypoxia, hypotension
    - Sedation and pain control
    - Treat ICP with hypertonic saline or mannitol (see Table 4.3)
  - Surgery
    - To stop bleeding in penetrating brain injury, epidural hematoma, and subdural hematoma
    - Evacuation of the blood and monitoring of ICP with a ventriculostomy may be required in the PICU.

Nursing Interventions

- Assess history of event and neurologic exam. Include the following questions in history:
  - Was the child wearing a helmet?
  - When did the injury occur?
  - What was the mechanism of injury?
  - Did the child lose consciousness? If so, how long?
  - Did the child have nausea or vomiting?
  - Has there been a change in mental status?
- Assessment of neurologic system includes:
  - Mental status
    - LOC
    - Interaction with environment
    - Oriented to person, place, and time
    - Speech clarity
  - Motor functions
    - Push and pull against hands of the healthcare provider with arms and legs
    - Balance
    - Active and passive movement of the joints
  - Sensory exam
    - Feel different instruments (e.g., sharp, soft, dull)
    - Feel difference between hot/cold
  - Reflexes (Chapter 2)
    - Newborn
      - Blinking
      - Babinski
      - Crawling
      - Moro's reflex
      - Palmar/plantar grasp
    - Older child
      - Reflex hammer
  - Cranial nerves
    - #1 Olfactory: smell
    - #2 Optic: vision
    - #3 Oculomotor: eye movements
    - #4 Trochlear: movement of the eyes
    - #5 Trigeminal: sensation of the face, inside the mouth, and muscles to chew
    - #6 Abducens: eye movements
    - #7 Facial nerve: movements of the face muscles and taste
    - #8 Acoustic: hearing
    - #9 Glossopharyngeal: taste, swallowing, gag reflex
    - #10 Vagus: swallow, gag reflex, some taste
    - #11 Accessory nerve: shoulders, neck
    - #12 Hypoglossal: tongue movements
  - Coordination exam
    - Walk on a line
    - Touch nose with eyes closed
- Maintain C-collar if cervical spine injury is suspected.
- Medicate as ordered for symptoms, such as headache, nausea, and pain.
- Monitor urine output, I/O, serum electrolytes, serum sodium osmolality, and urine osmolality.
- Monitor patient symptoms using the GCS trends.
- Monitor ICP, if applicable. It should be less than 20 mmHg.
- Monitor glucose and temperature.
- Monitor respiratory status and ventilatory effort.

 ALERT!

Risk of TBI is higher if is it is a fall over 3 feet, the head is struck by a high-speed object, a significant MVA, or if the mechanism is unknown.

Patient and Family Education

- Inform provider of any worsening symptoms.
  - Worsening headache
  - Vomiting
  - Cognition or behavior changes
  - Abnormal gait
  - Seizure
- Rest mentally and physically.
- Medicate for symptoms of headache, nausea, and sleeping problems.
- No sports or other strenuous activities until the patient is cleared by provider.
- Wear a helmet for sports and riding a bike.
- Wear seat belts and utilize appropriately sized car seats.

HYDROCEPHALUS

Overview

- *Hydrocephalus* is a condition where there is an imbalance in the production and absorption of CSF. This causes the accumulation of CSF within the cerebral ventricles and/or subarachnoid spaces. The result is either impaired absorption of CSF within the subarachnoid space, malfunction of the arachnoid villi (noncommunicating), or an obstruction to flow of CSF in the ventricular system (communicating hydrocephalus).
- This results in ventricular dilation and often-increased ICP.
- A *VP shunt* is a drain placed into the brain to relieve pressure caused by too much cerebral spinal fluid. It relieves pressure by draining excess CSF into the peritoneum.
- Risk factors for hydrocephalus include:
  - Brain hemorrhage or infections
  - Brain tumors
  - Birth weight less than 1,500 g
  - CNS malformations
  - Inherited genetic abnormalities
  - Intrauterine infections
  - Low socioeconomic status
  - Male sex
  - Maternal diabetes
  - Myelomeningocele
  - Race/ethnicity (decreased in Asians)
  - Various syndromes

Signs and Symptoms

Signs and symptoms of hydrocephalus (or increasing ICP) include:

- Abnormal gait
- Bulging anterior fontanel (infants)
- Cushing's triad (late sign)
- Enlarged head circumference
- Headache

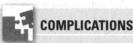

COMPLICATIONS

The most common complication of a VP shunt is shunt malfunction. Shunt malfunctions are caused by either infection or mechanical failure. If shunt malfunction or infection is suspected, refer for a neurologic assessment and neuroimaging. Keep patient NPO for possible surgical intervention.

ALERT!

Cushing's triad is a medical emergency that is a nervous system response to increased ICP, which affects three vital signs:

- Heart rate: bradycardia
- Respiration: irregular respirations (slow, deep respirations with periods of apnea)
- BP: Sudden hypertension or a widened pulse pressure (a large difference between the systolic and diastolic blood pressure)

Nurses should anticipate contacting a provider immediately if they note Cushing's triad, as this is a late sign of increased ICP.

- Hypertension
- Irritability
- Lethargy
- Papilledema
- Poor coordination
- Poor feeding
- Seizures
- Vomiting
- Visual disturbance

Diagnosis

Labs

There are no labs specific to diagnosing hydrocephalus. However, the following may be helpful when determining severity and treatment:

- Measurement of ICP through a lumbar puncture
- Screen for microbial agents, cytology, and antigen testing:
  - ABGs
  - Blood cultures
  - CBC
  - Serum electrolytes, calcium, magnesium
  - Urinalysis
  - Urine culture

Diagnostic Testing

- CT scan
- MRI
- MR venography

Treatment

- First-line treatment: placement of a VP shunt
  - The catheter is connected to a one-way valve that opens when pressure reaches a certain level.
  - The distal end of the catheter is placed in the peritoneal cavity; the proximal end is placed in the ventricle.
- Diuretics for short periods if patient is too unstable for surgery
- Asymptomatic patients: watchful waiting with monthly CTs and measuring head circumference in infants indicated
- Ventricle to atria shunt possible if VP shunt cannot be placed

Nursing Interventions

- Assess patient for signs of VP shunt malfunction:
  - Headache
  - Irritability
  - Lethargy
  - Papilledema
  - Vomiting
- Assess patient for signs of VP shunt infection:
  - Abdominal pain
  - Fever
- Monitor for infection.
  - Approximately 40% of shunts malfunction in the first year.
  - Infections are most common in the first 6 months after placement.
  - Antibiotics should be started immediately, but this is rarely the complete treatment.

 ALERT!

Shunt malfunctions are caused by either infection or mechanical failure. If shunt malfunction or infection is suspected, refer for a neurologic assessment and neuroimaging. Keep patient NPO for possible surgical intervention.

(continued)

Nursing Interventions *(continued)*

- Surgery to remove the infected shunt is needed in most cases.
  - If malfunction is caused by infection, the shunt may have to be externalized for a time while the infection is treated with IV antibiotics. If one of the components of the shunt is infected, that component may be replaced. If necessary, the entire shunt may be replaced.
- Mechanical failure malfunction is most common in the first year after placement.
  - Shunt mechanical failure malfunction is usually caused by obstruction of the catheter.
  - Other causes are broken tubing, shunt migration, and excessive drainage.

Patient and Family Education

- Child, family, and healthcare provider should collaborate to discuss options before participating in any sports.
- If shunt is programmable, this may need to be reprogrammed if the child has an MRI.
- Learn about hydrocephalus and the signs and symptoms of shunt malfunction.
- Utilize available community resources.
- Younger patients should have their shunt checked every year or as directed by their neurosurgeon. Remember a shunt placed as an infant or young child with need a revision as the child grows. Several shunt revisions may be needed throughout the patient's lifetime into adulthood.

 POP QUIZ 4.2

A 2-year-old child presents at the ED with extreme irritability, a decreased appetite, headache, and somnolence. Vital signs are HR 165, RR 24, BP 98/54 and temperature 98.06 °F (36.7 °C). The child's only health concern until now is the placement of a VP shunt soon after birth. What is the most likely cause of the child's symptoms?

LEAD POISONING

Overview

- Lead exposure can occur by contact, ingestion, or inhalation of lead or lead-based paint and dust.
  - Exposure:
    - Lead-containing paint: Lead was eliminated from paint in 1978, but older homes may not have been mitigated. Window edges painted with lead paint often contribute to the lead dust when they are opened and closed.
    - Soil
    - Contact with others who were exposed: Lead can be carried into the home on the clothes or shoes of others who have been exposed, such as caregivers who work in construction.
- Lead poisoning is most dangerous to children under 6 because their brains are still developing.
- It may take several years for serum lead levels to decrease once exposed.
- Risk factors for lead poisoning include:
  - Living in low-income housing
  - Living in older houses with lead paint
  - Living in a house with old plumbing containing lead
  - Using imported products that contain lead, including food and toys

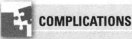 **COMPLICATIONS**

Lead exposure can affect any part of the body including renal, hematologic, and neurologic systems. Lead can damage the brain and nervous system, resulting in learning disabilities, behavioral problems, delayed growth, loss of hearing, and speech problems.

Signs and Symptoms

- Abdominal pain
- Coma
- Developmental delay
- Fatigue
- GI disturbances: constipation, nausea, vomiting
- Headaches
- Hearing loss
- Irritability
- Loss of appetite
- Neurologic changes
- Peripheral neuropathy
- Pica
- Seizures
- Weight loss

 ALERT!

Symptomatic lead intoxication should be treated as an emergency and confirmed with a repeat blood lead level. Hospitalization and chelation therapy should be initiated. If the patient has encephalopathy, they should be admitted to a pediatric ICU.

Diagnosis

Labs

- Blood test to measure lead level in blood
- Ongoing testing every 1 to 2 months for levels between 5 mcg/dL and 45 mcg/dL
- Treatment for levels 45 mcg/dL or higher in children
- Labs for iron deficiency, serum electrolytes, BUN and creatinine, serum calcium and magnesium, alanine and aspartate aminotransferases, and urinalysis

 ALERT!

The CDC advises that there is NO safe level of lead in the blood. If there is any level of lead in the blood, the source should be investigated.

Diagnostic Testing

There are no diagnostic tests specific to diagnose lead poisoning.

Treatment

- Chelation therapy to remove lead from blood, soft tissues, and the brain recommended for lead levels greater than 45 mcg/dL
- Optimized nutrition to improve outcomes, but no iron supplements simultaneously with chelation therapy

 ALERT!

Extreme care must be taken when using chelation agents. Death can occur from hypocalcemia when Na$_2$EDTA is used vs. calcium disodium versenate (CaNa$_2$EDTA). Adequate oral fluid intake and urine output are imperative when giving CaEDTA.

Nursing Interventions

- Identify whether other children in the household are at risk and, if so, let family know that they should also be tested.
- Notify public health authority.
- Provide information on home checks.
- Provide resources for eliminating exposure to lead.

Patient and Family Education

- Identify possible sources of lead in the home and neighborhood.
- Learn the sources of lead and the health effects of lead exposure.
- Obtain support information from the local health department.
- Review the signs and symptoms of lead poisoning.
- Toys for small children should be safety tested. Look for safety seals and learn what to look for on toy packages.

Overview

- *Meningitis* is inflammation of the meninges of the brain.
- The majority of cases are either viral or bacterial.
  - Bacterial is generally more severe and has almost 100% mortality rate if untreated.
  - All cases need to be treated as bacterial until proven otherwise.
- Presentation depends on age, immune status, and causing agent.
- Some common bacteria are:
  - Most common bacteria (protective vaccines):
    - ○ *Streptococcus pneumoniae* (pneumococcal conjugate vaccine)
    - ○ *Meningococcal* (polysaccharide diphtheria toxoid conjugate vaccine)
    - ○ *Haemophilus influenzae* (HIB)
  - Others
    - ○ *Pneumococcal* (infants)
    - ○ *Neisseria meningitides*
    - ○ *Staphylococcal*
    - ○ *Escherichia coli*
    - ○ *Group β streptococci*
- Some viral causes that may require treatment are:
  - Enteroviruses (90% caused by enteroviruses, coxsackie, and echoviruses)
  - Herpes viruses (types 1 and 2)
  - Arboviruses (West Nile virus)
  - Cytomegalovirus
  - Influenza
  - Coronavirus (including SARS-CoV-2)
  - Varicella zoster virus
  - Mumps

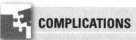

COMPLICATIONS

Complications of bacterial meningitis can be systemic or neurologic.

- Systemic
  - ○ Septic, hypovolemic shock
  - ○ SIADH
  - ○ DIC
  - ○ ARDS
- Neurologic (sudden or gradual)
  - ○ Ataxia
  - ○ Developmental delay
  - ○ Hearing loss
  - ○ Hemiparesis, quadriparesis
  - ○ Hydrocephalus
  - ○ Impaired mental status
  - ○ Palsies
  - ○ Seizures
  - ○ Subdural effusion

Signs and Symptoms

- Infants
  - Bulging fontanel
  - Decreased oral intake
  - Fever
  - Nuchal rigidity
- Older children
  - Fever
  - Headache
  - Nausea/vomiting
  - Nuchal rigidity
  - Photophobia

Diagnosis

Labs
- Blood tests
  - CBC with Diff
  - Coagulation studies (PT, PTT)
  - Cultures (shows pathogen)
  - Glucose (normal, viral; less than 45 mg/dL, bacterial)
  - Inflammation markers (CRP, procalcitonin)
  - Platelet count
  - Serum electrolytes, BUN, creatinine
- CSF
  - Cell count and differential (WBC 100–10,000 or more, bacterial; 1,000 or less, viral)
  - Glucose (decreased or greater than 40, bacterial; normal to less than 40, viral)
  - Protein (100–500, bacterial; 50–200, viral)
  - Gram stain, bacterial cultures
  - Viral PCR studies

Diagnostic Testing
Brain MRI.

Treatment

- Supportive care
  - Acetaminophen or ibuprofen (Table A.2)
  - Hydration
  - Rest
    - ○ Avoid watching television or playing video games
    - ○ Keep lighting dim/dark
    - ○ Provide quiet environment
  - Adequate hydration, but not over-hydration, as too much fluid can increase ICP
- Hospital
  - Antibiotics (vancomycin, ceftriaxone) for bacterial meningitis
  - Antiviral (acyclovir) for viral meningitis
  - IV hydration
  - Pain control
  - Steroids (dexamethasone) to reduce inflammation, tissue repair

 ALERT!

It is crucial that the lumbar puncture is performed before administering antibiotics so that the bacteria can be identified and treated with the appropriate antibiotic.

 NURSING PEARL

Since the causative organism is unknown initially, antibiotics should provide coverage for meningococcal and PCN-resistant pneumococcus because they are the most common causes. Antibiotics are given until 48 to 72 hours after a negative blood culture.

 ALERT!

Fluid management in bacterial meningitis must be monitored very carefully. Avoid hypotonic fluids because they deliver too much free water and can cause hyponatremia and exacerbate cerebral edema.

Nursing Interventions

- Elevate HOB 30 degrees with head in neutral position.
- Keep patients and family informed and explain rationales for interventions.
- Maintain a quiet environment with dim lighting.
- Medicate as ordered. Use antibiotics for bacterial infections only.
- Monitor neurologic status and symptoms including temperature, pain, consciousness, protective reflexes (gag, swallowing, cough, blink), and pupils.
- Use seizure precautions if necessary.

Patient and Family Education

- Keep the environment as quiet as possible.
- Learn about the condition and what needs reported to the physician.
- Monitor the patient's hearing acuity and developmental progress, as both can be affected by meningitis.
- Recognize importance of immunizations (Chapter 2).
- Rest mentally as well as physically, restricting video games, TV, too many friends, and so on.

SEIZURES

Overview

- Seizures are caused by abnormal, excessive, or synchronous discharges of neurons in the cerebral cortex.
- An *acute symptomatic seizure* is one that is caused by an acute illness or brain injury.
- Unprovoked seizures occur in absence of a clinical condition.
- *Status epilepticus* are seizures that are prolonged (usually lasting from 5 to 30 minutes) or a series of seizures that occur without the child regaining their previous LOC. This is a medical emergency that can lead to permanent brain damage or death.
- Types of seizures include focal and generalized.
  - Focal seizures are focused in one hemisphere.
    - Autonomic seizures include autonomic reflexes.
    - Motor seizures have motor activity on one side.
    - Patient may or may not be aware of the seizure.
    - Sensory seizures are internal to the patient.
  - Generalized seizures involve both hemispheres and are subdivided into two categories.
    - *Absence seizures*: brief, sudden lapses in consciousness, more common in infants and children than adults
    - *Generalized tonic-clonic seizures*: bilateral, convulsive tonic-clonic muscle contractions
- *Epilepsy* is a disorder where the child has a predisposition to recurrent seizures. It is not one isolated seizure event.
  - Epilepsy is diagnosed when a child has had two or more seizures, disregarding febrile seizures.
  - Epilepsy may be caused by genetic, structural, metabolic, immune disorders, or infectious agents. The cause of epilepsy may be unknown.

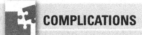 **COMPLICATIONS**

Complications of seizures include:
- Aspiration of food or saliva into the lungs while seizing
- Injury from falling, bumping into things while seizing
- Driving or operating machinery when a seizure happens
- Brain damage from a stroke

 NURSING PEARL

Febrile seizures are generally benign and occur in approximately 4% of children under 5 years of age. The occurrence of a febrile seizure happens with high fevers and does not predispose the child to epilepsy later in life. Children who have febrile seizures may have a strong family history of febrile seizures or have. They are treated if they last over 5 minutes.

Signs and Symptoms

- Focal seizures
  - Motor symptoms
    - Brief twitching
    - Jerking (clonic)
    - Repeated movements such as lip-smacking, chewing, or clapping
    - Weak muscles (atonic)
  - Nonmotor symptoms include changes in the following:
    - Autonomic functions
    - Emotions

 ALERT!

Seizure signs in infants include apnea, repetitive facial movements (rhythmic blinking and lip-smacking), staring, and unusual bicycling or pedaling movements.

- ○ Sensation
- ○ Thinking
- Generalized seizures
  - Motor symptoms
    - ○ Difficulty breathing
    - ○ Loss of bladder control
    - ○ Sustained jerking movements
    - ○ Tense or rigid muscles
  - Nonmotor symptoms
    - ○ Absence/staring spells
    - ○ Cessation of activity
    - ○ Lack of response when touched
    - ○ May happen many times in a day

Diagnosis

Labs

There are no labs specific to diagnosing seizures. However, the following may be helpful when determining severity and treatment:
- BMP
- CBC with attention to the white blood cell count (to rule out infection)
- CSF analysis
- Liver function tests
- Ammonia and urine organic acids may indicate metabolic disturbances
- Urinalysis and toxicology

Diagnostic Testing
- EEG
- Head CT, and MRI

Treatment

- Medication first-line agents:
  - Benzodiazepines (lorazepam and diazepam) for initial treatment (Table A.2)
  - Phenobarbital: used for most infant seizures
  - Phenytoin (see Table 4.3)
  - Fosphenytoin (see Table 4.3)
- Maintenance medications:
  - Levetiracetam, phenytoin, valproate, carbamazepine (therapeutic level 4–12 mcg/mL)
  - Valproic acid, gabapentin, lamotrigine, topiramate (see Table 4.3)
- Emergent medications:
  - Diazepam: rectal gel that can be given at home or in the hospital at the start of a seizure; comes in various doses and should be kept in refrigerator
  - Buccal or intranasal midazolam: alternate rescue medications
- Ketogenic diets: patients with medication-resistant epilepsy
  - High-fat, low carbohydrate diet producing metabolic changes in the brain is like starvation: 70% to 80% fats, 20% proteins, and 5% to 10% carbohydrates
  - Changes in ketones, insulin, glucose, glucagon, and fatty acids when the body is retrained to burn fat for energy
  - Ketones are theoretically anticonvulsants when crossing the BBB
  - Ketogenic formulas available
  - Side effects of the diet:
    - ○ Bone disease
    - ○ Constipation
    - ○ High cholesterol
    - ○ Kidney stones

(continued)

Treatment *(continued)*

- ○ Slower growth
- ○ Tiredness
- Other options: vagal nerve stimulators, responsive neurostimulation, and deep brain stimulation
  - Vagal nerve stimulators generally implanted in patient's chest
  - When activated, device sends electrical signals along the left vagal nerve to brainstem and then to brain
  - May take up to a year before differences in frequency and intensity of seizures noticed
- Surgery possible if medications not effective

Nursing Interventions

- Maintain seizure precautions.
  - Add padded side rails.
  - Keep the bed at the lowest height.
  - Keep suction and O_2 available at bedside.
  - Refer child to social services and report to children and youth services if a head injury and seizures occur together and abuse is suspected (Chapter 16).
- Maximize patient's safety when actively seizing:
  - Do not put anything in the patient's mouth.
  - Ensure the airway is patent.
  - Ease the patient to the floor or a chair if patient is not lying down when seizure occurs.
  - Place the patient on their left side.
  - Loosen restrictive clothing.
  - Protect the patient's head.
  - Move items away from the patient to prevent injury.
  - Stay with the patient and observe activity.
  - Time the duration of the seizure.
  - After seizure, observe postictal behavior. Reassure and comfort the patient.
- Encourage adherence in taking medications.
- Encourage patient to keep all follow-up appointments.
- If the patient is on a ketogenic diet, refer family to a dietician to monitor.
- Evaluate patient's labs to verify that seizure medications are within the therapeutic range.

Patient and Family Education

- Call the doctor's office 2 weeks before the prescription runs out for a refill.
- Learn the side effects of medications and the importance of taking medications at the same time every day (see Table 4.3).
- Learn the signs and symptoms of seizures.

 NURSING PEARL

There are three main phases of a seizure: the aura, ictal, and postictal phases.

- Aura:
  - ○ The early part of the seizure. Symptoms include:
    - Odd smells, sounds, or tastes
    - Déjà vu (the feeling that something has happened before, but it has not)
    - Dizziness
    - Vision difficulties
    - Numbness in parts of the body
    - Headache
    - Feeling panic, intense fear
  - ○ Some people will have the aura and no seizure. Not all people have the aura period before the seizure begins.
- Ictal:
  - ○ The middle phase
  - ○ Lasts until the seizure is over, the period where electrical activity happens in the brain
  - ○ Symptoms of this phase:
    - Loss of awareness
    - Loss of memory
    - Confusion
    - Repeated movements like lip-smacking
    - Uncontrolled body movements
- Postictal:
  - ○ Period immediately following the seizure
  - ○ Can last between 5 and 30 minutes and ends when patient returns to baseline
  - ○ Symptoms of this phase include:
    - Confusion
    - Drowsiness
    - Headache
    - Nausea

 NURSING PEARL

Be sure to instruct family not to put anything in the patient's mouth during a seizure. This is not necessary and can be potentially dangerous.

- Family should learn what to do when a patient has a seizure:
  - Call 911 if seizure lasts more than 5 minutes or if the patient does not wake up after seizure.
  - Give prescribed seizure rescue medication (i.e., rectal valium, intranasal midazolam).
  - Place the patient on their side.
  - Make sure the environment is safe to prevent injury.
  - Write down what happens to the patient during a seizure to report to the doctor or provider.
- Obtain appropriate education for patients on a ketogenic diet.
  - Multiple sugar-free food options are available.
  - Return to the physician's office for blood and urine tests.
  - Adhere to the diet, as one "cheat" meal can alter ketone levels.

POP QUIZ 4.3

A child with seizures is admitted to the hospital for surgical repair of a humerus fracture. This patient has been following a ketogenic diet hoping to reduce the number of seizures she has been having. When putting in the lunch order with the cafeteria, the child requests a cheeseburger with bun, french fries, broccoli, and ice cream. Which of these foods should the nurse allow the child to have?

Overview

- Trisomy 21, or Down syndrome, is a common genetic disorder caused by inheriting an extra 21st chromosome.
- There are multiple health issues associated with Down syndrome, and there is a wide range of disability among patients (Table 4.2).
- The primary risk factor for having a trisomy 21 child is advanced maternal age, although children with Down syndrome can be born to parents of all ages.

COMPLICATIONS

Children with Trisomy 21 have an increased risk of having obstructive sleep apnea because of soft tissue and skeletal differences in the neck that cause upper airway obstruction. Symptoms include snoring and restless sleep. An evaluation includes a sleep study with oxygen saturation monitoring.

Signs and Symptoms

- Head and neck
  - Abnormal teeth
  - Flat nose bridge
  - Folded ears
  - High, arched, narrow palate
  - Large, protruding tongue
  - Low-set small ears and narrow canals
  - Short neck
  - Up-slanting palpebral fissures
- Extremities
  - Hyper-flexibility of joints
  - Short, broad hands and fingers
  - Transverse palmar crease (Simian crease)
- Intellectual disability
  - Language delays
  - IQ anywhere between 20 and 70

Table 4.2 Health Concerns for Trisomy 21 Patients

Concern	Clinical Features
Cardiovascular disease	• Complete atrioventricular septal defect: most common congenital heart defect in Down syndrome patients • Cardiovascular involvement: half of all Down syndrome patients • Pulmonary hypertension common
GI abnormalities	• Celiac disease • Duodenal atresia or stenosis • Hirschsprung disease
Endocrine disorders	• Low birth weight, smaller head circumference, and length • Shorter stature • Diabetes type 1 • Hypo- and hyperthyroidism • Higher BMI • Slower metabolism
Vision problems	• Nearsightedness, farsightedness, astigmatism • Nystagmus • Strabismus
Hearing loss	• Congenital hearing loss • Secondary hearing loss from recurrent otitis media
Hematologic disorders	• Acute lymphoblastic leukemia • Leukopenia • Macrocytosis • Polycythemia • Thrombocytosis • Transient leukemia • Immune deficiency
Pulmonary disorders	• Asthma • Chronic aspiration • Obstructive sleep apnea • Parenchymal lung disease • Upper and lower airway disorders
Skin disorders	• Most benign • Alopecia • Fissured tongue • Hyperkeratosis of the palms • Seborrheic dermatitis
Reproduction disorders	• Females are fertile; may experience early menopause • Nearly all males infertile, usually with abnormally low sperm counts, though some have fathered children
Urologic abnormalities	• Hypospadias • Kidney malformations • Testicular cancer • Undescended testicles
Atlantoaxial instability	• Gait abnormalities • Loss of bowel or bladder control • Subluxation of cervical spine • Spinal cord compression • Torticollis

Source: Data from Ostermaier, K. (2020). Down syndrome: Clinical features and diagnosis. *UpToDate*. https://www.uptodate.com/contents/down-syndrome-clinical-features-and-diagnosis

Diagnosis

Labs
Blood karyotype testing.

Diagnostic Testing
Prenatal diagnostic tests:
- Amniocentesis
- Chorionic villus sampling
- Ultrasound

Treatment

- Newborns referred to specialists:
  - Cardiologist
  - Hearing test using brain-evoked response
  - Ophthalmologist
- Ophthalmology and hearing evaluations annually after newborn period
- Childhood management includes:
  - Evaluate possible psychiatric and behavioral problems.
  - Maximize cognitive ability.
  - Monitor for possible sleep apnea.
  - Monitor CBC for possible anemia and leukemia.
  - Monitor for growth disturbances.
  - Refer to frequent dental visits.
  - Screen for celiac starting at age 1 and annually throughout childhood.
  - Screen for thyroid imbalances throughout childhood.

Nursing Interventions

- Advocate for the patient and provide family with emotional support.
- Educate family regarding prenatal screening and support decisions they make.
- Provide information to family about Down syndrome.
- Offer information for community groups that support families of Down syndrome children.

Patient and Family Education

- Consider contacting a support group. There are many organizations that offer support, including the March of Dimes, the National Association for Down Syndrome, and the Association for Children with Down Syndrome.
- Keep all appointments with the medical team to ensure early detection of any possible abnormalities.

 POP QUIZ 4.4

A 40-year-old woman has just had her first baby. She did not have prenatal care. The baby is small for gestational age, has a palmar crease, low-set ears, and a thick neck. How should the nurse prepare the mother?

Table 4.3 Neurologic Medications

Indications	Mechanism of Action	Contraindications, Precautions, and Adverse Effects
Alpha 2A-adrenergic receptor agonists (guanfacine)		
• Treat ADHD • Used in patients in which stimulants are not effective	• Reduce sympathetic nerve impulses, which decreases sympathetic vasomotor tone and heart rate • Not a CNS stimulant	• Precaution is needed in patients with heart conduction and other heart abnormalities, cardiovascular disease, or hepatitis and renal impairment. • The American Heart Association and American Academy of Pediatrics recommend a thorough heart disease risk factor examination prior to taking. • Adverse effects include drowsiness, headache, insomnia, abdominal pain, and decrease in appetite. • Take immediate release at bedtime. • Do not stop suddenly.
Anticonvulsants (carbamazepine)		
• Treats focal • Temporal lobe seizures	• Limit the influx of sodium ions across the cell membrane	• Medication is contraindicated for use in patients with bone marrow depression and in those taking MAO inhibitors in the past 14 days. • Precautions include the risk of developing anemia or agranulocytosis during treatment. Monitor platelets and WBC closely. • Substitution of a different carbamazepine product may cause changes in the blood concentration. If required, monitor closely. • Precautions related to hepatic injury require monitoring liver function. • Adverse effects include hyponatremia, psychiatric effects, renal toxicity, and suicidal ideation. • Adverse effects also include toxic epidermal necrolysis, Stevens–Johnson syndrome, aplastic anemia, agranulocytosis, dizziness, drowsiness, ataxia, nausea, and vomiting.

Table 4.3 Neurologic Medications (continued)

Indications	Mechanism of Action	Contraindications, Precautions, and Adverse Effects
Anticonvulsants (fosphenytoin)		
• Treat focal, complex partial seizures, refractory, generalized seizures, tonic-clonic seizures • Treat status epilepticus	• Limit the spread of seizure activity by reducing seizure propagation • Decrease seizure activity by decreasing influx of sodium ions across cell membranes in motor cortex	• Medication is contraindicated in patients with bradycardia, sinoatrial block, second- and third-degree heart blocks, or Adams–Stokes syndrome. • Precautions include monitoring CV during administration for possible arrhythmias, hypotension, or ventricular defibrillation. • Monitor vitamin D levels, especially in chronic therapy. • Hematologic reactions have also been reported. Patients with a history of blood conditions may be at higher risk. • Adverse reactions include pruritus, ataxia, dizziness, drowsiness, and nystagmus. • Medication is compatible with dextrose and NSS IV solution. • For status epilepticus, dilute and give as an IV push no faster than 150 PE/min.
Anticonvulsants (gabapentin)		
• Treat seizures • Treat focal and complex partial seizure	• Has affinity to calcium channels, which modulate the release of excitatory neurotransmitters	• Contraindications include hypersensitivity to gabapentin. • Precautions include monitoring patients with renal impairment, seizure disorder (ER only), and substance abuse. • Adverse effects include viral infections, dizziness, drowsiness, and fatigue. • IR and ER formulas are not interchangeable. • Do not stop suddenly.
Anticonvulsants (lamotrigine)		
• Treat focal, complex partial seizures, and generalized tonic-clonic and refractory seizures	• Inhibit the release of glutamate and inhibit sodium channels to stabilize neuronal membranes	• Precautions include possible CNS depression. Patient should be warned. • Use caution in patients with structural or functional heart abnormalities. Medication may cause arrhythmias; monitor closely. • Use caution in patients with hepatic and renal impairment. Dosage may need to be adjusted in both cases. • Adverse effects include nausea.

(continued)

Table 4.3 Neurologic Medications *(continued)*

Indications	Mechanism of Action	Contraindications, Precautions, and Adverse Effects
Anticonvulsants (levetiracetam)		
• Commonly used as a first-line treatment medication for early epilepsy • Used for focal, simple partial seizures	• Mechanism of action unknown • Possibly inhibit sodium channels • Possibly facilitate GABA • Possibly decrease K+ current • Possibly bind to synaptic proteins, which modulate neurotransmitter release	• Use with caution in patients with hepatic disease. • Use with caution in patients with preexisting psychosis or schizophrenia. • Precautions include monitoring blood pressure in children less than 4 years old for higher-than-normal diastolic pressure. • Give smaller doses to patients with renal disease or impairment. • Do not stop suddenly. • Adverse effects include drowsiness, headache, fatigue, increased blood pressure, dizziness, somnolence, behavioral disturbances, psychotic symptoms, and vomiting. • Monitor for suicide and depression.
Anticonvulsant, barbiturate (phenobarbital)		
• Treat focal, complex partial seizures • Generalized tonic-clonic seizures • Refractory seizures	• Depress sensory cortex, decrease motor activity, and alter cerebellar function • Has sedative, hypnotic, and anticonvulsant properties	• Contraindications include severe hepatic impairment, dyspnea, and porphyria. • Precautions include CNS depression, paradoxical stimulation, respiratory depression, and asthma. • Use caution in patients with anemia, cardiac disease, depression, diabetes, hepatic impairment, hyperthyroidism, and renal impairment. • In children, medication can cause cognitive deficits. • Do not stop suddenly. • Adverse effects include nausea, rash, apnea, bradycardia, syncope, hypotension, anxiety, nightmares, headache, and lethargy. • Give slowly using a large vein to avoid the possibility of respiratory depression, laryngospasm, hypertension, and severe hypotension.

Table 4.3 Neurologic Medications *(continued)*

Indications	Mechanism of Action	Contraindications, Precautions, and Adverse Effects
Anticonvulsants (phenytoin)		
• Treat focal, complex partial seizures, and generalized tonic-clonic seizures • Treat refractory seizures	• Limit the spread of seizure activity by reducing seizure propagation • Decrease seizure activity by decreasing influx of sodium ions across cell membranes in motor cortex	• Contraindications include sinus bradycardia, SA block, second- and third-degree heart block, and Adams–Stokes syndrome. • Caution must be used with hematologic patients, as reactions have been reported. Patients with a history of blood conditions may be at higher risk. • Monitor CV during administration for possible arrhythmias, hypotension, or ventricular fibrillation. • Monitor liver function, as acute hepatic failure has occurred. • Use caution in patients with diabetes, hypoalbuminemia, hypothyroidism, renal impairment, and porphyria. • Adverse reactions include cardiac rhythm abnormalities, CNS dysfunction, dermatitis, constipation, and nausea/vomiting. • Medication may cause depression and suicidal ideation. • Give slowly over a minimum of 30 minutes. • Medication is compatible in only NSS IV solution and will precipitate if mixed with dextrose.

(continued)

Table 4.3 Neurologic Medications *(continued)*

Indications	Mechanism of Action	Contraindications, Precautions, and Adverse Effects
Anticonvulsants (sodium valproate)		
• Treat seizures • Used specifically in myoclonic epilepsy	• Increase GABA • Block sodium channels to suppress repetitive neuronal firing	• Contraindications include significant hepatic impairment, acute head trauma, mitochondrial disease, pancreatitis, and urea cycle disorders. • Precautions must be taken before surgery. Monitor CBC and coagulation parameters. • Use with caution in patients with renal failure, impairment, and HIV. • Do not stop suddenly. • Medication may cause drug reaction with eosinophilia and systemic symptoms and be life-threatening or fatal. • Use with caution in patients with renal failure, impairment, and HIV. • Adverse effects include alopecia, dizziness, drowsiness, headache, GI disturbance, infection, thrombocytopenia, and tremor.
Anticonvulsants (topiramate)		
• Treat all types of seizures	• Block neuronal sodium channels • Enhance GABA • Antagonize glutamate receptors • Inhibit carbonic anhydrase	• Precautions must be used for patients with hepatic and renal impairment. • Do not stop suddenly. • Monitor for signs of kidney stone development, which has happened in the pediatric population. • Medication has caused metabolic acidosis in pediatric patients. • Adverse effects include anorexia, agitation, confusion, dizziness, hyperthermia, suicidal ideation, hypotension, rash, diarrhea, agitation, confusion, headache, dizziness, and nasal congestion.

Table 4.3 Neurologic Medications *(continued)*

Indications	Mechanism of Action	Contraindications, Precautions, and Adverse Effects
Diuretic osmotic (mannitol)		
• Treat high ICP with cerebral edema	• Decrease blood viscosity and increase cerebral blood flow and O_2 transport, which decreases cerebral blood volume and ICP	• Contraindications include active intracranial bleeding, anuria, hypersensitivity to mannitol, preexisting severe pulmonary vascular congestion, or pulmonary edema. • Medication is contraindicated in patients with severe renal impairment. • Precautions include an increase in cerebral blood flow, which would increase the risk of postop bleeding in neurologic patients. This could also worsen intracranial hypertension in children who develop cerebral hyperemia in the first 24–48 hours after TBI. • High doses may cause renal dysfunction. • For cerebral edema, boluses are better than continuous infusions. • Monitor urine output, intake and output, serum electrolytes, and serum and urine osmolality. • Adverse effects include electrolyte imbalance, hypertension, tachycardia, chills, confusion, dizziness, diaphoresis, dehydration, nausea/vomiting, anuria, urinary retention, blurry vision, and dyspnea.
Muscle relaxants (baclofen)		
• Treat muscle contractures	• Inhibit transmission of reflects at the spinal cord level	• Caution should be used in patients with urinary obstruction, peptic ulcers, decreased GI mobility, psychiatric disease, renal impairment, respiratory disease, and seizure disorders. • Do not stop abruptly. • Adverse effects include nausea/vomiting, confusion, headache, fatigue, confusion, deep vein thrombosis, and transient ischemic attacks.

(continued)

Table 4.3 Neurologic Medications *(continued)*

Indications	Mechanism of Action	Contraindications, Precautions, and Adverse Effects
Neurotoxins (OnabotulinumtoxinA)		
• Used to treat muscle contractures	• Neurotoxin to prevent calcium release of acetylcholine and produce a state of denervation • Muscle inactivation until new fibrils grow from nerve	• Contraindications include infection at proposed injection site. • Use caution if patient is using any other agents that interfere with neuromuscular transmission. • Use caution in patients with bleeding disorders. • Adverse effects include decreased appetite, fatigue, nausea, and constipation. • Myocardial infarct has occurred with medication use. • Adverse effects include the effects of toxin may spread from the area of injection, causing muscle weakness, ptosis, dysphagia, urinary incontinence, and breathing difficulties. • Store in a refrigerator.
Selective norepinephrine reuptake inhibitor (atomoxetine)		
• Treat ADHD in patients 6 and older	• Selectively inhibit the reuptake of norepinephrine	• Contraindications include use with MAO inhibitors, patients with narrow-angle glaucoma, severe cardiac or vascular disorders, or a history of pheochromocytoma. • Has caused sudden death in children with preexisting cardiac abnormalities. • Precautions needed as atomoxetine can cause aggression and hostility, particularly at the beginning of treatment. • Precaution needed in patients with cardiac history and hepatic conditions. Medication has also caused priapism and psychiatric events. • Adverse reactions include headache, insomnia, nausea/vomiting, palpitations, syncope, weight loss, tremor, blurred vision, weakness, anxiety, and growth suppression.

Table 4.3 Neurologic Medications *(continued)*

Indications	Mechanism of Action	Contraindications, Precautions, and Adverse Effects
Stimulant (amphetamine)		
• Treat ADHD • First-line treatment for uncomplicated ADHD	• Noncatecholamine agents that stimulate the release of dopamine and norepinephrine	• Medication is contraindicated if used during or within 14 days following MAO inhibitor. • Medication is contraindicated in patients with moderate hypertension, hyperthyroidism, history of drug abuse, heart dysfunction, or agitated states. • Medication is contraindicated in combination with serotonergic agents. • Precautions indicated in patients with bipolar disorder or agitation. • Use caution in patients with cerebrovascular conditions, hyperthyroidism, and Tourette's. • Adverse effects include depression, suicidal ideation, hypertension, tachycardia, and peripheral vasculopathy. • This medication is a controlled substance. Use caution to prevent unauthorized usage. It has a high risk for abuse, dependency, and for nontherapeutic use.

RESOURCES

American Academy of Pediatrics. (2018). *Developmental and behavioral pediatrics* (2nd ed.). Author.

Brazelton, T., & Gosain, A. (2020). Classification of trauma in children. *UpToDate*. https://www.uptodate.com/contents/classification-of-trauma-in-children?search=pediatric%20glasgow%20coma%20scale&source=search_result&selectedTitle=1~125&usage_type=default&display_rank=1

Centers for Disease Control and Prevention. (2021, February 10). *Childhood lead poisoning prevention*. U.S. Department of Health and Human Services, Centers for Disease Control and Prevention. http://www.cdc.gov/nceh/lead/p

Hockenberry, M., Wilson, D., & Rogers, C. (2019). *Wong's nursing care of infants & children* (11th ed.). Elsevier.

Kemp, C. (2018, January 4). Most children as young as 6 can use 0–10 scale to rate pain. *American Academy of Pediatrics*. https://publications.aap.org/aapnews/news/12054?autologincheck=redirected

Lexicomp. (2021a). Baclofen: Pediatric drug information [Drug Information]. *UpToDate*. https://www.uptodate.com/contents/baclofen-pediatric-drug-information?search=baclofen&source=panel_search_result&selectedTitle=1~93&usage_type=panel&kp_tab=drug_pediatric&display_rank=1

Lexicomp. (2021b). Botox: Pediatric drug information [Drug Information]. *UpToDate*. https://www.uptodate.com/contents/onabotulinumtoxina-botox-pediatric-drug-information?search=botox&selectedTitle=1~138&usage_type=panel&display_rank=1&kp_tab=drug_pediatric&source=panel_search_result

Lexicomp. (2021c). Carbamazepine: Pediatric drug information [Drug Information]. *UpToDate*. https://www.uptodate.com/contents/search?search=carbamazepine&sp=0&searchType=PLAIN_TEXT&source=USER_INPUT&searchControl=TOP_PULLDOWN&searchOffset=1&autoComplete=true&language=en&max=10&index=0~6&autoCompleteTerm=carb

Lexicomp. (2021d). Dexmethylphenidate: Pediatric drug information [Drug Information]. *UpToDate*. https://www.uptodate.com/contents/dexmethylphenidate-pediatric-drug-information?search=dexmethylphenidate&selectedTitle=1~25&usage_type=panel&display_rank=1&kp_tab=drug_pediatric&source=panel_search_result

Lexicomp. (2021e). Guanfacine: Pediatric drug information [Drug Information]. *UpToDate*. https://www.uptodate.com/contents/search?search=guanfacine&sp=0&searchType=PLAIN_TEXT&source=USER_INPUT&searchControl=TOP_PULLDOWN&searchOffset=1&autoComplete=true&language=en&max=10&index=0~6&autoCompleteTerm=guan

Lexicomp. (2021f). Lamotrigine: Pediatric drug information [Drug Information]. *UpToDate*. https://www.uptodate.com/contents/search?search=lamotrigine&sp=0&searchType=PLAIN_TEXT&source=USER_INPUT&searchControl=TOP_PULLDOWN&searchOffset=1&autoComplete=true&language=en&max=10&index=0~6&autoCompleteTerm=lamo

Lexicomp. (2021g). Levetiracetam: Pediatric drug information [Drug Information]. *UpToDate*. https://www.uptodate.com/contents/search?search=levetiracetam&sp=0&searchType=PLAIN_TEXT&source=USER_INPUT&searchControl=TOP_PULLDOWN&searchOffset=1&autoComplete=true&language=en&max=10&index=0~6&autoCompleteTerm=levet

Lexicomp. (2021h). Methylphenidate: Pediatric drug information [Drug Information]. *UpToDate*. https://www.uptodate.com/contents/search?search=methylphenidate&sp=0&searchType=PLAIN_TEXT&source=USER_INPUT&searchControl=TOP_PULLDOWN&searchOffset=1&autoComplete=true&language=en&max=10&index=1~6&autoCompleteTerm=methyl

Lexicomp. (2021i). Phenobarbital: Pediatric drug information [Drug Information]. *UpToDate*. https://www.uptodate.com/contents/search?search=phenobarbital&sp=0&searchType=PLAIN_TEXT&source=USER_INPUT&searchControl=TOP_PULLDOWN&searchOffset=1&autoComplete=true&language=en&max=10&index=1~6&autoCompleteTerm=phen

Lexicomp. (2021j). Phenytoin: Pediatric drug information [Drug Information]. *UpToDate*. https://www.uptodate.com/contents/search?search=phenytoin&sp=0&searchType=PLAIN_TEXT&source=USER_INPUT&searchControl=TOP_PULLDOWN&searchOffset=1&autoComplete=false&language=en&max=10&index=&autoCompleteTerm=

Lexicomp. (2021k). Sucrose: Pediatric drug information [Drug Information]. *UpToDate*. https://www.uptodate.com/contents/search?search=sucrose&sp=0&searchType=PLAIN_TEXT&source=USER_INPUT&searchControl=TOP_PULLDOWN&searchOffset=1&autoComplete=false&language=en&max=10&index=&autoCompleteTerm=

Lexicomp. (2021l). Topiramate: Pediatric drug information [Drug Information]. *UpToDate*. https://www.uptodate.com/contents/search?search=topiramate&sp=0&searchType=PLAIN_TEXT&source=USER_INPUT&searchControl=TOP_PULLDOWN&searchOffset=1&autoComplete=true&language=en&max=10&index=1~6&autoCompleteTerm=top

Lexicomp. (2021m). Valproate: Pediatric drug information [Drug Information]. *UpToDate*. https://www.uptodate.com/contents/search?search=valproate&sp=0&searchType=PLAIN_TEXT&source=USER_INPUT&searchControl=TOP_PULLDOWN&searchOffset=1&autoComplete=true&language=en&max=10&index=0~6&autoCompleteTerm=valproate

Lexicomp. (n.d.[a]). Acyclovir: Pediatric drug information [Drug Information]. *UpToDate*. https://www.uptodate.com/contents/acyclovir-systemic-pediatric-drug-information?search=acyclovir&source=panel_search_result&selectedTitle=1~142&usage_type=panel&display_rank=1#F7808308

Lexicomp. (n.d.[b]). Amphetamine: Pediatric drug information [Drug Information]. *UpToDate*. https://www.uptodate.com/contents/search?search=amphetamine&sp=0&searchType=PLAIN_TEXT&source=USER_INPUT&searchControl=TOP_PULLDOWN&searchOffset=1&autoComplete=true&language=en&max=10&index=0~6&autoCompleteTerm=ampheta

Lexicomp. (n.d.[c]). Atomoxetine: Pediatric drug information [Drug Information]. *UpToDate*. https://www.uptodate.com/contents/search?search=atomoxetine&sp=0&searchType=PLAIN_TEXT&source=USER_INPUT&searchControl=TOP_PULLDOWN&searchOffset=1&autoComplete=true&language=en&max=10&index=0~4&autoCompleteTerm=atom

National Institute of Neurological Disorders and Stroke. (2021). *Cerebral palsy: hope through research*. U.S. Department of Health and Human Services, National Institute of Neurological Disorders and Stroke. https://www.ninds.nih.gov/Disorders/Patient-Caregiver-Education/Hope-Through-Research/Cerebral-Palsy-Hope-Through-Research#3104_12

National Institute of Neurological Disorders and Stroke. (2021). *What is hydrocephalus?*. U.S. Department of Health and Human Services, National Institute of Neurological Disorders and Stroke. https://www.ninds.nih.gov/Disorders/Patient-Caregiver-Education/Fact-Sheets/Hydrocephalus-Fact-Sheet

Ostermaier, K. K. (2020a). Down syndrome: Clinical features and diagnosis. *UpToDate*. https://www.uptodate.com/contents/down-syndrome-clinical-features-and-diagnosis

Ostermaier, K. K. (2020b). Down syndrome: Management. *UpToDate*. https://uptodate.com/contents/down-syndrome-management

Pentima, C. D. (2021). Viral meningitis in children; Clinical features and diagnosis. *UpToDate*. https://www.uptodat
e.com/contents/viral-meningitis-in-children-clinical-features-and-diagnosis?search=meningitis&source=search
_result&selectedTitle=2~150&usage_type=default&display_rank=2#H19

Varghese, R., Chakrabarthy, J., & Menon, G. (2017). Nursing management of adults with severe traumatic brain
injury: A narrative review. *Indian Journal of Critical Care Medicine, 21*(10), 684–697. https://www.ncbi.nlm.nih
.gov/pmc/articles/PMC5672675/

Vasudeva, S. S. (2021). Medscape. *Meningitis*. https://emedicine.medscape.com/article/232915-overview

Vetter, V. L., Elia, J., Erikson, C., Berger, S., Blum, N., Uzark, K., & Webb, C. L. (2008). Cardiovascular monitoring
of children and adolescents with heart disease receiving medications for attention deficit hyperactivity disorder.
American Heart Association Journals, 117, 2407–2423. https://www.ahajournals.org/doi/10.1161/circulationaha
.107.18

EYES, EARS, NOSE, AND THROAT

EYES

ASSESSMENT

- Inspect the eyes, eyelids, sclerae, irises, pupils, and conjunctivas.
  - Eyelids should open and close completely.
  - Sclera should be white in appearance.
  - Iris should be round with the appropriate color (permanent color at 6–12 months of age).
  - Pupils should be equal, round, and assessed for reactivity to light and accommodation.
  - Conjunctivas should be pink.
- Nystagmus is evaluated by noting extraocular movements in the six cardinal fields of gaze.
- The corneal light reflex test assesses alignment.
- Peripheral vision is assessed using the confrontation test.
- Abnormal findings include strabismus, anisocoria, and nystagmus.
- Further testing includes testing color vision, visual acuity, and internal structures.
- Red reflex should be present in infants.

AMBLYOPIA

Overview

- *Amblyopia* is decreased visual acuity in one eye due to abnormal vision development. It occurs when nerve pathways between the brain and the eye are not adequately stimulated.
- Amblyopia is also known as lazy eye because, over time, the brain relies on the stronger eye.
- It is the most common cause of visual impairment in childhood.
- Risk factors include premature birth, nearsightedness, farsightedness, strabismus, ptosis, and a family history of amblyopia or cataracts.

 COMPLICATIONS

Strabismus is a misalignment of the eye, or when one eye deviates from the point of fixation; if uncorrected by ages 4–6, amblyopia may result.

Signs and Symptoms

- Poor vision in the affected eye
- Shutting one eye
- Squinting
- Tilting head

Diagnosis

Labs
There are no labs specific to diagnose amblyopia.

Diagnostic Testing
- Corneal light reflex test for identifying strabismus or amblyopia
- Eye alignment testing for strabismus
- Visual screening for acuity in both eyes
  - For children ages 3 and older only

Treatment

- Atropine eye drops to blur stronger eye's vision (Table 5.1*)
- Eye patch covering stronger eye to increase amblyopic eye stimulation
- Eyeglasses or corrective lenses for nearsightedness and farsightedness
- Surgery for cataracts

Nursing Interventions

- Assess vision impairment signs in infants and children.
- Detect amblyopia symptoms early to improve vision outcomes and eye development prognosis.
- Encourage proper eye patch use on the unaffected or stronger eye.
- Encourage properly prescribed eye drop use in the unaffected eye.
- Screen for eye issues by asking family about the child's vision.

Patient and Family Education

- Ensure proper eye specialist follow-up.
- Instill eye drops into the lower conjunctival sac by tilting head back, looking up, and gently pulling lower eyelid down.
- Instill eye drops without touching the dropper to the eye.
- Recommend screening for amblyopia and strabismus at 3, 4, and 5 years old.
- Use an eye patch to prevent the stronger eye from compensating and to stimulate the affected, amblyopic eye.

CONJUNCTIVITIS

Overview

- *Conjunctivitis* is inflammation of the conjunctiva, also known as pink eye.
- In children, causes can be viral, bacterial, allergic, or from a foreign body.
- In neonates, causes include infections from birth such as chlamydia, gonorrhea, and HSV.

Signs and Symptoms

- Allergic
  - Bilateral eye redness
  - Itchy eyes
  - Swollen eyelids
  - Watery, stringy drainage

COMPLICATIONS

If untreated, neonatal conjunctivitis can lead to severe illness, pneumonia, and permanent visual impairment.

ALERT!

Instruct patients to clean contact lenses with contact lens disinfecting solution after every wear. Do not use water or saliva.

---

* Table 5.1 is located at the end of this chapter.

- Bacterial
  - Crusting of eyelids
  - Purulent drainage
  - Swollen eyelids
- Foreign body
  - Pain
  - Specific to one eye
  - Tearing
- Viral
  - Current upper respiratory infection
  - Swollen eyelids
  - Watery drainage

Diagnosis

Labs
- Drainage cultures for pathogen identification and confirmation
- Viral PCR for identifying the viral cause, such as adenovirus or enterovirus

Diagnostic Testing
- Conjunctivitis eye exam

Treatment

- Antibiotic drops or antibiotic ointment administered at night for bacterial conjunctivitis
- Erythromycin (Table 5.1) drops or ointment in newborns' eyes immediately after birth for neonatal conjunctivitis prevention
- Olopatadine (Table 5.1) drops and artificial tears for allergic symptoms
- Supportive treatment, including removal of drainage and good hand hygiene, for viral infection management

Nursing Interventions

- Administer ophthalmic eye drops as prescribed.
- Apply warm, wet compresses to remove drainage from the eyes.
- Use cold compresses to relieve discomfort and redness.
- Wipe eyes clean from inner canthus downward and outward.

Patient and Family Education

- Avoid contact with known allergens.
  - For animal dander allergens, avoid contact with animals. Wash clothing.
  - For dust mite allergens, vacuum frequently, dust with a moist cloth, and replace/wash bedding.
  - Limit outdoor activity and avoid allergens such as trees, grass, and pollen.
- Avoid wearing contact lenses until conjunctivitis has resolved.
- Discard used tissues after wiping the eyes.
- Encourage children to stay home from school until they are symptom-free from bacterial or viral conjunctivitis.
- Prevent infecting other family members by using proper hand hygiene and avoid sharing personal items.
- Refrain from scratching and rubbing the affected eye to prevent spreading the infection to the other eye.
- Wash hands before and after touching eyes.
- Wash pillowcases, washcloths, and towels to prevent spreading.
- Wear safety gear, such as helmets and safety glasses, to prevent foreign body injury.

 POP QUIZ 5.1

How can the nurse educate a 5-year-old patient and their parent who are asking why the provider told them to wear an eye patch covering the right eye when the left eye is the lazy eye?

EARS

ASSESSMENT

- External structures
  - Inspect the pinna on each side of the head.
    - Assess ear alignment by visualizing a horizontal line from the outer orbit of the eye. The pinna should reach the horizontal line.
    - Measure the angle of the ear by visualizing a perpendicular vertical line across that horizontal line. The pinna should be within 10° of the vertical line.
  - Note that cerumen may be visualized.
  - Palpate pinna for tenderness.
- Internal structures
  - Assess the internal structures with an otoscope.
  - Inspect the tympanic membrane.
    - The tympanic membrane should be a light pearly pink or gray color.
    - Light reflex is a cone-shaped reflection and will be seen at 5 o'clock in the right ear or 7 o'clock in the left ear.
  - If the patient is experiencing pain, assess the unaffected ear before examining the painful ear.

> **ALERT!**
>
> Low-set ears are commonly associated with renal anomalies. The kidneys and ears develop at the same time prenatally.

ACUTE OTITIS MEDIA

Overview

- *Acute otitis media* is an infection of the middle ear characterized by inflammation of the middle ear and rapid onset of fever and pain.
- Acute otitis media occurs more frequently in children having shorter and more horizontal eustachian tubes.
- Risk factors include a recent viral respiratory infection and bottle propping or bottle-feeding an infant in the supine position.

> **COMPLICATIONS**
>
> Chronic or recurrent otitis media can lead to hearing loss, difficulty communicating, and tinnitus. Ear tubes may be placed to help prevent the accumulation of fluids.

Signs and Symptoms

- Bulging, red tympanic membrane
- Crying
- Drainage from the external ear canal
- Ear pain
- Fever
- Irritability
- Lethargy
- Rubbing or pulling the ear

Diagnosis

Labs
There are no labs specific to diagnose acute otitis media.

Diagnostic Testing
Visualization of the tympanic membrane using an otoscope to confirm acute otitis media

> **NURSING PEARL**
>
> To assess the tympanic membrane for children under 3, gently pull the pinna down and back. For children over the age of 3, gently pull the pinna up and back.

Treatment

- Antibiotics
  - Amoxicillin (Table A.1)
- Comfort measures
- Management of fevers and pain

Nursing Interventions

- Administer antipyretics as needed for fevers and pain.
- Assess ears using the appropriate technique for patient's age.

Patient and Family Education

- Avoid secondhand smoke and allergens.
- Complete the entire course of antibiotics, even if symptoms resolve.
- Feed infants in an upright position to avoid pooling milk from the bottle.
- Remain up to date on immunizations.

HEARING LOSS

Overview

- The location of the defect characterizes the hearing impairment.
  - *Conductive* hearing loss originates in the middle ear and can result from recurrent otitis media. It affects the loudness of sounds.
  - *Sensorineural* hearing loss is related to an inner ear or auditory nerve (CN VIII) problem. It is a result of congenital disabilities, ototoxic drugs, and exposure to excessive noise.
- The severity of hearing impairment is classified from slight to profound based on the hearing level in decibels.

COMPLICATIONS

Commonly used ototoxic drugs include aminoglycosides, such as gentamicin, and high-dose loop diuretics, such as furosemide. These can cause acquired sensorineural hearing loss

Signs and Symptoms

- Absence of babble by 7 months old
- Lack of startle to loud sounds during infancy
- Lack of speech development in toddler years
- Frequently asking to repeat what was said or responding incorrectly

ALERT!

Children missing speech milestones or struggling with articulation should have their hearing tested.

Diagnosis

Labs
There are no labs specific to diagnose hearing loss.

Diagnostic Testing
- Auditory screening for hearing loss and confirm whether a full hearing test is needed
- BAER to confirm hearing loss
- ABR to confirm hearing loss

Treatment

- Conductive treatment: antibiotics for ear infections, ear tubes, and hearing aids
- Sensorineural treatment: cochlear implants and hearing aids

Nursing Interventions

- Assess infants and children for signs of hearing impairment.
- Connect family with a multidisciplinary team to support language learning and management of hearing loss.
- Use caution when administering ototoxic medications.

Patient and Family Education

- Remain up to date on immunizations.
- Wear ear protection or earplugs around loud noises.

POP QUIZ 5.2

The nurse is assessing an 8-month-old baby who is not babbling or imitating sounds and has a history of completing a course of gentamicin. What should the nurse be concerned for and why?

NOSE

ASSESSMENT

- Abnormal findings include discharge, redness, or septum deviation.
- Inspect nose.
    - Internal mucosa and turbinates should be pink and free of swelling.
    - Nostrils should be present and patent.
    - Septum should be midline and intact.
    - The nose should be midline and skin color consistent throughout the head and face.

ALLERGIC RHINITIS

Overview

- *Allergic rhinitis*, or hay fever, is a reaction to seasonal allergens, most often in the autumn or spring months.
- Risk factors include having a family history of allergies, asthma, and eczema.
- The most common allergens are pollen, dust mites, and animal dander.

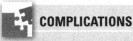

COMPLICATIONS

Inflammation caused by allergic rhinitis can lead to sinusitis, acute otitis media, and worsening asthma symptoms.

Signs and Symptoms

- Fatigue
- Headache
- Itchy nose, eyes, and throat
- Nasal obstruction and snoring
- Rhinorrhea
- Sneezing

Diagnosis

Labs
There are no labs specific to diagnose allergic rhinitis.

Diagnostic Testing
Skin prick allergy test to confirm reaction and identify specific allergens.

Treatment

- Antihistamines (Table 5.1)
  - Cetirizine
  - Fexofenadine
  - Loratadine
- Inhaled corticosteroids (Table 5.1)
  - Budesonide
  - Fluticasone
- Mast cell stabilizers (Table 5.1): cromolyn

Nursing Interventions

- Administer allergy medications as ordered.
- Educate family on allergy medications and allergens.
- Encourage nasal saline irrigation before administering nasal medications and as needed to remove allergens from the nares.

Patient and Family Education

- Avoid known allergens.
- Change clothes and take a shower after being outside during pollen season and after exposure to animals or secondhand smoke.
- Change HVAC filters frequently.
- Keep windows closed during allergy season.
- Mop, vacuum, and dust frequently inside the home, and consider hard flooring instead of carpet.
- Wash bedding in hot water, limit or frequently wash stuffed animals, and place mattress in an encased cover to control dust mites.

EPISTAXIS

Overview

- *Epistaxis* refers to short, isolated episodes of nosebleeds.
- Bleeding usually results from trauma or irritation from allergies.
- Nose bleeds are common during childhood.
- Risk factors include picking nose, low humidity, injury, or medications such as anticoagulants.

> **COMPLICATIONS**
>
> Recurrent epistaxis may indicate an underlying bleeding disorder such as hemophilia, leukemia, or idiopathic thrombocytopenic purpura.

Signs and Symptoms

- Bleeding from nostril
- Nose pain

Diagnosis

Labs

- CBC to evaluate for low platelet count or low hemoglobin and hematocrit for severe or recurrent episodes
- PT, PTT, INR to rule out a bleeding or clotting disorder

Diagnostic Testing

There are no diagnostic tests specific to diagnose epistaxis.

Treatment

Supportive measures to stop bleeding.

Nursing Interventions

- Apply continuous pressure by pinching the nose for at least 5 to 10 minutes.
- Ask the child to sit up and lean forward to avoid swallowing blood.
- Help keep the child calm and encourage breathing through the mouth.
- Notify provider of abnormal low lab values or a large number of estimated blood loss.

Patient and Family Education

- Avoid picking or blowing the nose and bending over with the head lower than the heart to prevent rebleeding.
- Use humidification in the child's bedroom and moisten the nares with saline spray.

POP QUIZ 5.3

A 16-year-old patient with seasonal allergies to pollen states they heard they should check the weather for high pollen count days, but is asking what they should do when the pollen count is high. How can the nurse educate this patient about pollen and allergens?

THROAT

ASSESSMENT

Inspect inside of the mouth.
- Cheeks, tongue, gums, teeth, hard and soft palate, uvula
- Tonsils
  - Can be visualized at 6 to 9 months of age
  - Symmetric and color consistent with surrounding mucosa
  - Abnormal findings: asymmetry, enlargement causing obstruction, and exudate
- Pharynx
  - Pink and moist
  - No erythema

CLEFT LIP AND PALATE

Overview

- *Cleft lip* and *cleft palate* are birth defects where the lip and/or palate does not close properly.
- Infants may have one condition or both.
- The cause is unknown but thought to be genetic and/or the baby's environment in utero.
- Risk factors include maternal smoking, gestational diabetes, and maternal exposure to certain medications while pregnant.
- The primary preventative measure is to take 400 mcg of folic acid during pregnancy.
- A cleft lip and palate patient will have a team of specialists, including:
  - Audiologist
  - Dentist

COMPLICATIONS

Cleft lip and palate can lead to other issues with the following:

- Feeding
- Hearing, recurrent ear infections
- Speaking
- Teeth

- Ears, nose, throat physician (otolaryngologist)
- Orthodontist
- Pediatrician
- Plastic surgeon
- Psychologist
- Social worker
- Speech-language pathologist

Signs and Symptoms

- Cleft lip may be a small notch in the lip.
- Cleft palate is characterized by an opening in the roof of the mouth connecting the mouth and nasal cavity.
- In more severe cases, there is a separation from the upper lip toward the nose.

Diagnosis

Diagnostic Testing

- Ultrasound during pregnancy to show defects; harder to see the cleft palate
- Amniocentesis if suspected during pregnancy to detect inherited genetic syndromes that could cause other birth defects
- Provider examination at birth to feel for cleft palate

Treatment

- Surgery:
  - Individualized timing and types of surgeries
    - ○ Cleft lip: usually around 3 months old, but within first year of life
    - ○ Cleft palate: usually 10 to 12 months old, but before 18 months
  - Bone marrow graft to palate, usually from hip
  - Additional surgeries as needed

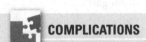

COMPLICATIONS

Notify the surgeon of any postsurgical complications, including:

- Fever above 101.3 °F (37 °C)
- Heavy bleeding from nose or mouth
- No wet diapers
- Pain not controlled with medication
- Refusing fluids

Nursing Interventions

- Before surgery:
  - Assess the family's reaction to patient's appearance, their understanding of instructions, and any other concerns.
  - Encourage bonding with infant.
  - Provide information about support groups for the family.
- Postsurgery:
  - Assess the patient's skin color and cap refill to assure that the baby is properly oxygenated after surgery with changes in the mouth/upper airway.
  - Provide arm immobilizers, if needed, to prevent infants from putting things in their mouth while it is healing.
  - Feeding:
    - ○ Assess the patient's respiration rate and effort during feeding or while eating.
    - ○ Monitor weight gain.
    - ○ Place patient at a 30° to 45° angle when feeding and suction as needed.
    - ○ Provide special nipples for bottle-feeding.
    - ○ Provide post-op care instructions for feeding and suture care.
    - ○ Teach family about the condition(s), review the signs and symptoms of choking and aspiration, and advise on how to respond.

Patient and Family Education

Education is primarily for the patient's family:

- Consider support groups.
- Do not let child put objects into mouth while the mouth is healing.
- Follow all postsurgery instructions, including pain medication administration and proper feeding techniques.
- Learn about the surgeries that will be done and the timetable.
- Use appropriate feeding techniques and the appropriate bottles or nipples. Nursing mothers can provide breast milk through pumping.
- Seek psychological intervention for the child, when older, if having issues with self-esteem.

INFECTIOUS MONONUCLEOSIS

Overview

- *Infectious mononucleosis* is an acute, self-limiting, contagious infection most commonly caused by the Epstein-Barr virus.
- It typically affects adolescents and is transmitted through saliva or direct contact.

COMPLICATIONS

The spleen may become enlarged when infected with mononucleosis. Contact sports should be avoided until fully recovered to avoid splenic rupture.

Signs and Symptoms

- Exudative pharyngitis
- Fatigue
- Fever
- Hepatosplenomegaly
- Loss of appetite
- Lymphadenopathy
- Sore throat
- Swollen glands

Diagnosis

Labs

- CBC to evaluate for elevated WBC
- Positive spot test confirms mononucleosis infection

Diagnostic Testing

There are no diagnostic tests specific to diagnose infectious mononucleosis.

Treatment

Supportive measures:
- Antipyretics for pain and fever
- Water and fluid intake for hydration

Nursing Interventions

- Encourage hydration.
- Maintain standard precautions.
- Promote rest.

Patient and Family Education

- Avoid contact sports for 3 to 4 weeks.
- Do not share drinks or personal items such as toothbrushes.
- Follow hand hygiene guidelines to prevent the spread of infection.

STREPTOCOCCAL PHARYNGITIS

Overview

- *Streptococcal pharyngitis*, or strep throat, is an infection of the pharynx.
- It is caused by *Streptococcus pyogenes* pathogen.

Signs and Symptoms

- Abdominal pain
- Fever
- Headache
- Nausea
- Pharyngeal erythema
- Sudden onset sore throat
- Tonsillar hypertrophy with or without exudate
- Vomiting

Diagnosis

Labs

- Rapid antigen detection test for GABHS
- Throat culture for pathogen identification

Diagnostic Testing

There are no diagnostic tests specific to diagnose streptococcal pharyngitis.

Treatment

- Oral antibiotics
  - Amoxicillin (Table A.1)
- Supportive management
  - Adequate hydration
  - Antipyretics
  - Rest
  - Warm saltwater gargles

Nursing Interventions

- Encourage hydration with ice chips or ice pops.
- Obtain throat swab for culture.

Patient and Family Education

- Do not share drinks, food, or utensils.
- Encourage children to stay home from school or daycare until they are afebrile, or it has been 12 to 24 hours since starting antibiotics.
- Prevent spread of infection with proper hand hygiene. Cover coughs and sneezes.
- Replace toothbrush after 24 hours of antibiotics to prevent re-infection.
- Take the entire course of antibiotics, even if symptoms have resolved.
- Wash any toys that toddlers place in their mouths.

COMPLICATIONS

Untreated GAS can lead to acute rheumatic fever and poststreptococcal glomerulonephritis. Symptomatic children over the age of 3 should be tested to confirm and treated with antibiotics.

POP QUIZ 5.4

A child's rapid antigen detection test is positive for streptococcal pharyngitis. What back-to-school instructions should the nurse give the family?

TONSILLECTOMY

Overview

- The most common indication for a tonsillectomy is recurrent throat infections, which fall into three categories:
  - Five or more infections in the previous 2 years
  - Seven infections in the previous year
  - Three infections per year in the previous 3 years
- The second most common indication for a tonsillectomy is obstructive sleep apnea.
- *Tonsillectomy* is the surgical removal of the palatine tonsils. The procedure may include an adenoidectomy.

Signs and Symptoms

Tonsillitis signs and symptoms include:
- Difficulty breathing
- Difficulty swallowing
- Inflammation of tonsils

Diagnosis

Labs
- CBC to rule out anemia prior to surgery
- Throat cultures for throat infection identification
- Type and screen as a preoperative lab

Diagnostic Testing
Polysomnography before tonsillectomy in children with sleep-disordered breathing.

Treatment

- Analgesics (Table A.2)
  - Acetaminophen
  - Opioids if needed
- Ice collar for discomfort

Nursing Interventions

- Assess any secretions and vomit for blood. If blood is visible, document the color and quantity.
- Assess pain levels and administer pain medications, both scheduled and as needed.
- Avoid offering juice or colored ice pops that could discolor vomit or secretions and be confused with blood.
- Avoid suctioning to prevent bleeding and trauma.
- Monitor for postoperative airway obstruction.
- Monitor for postoperative bleeding signs.

 COMPLICATIONS

Postoperative bleeding is a potentially life-threatening complication of a tonsillectomy. It typically occurs within the first 24 hours but may happen up to 5 to 10 days after the procedure. Monitor for symptoms of bleeding, such as tachycardia, pallor, frequent swallowing, and vomiting bright red blood. Educate family and patients about the risk of postoperative bleeding and its symptoms before discharge.

 NURSING PEARL

Polysomnography is used to diagnose obstructive sleep apnea. Children should be encouraged to bring comforting personal items such as blankets or stuffed animals from home.

 ALERT!

Monitor for postoperative respiratory distress, stridor, and drooling. These can be signs of airway obstruction due to edema and accumulated secretions.

Patient and Family Education

- Avoid coughing and blowing the nose.
- Do not use straws.
- Drink fluids and eat soft foods for 1 to 2 days after surgery.
- Expect to have pain or discomfort for up to 2 weeks after surgery.
  - Do not take ibuprofen or aspirin.
  - It is helpful to take pain medications prior to eating.
  - Take pain medications as prescribed to help avoid readmissions for pain control.
- Limit activity for 1 to 2 weeks after surgery.
- Monitor for any bleeding, frequent swallowing, vomiting, or not feeling well up to 10 days after the tonsillectomy. Contact provider for any bleeding or fever.
- Take antibiotics as prescribed.

 POP QUIZ 5.5

What signs would the nurse need to monitor for on a post-op tonsillectomy patient that would indicate a need for immediate intervention?

Table 5.1 EENT Medications

Indications	Mechanism of Action	Contraindications, Precautions, and Adverse Effects
Antihistamines (cetirizine, fexofenadine, loratadine)		
• Management of allergic rhinitis and seasonal allergy symptoms	• Compete with histamine for H1 receptor sites on effector cells	• Medication is contraindicated in children less than 2 years old. • Use caution in children less than 4 years old. • Use caution with other OTC cough or cold medications.
Anticholinergic (atropine)		
• Pupillary dilation of a stronger eye for treatment of amblyopia	• Reduce ability to accommodate and focus of the stronger eye, thereby encouraging the use of the amblyopic eye	• Adverse effects include light sensitivity, conjunctival irritation, eye pain, and anticholinergic effects.
Inhaled corticosteroid (budesonide, fluticasone)		
• Decrease airway inflammation and bronchoconstriction	• Reduce allergic responses associated with allergies	• Adverse effect includes thrush; rinse mouth after each use. • Adverse effects include growth suppression. • Use with caution in immunocompromised patients. • Use with caution in long-term use for nasal septum perforation or ulcers. • Do not abruptly discontinue, and monitor for adrenal insufficiency.

(continued)

Table 5.1 EENT Medications *(continued)*

Indications	Mechanism of Action	Contraindications, Precautions, and Adverse Effects
Mast cell stabilizers (cromolyn)		
• Relieve nasal symptoms of hay fever	• Decrease histamine from mast cells	• Medication is contraindicated in children less than 2 years old.
Ocular antihistamine (olopatadine)		
• Treatment of symptoms of allergic conjunctivitis	• Inhibit histamine release from mast cells and relieve ocular pruritus symptoms	• Medication is contraindicated while wearing contact lenses. • Medication is contraindicated in children less than 2 years old.
Ophthalmological anti-infectives (erythromycin)		
• Prevention of conjunctivitis of the newborn • Treatment of superficial eye infections	• Inhibit bacterial protein synthesis	• Adverse effects include eye irritation. • There are no contraindications.

RESOURCES

Centers for Disease Control and Prevention. (2018, November). *Pharyngitis.* U.S. Department of Health and Human Services, Centers for Disease Control and Prevention. https://www.cdc.gov/groupastrep/diseases-hcp/strep-throat.html

Centers for Disease Control and Prevention. (2019, January). *Conjunctivitis.* U.S. Department of Health and Human Services, Centers for Disease Control and Prevention. https://www.cdc.gov/conjunctivitis/index.html

Centers for Disease Control and Prevention. (2020a, June). *Common eye disorders and diseases.* U.S. Department of Health and Human Services, Centers for Disease Control and Prevention. https://www.cdc.gov/visionhealth/basics/ced/index.html

Centers for Disease Control and Prevention. (2020b, September). *About infectious mononucleosis.* U.S. Department of Health and Human Services, Centers for Disease Control and Prevention. https://www.cdc.gov/epstein-barr/about-mono.html

Lexicomp. (n.d.). Cromolyn [Drug information]. *UpToDate.* https://www.uptodate.com/contents/cromolyn-sodium-cromoglicate-nasal-pediatric-drug-information?search=cromolyn&source=panel_search_result&selectedTitle=2~61&usage_type=panel&display_rank=2#F8012093

Lexicomp. (2021a). Budesonide (oral inhalation): Pediatric drug information [Drug information]. *UpToDate.* https://www.uptodate.com/contents/budesonide-oral-inhalation-drug-information?search=budesonide&source=panel_search_result&selectedTitle=1~140&usage_type=panel&display_rank=1

Lexicomp. (2021b). Cetirizine: Pediatric drug information [Drug information]. *UpToDate.* https://www.uptodate.com/contents/cetirizine-systemic-pediatric-drug-information?search=cetirizine&source=panel_search_result&selectedTitle=1~92&usage_type=panel&display_rank=1

Lexicomp. (2021c). Erythromycin (ophthalmic): Pediatric drug information [Drug information]. *UpToDate.* https://www.uptodate.com/contents/erythromycin-ophthalmic-pediatric-drug-information?search=erythromycin&source=panel_search_result&selectedTitle=2~142&usage_type=panel&display_rank=2

Lexicomp. (2021d). Olopatadine (ophthalmic): Drug information [Drug information]. *UpToDate.* https://www.uptodate.com/contents/olopatadine-ophthalmic-drug-information?search=olopatadine&source=panel_search_result&selectedTitle=1~16&usage_type=panel&display_rank=1

National Eye Institute. (2019, July 2). *Amblyopia.* U.S. Department of Health and Human Services, National Eye Institute. https://www.nei.nih.gov/learn-about-eye-health/eye-conditions-and-diseases/amblyopia-lazy-eye

Smith, R., & Gooi, A. (2021). Hearing loss in children. *UpToDate.* https://www.uptodate.com/contents/hearing-loss-in-children-etiology?search=ototoxic%20drugs&source=search_result&selectedTitle=4~150&usage_type=default&display_rank=4#H29

CARDIOVASCULAR SYSTEM

CONGENITAL HEART DEFECTS

Overview

- *Congenital heart defects*, or *malformations*, are the most common type of birth defect. Although many are diagnosed in utero, they are still a leading cause of infant death.
- Defects can be in structure or in function, involving the wall of the heart, the valves of the heart, and/or the arteries and veins surrounding the heart.
- Defects can also affect blood flow, causing the blood to flow in the wrong direction, flow to the wrong place, or flow too slowly.
- The congenital heart defects are categorized as cyanotic or acyanotic.
  - Cyanotic heart defects:
    - Hypoplastic left heart syndrome
    - Pulmonary atresia
    - TOF
    - Transposition of the great arteries
  - Acyanotic heart defects:
    - Atrial septal defect
    - Atrioventricular septal defect
    - Aortic valve stenosis
    - Coarctation of the aorta
    - Pulmonary valve stenosis
    - Patent ductus arteriosus
    - Ventricular septal defect
- The defects can further be characterized by how they affect blood flow:
  - Cyanotic:
    - Decreased pulmonary blood flow: TOF, tricuspid atresia
    - Mixed blood flow: HLHS, transposition of great arteries
  - Acyanotic:
    - Increased pulmonary blood flow: ASD, VSD, PDA, AV canal defect
    - Obstruction to blood flow: coarctation of aorta, pulmonary stenosis, aortic stenosis
- Causes of congenital heart defects include:
  - Exposure of the fetus to maternal illnesses such as diabetes, rubella, fevers from other illnesses, and phenylketonuria

 COMPLICATIONS

Patients with congenital heart defects are at an increased risk of developing bacterial endocarditis. Frequently, prophylactic antibiotics are prescribed prior to dental visits or procedures.

 NURSING PEARL

Transposition of the great arteries is a defect where the two main arteries of the heart, the pulmonary artery and the aorta, are reversed. The aorta leaves the right ventricle, and the pulmonary artery leaves the left ventricle, thereby leading to inadequate oxygenated blood flowing to the body.

 ALERT!

The ductus arteriosus is a vascular opening between the aorta and the pulmonary artery that diverts blood from the pulmonary bed prenatally. After the baby is born, this opening normally closes within 72 hours. If the opening does not close, the patient has a PDA. However, multiple complex congenital heart defects require the PDA to remain open to supply oxygenated blood to the body for perfusion. To do this, the patient is administered Prostaglandin E1 (see Table 6.2*) to reopen or keep open the ductus arteriosus.

---

*Table 6.2 is located at the end of this chapter.

(continued)

Overview *(continued)*

- Smoking, alcohol, recreational drug use during pregnancy
- Some therapeutic drugs
- Environmental factors such as air pollution, pesticides, and extreme heat waves
- Certain inherited genetic defects and chromosomal abnormalities
- Research has shown that some congenital heart defects may be preventable:
  - Prenatal diets rich in vitamin B12, folic acid, riboflavin, and B3 have been shown to protect the fetus from congenital heart disease.
  - Vaccines to prevent flu and pneumonia protect the mother from serious infection, which could lead to a pregnancy complication and harm the fetus's heart.
- Many infants and children will not need intervention while others will need surgery, medications, transplant, catheterization, NICU admission, or a hospital stay. The family must be educated and supported as they face a congenital heart defect diagnosis.
  - NICU discharge criteria includes:
    - Ability to maintain a stable body temperature in an open crib
    - Breathing on their own
    - Consistent weight gain
    - Free of infection
    - Hemodynamic stability
    - Prepared family and adequate home care supplies.
    - Stable bilirubin levels

ALERT!

Families with children who have heart defects must learn CPR before leaving the hospital.

ATRIAL SEPTAL DEFECT

Overview

- An *ASD* is a hole, or opening, between the atria, or the top chambers of the heart.
- ASD is a heart defect with increased pulmonary flow, allowing blood from the left atrium (higher pressure) to flow into the right atrium (lower pressure). This is called a left-to-right shunt.
- The size of the ASD determines treatment.
  - Trivial: less than 3 mm in diameter
  - Small: 3 mm to less than 6 mm
  - Moderate: 6 mm to 8 mm
  - Large: greater than 8 mm
- Small ASDs will often close spontaneously.
- ASDs are usually diagnosed prenatally or in infancy; however, sometimes they are not diagnosed until adulthood.

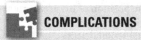

COMPLICATIONS

Postoperative complications of ASD include:
- Arrhythmias
- Bleeding
- Pericardial effusion
- Pleural effusions
- Pneumothorax
- Wound infection

Signs and Symptoms

- Failure to thrive
- Murmur: loud, harsh, with fixed split-second heart sound
- Palpitations
- Recurrent upper respiratory illnesses
- Shortness of breath
- Swelling of legs, feet, abdomen
- Tachypnea

Diagnosis
Labs
There are no labs specific to diagnose ASD.

Diagnostic Testing
- Chest x-ray to rule out other causes for the patient's symptoms
- Echocardiography to confirm the ASD
- EKG to assess for heart rhythm abnormalities
- MRI to evaluate parts of the heart that may not be visible on the echocardiogram
- Prenatal ultrasounds to diagnose defect before birth to alert provider

Treatment
- Medications to reduce signs and symptoms of ASD
  - Beta-blockers (see Table 6.2)
  - Anticoagulants (see Table 6.2)
- Mild cases managed by monitoring for complications
- Transcatheter patching:
  - For uncomplicated cases
  - Performed in the cardiac catheterization lab
- Surgery indicated for:
  - Large left-to-right shunt
  - Pulmonary over circulation
  - Right-sided heart enlargement
- Surgical options:
  - Suturing the opening
  - Transcatheter closure during cardiac catheterization with a septal occluded
  - Placing a patch (pericardial or Dacron)
  - Open repair with cardiopulmonary bypass for serious defects

Nursing Interventions
- Educate family on the condition, using pictures of the heart, and treatment plan.
- Encourage using support system during diagnosis, hospitalization, and postsurgery.
- Supply family with support group information to meet other families who have children with heart defects.
- Monitor patient postoperatively for any complications.
  - Medicate as needed for pain.
  - Aspirin (Table A.2) may be given to thin the blood and prevent complications.
- Monitor the patient's nutrition and consult a dietitian if needed.
- Monitor vital signs as well as heart rhythm, heart sounds, and lung sounds.
- Monitor strict I/O.

Patient and Family Education
- Consult with provider regarding activity restrictions prior to surgery.
- Discuss the need to report respiratory infections to physician.
- Discuss time frame for resuming activity after open-heart surgery.
  - Follow the provider's recommendation for physical activity. Common recommendations include:
    - If the surgery is successful without complications, the daily physical goals are the same as those of the general population.
    - If there has been ventricular dysfunction, elevated pulmonary artery pressure, right or left ventricular obstruction and/or dilation of the aorta, this amount of activity will be decreased depending on the severity of the dysfunction.
  - Patients with hypoxia will test the intensity of exercise by using the talking test.
  - Patients with arrhythmias may have low daily activity.

(continued)

Patient and Family Education *(continued)*

- Patients with syncope need to avoid areas that may be dangerous for them.
    - Patients who receive anticoagulants need to avoid sports that involve intense body contact.
- Educate patients with a heart defect that they may need palivizumab prophylactically to reduce hospitalization due to RSV.
- Explain that there will be lifelong follow-up visits after surgery to check for possible complications such as pulmonary hypertension, arrhythmias, heart failure, or valve problems.
- Recognize symptoms of heart failure, arrhythmias, and stroke.
- Notify provider for symptoms of:
    - Bluish color around the mouth, lips, or tongue
    - Decrease in activity
    - Failure to thrive
    - Increase in pain, fever, purulent drainage at incision site
    - Poor appetite or difficulty feeding
- Stress the importance of nutrition and the need to monitor weight.

ATRIOVENTRICULAR CANAL DEFECT

Overview

- *AVSD* is characterized by a group of congenital heart defects involving the AV septum and AV valves.
- This heart defect (along with VSD, PDA, and TOF) is common in children with trisomy 21.
- Types:
    - Complete AVSD
        - Blood flows freely between all four chambers
        - Basically, a hole in the middle of the heart
        - One valve instead of two
    - Partial AVSD
        - A hole in the atrial or ventricle septum near the center of the heart
        - Both valves usually present but may leak and cause blood backflow
        - May not be diagnosed until later in life due to lack of symptoms

> **COMPLICATIONS**
>
> Complications of AVSD include:
> - Arrhythmias
> - Congestive heart failure
> - Pulmonary hypertension

Signs and Symptoms

- Ashen/blue skin color
- Edema of legs, abdomen
- Fatigue
- Heart failure
- Murmur
- Pallor
- Pulmonary vascular disease
- Poor feeding
- Slow weight gain
- Sweating
- Tachypnea

Diagnosis

Diagnostic Testing

- EKG
- Chest x-ray

Treatment
- Surgery: definitive treatment
  - Timing is determined by the severity of the AV defect.
  - If the defect is complete, surgery will be done early in infancy.
- Medications (Table 6.2):
  - Diuretics, furosemide
  - Inotropic agent, digoxin
  - Ace inhibitor, enalapril
  - Beta-blockers, propranolol

Nursing Interventions
- Administer medications as ordered.
- Explain the condition to family using diagrams and answer questions.
- Monitor vital signs, watching especially for cardiac symptoms.
- Monitor strict I/O.
- Weigh patient daily.

Patient and Family Education
- Air travel may be restricted.
- All respiratory infections should be treated promptly.
- Attend yearly follow-up visits.
- Heart symptoms to watch out for include:
  - Blue cast to lips, fingernails
  - Dyspnea
  - Fatigue
  - Jugular venous distention
  - Noisy breathing
- Learn the balance of rest and activity.
- Prophylaxis antibiotics will be needed before dental visits and other procedures.
- Recognize the importance of immunizations for a child with a heart defect.

COARCTATION OF THE AORTA

Overview
- *Coarctation of the aorta* is an obstructive heart defect characterized by narrowing of the aorta, most often at or near the ductus arteriosus (Figure 6.1).
- The narrowing causes increased pressure proximal to the defect (the head and upper extremities) and decreased pressure distal to the defect (the lower extremities).
  - Discrepancies in four-extremity blood pressures are an indication of this heart defect.
  - Usually presents after the PDA closes in an infant.
- The obstruction causes the left ventricle to be overloaded.
- Usually, it occurs in addition to another heart abnormality, including:
  - ASD
  - Bicuspid aortic valve
  - Congenital mitral valve stenosis
  - PDA
  - Subaortic stenosis
  - Ventricular septal defect

 COMPLICATIONS

If left untreated, coarctation of the aorta can lead to heart failure or death in infants. It can also lead to an aneurysm in the brain or in the aorta. Hypertension is the most common long-term complication.

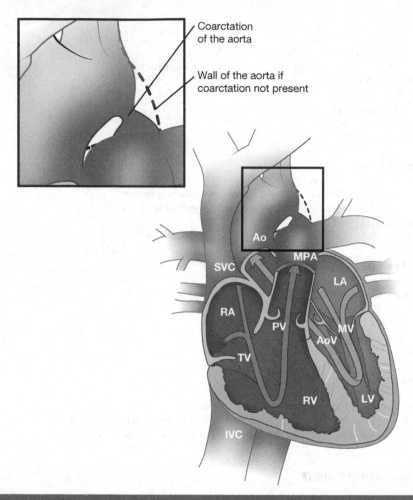

Figure 6.1 Coarctation of the aorta.

Ao, aorta; AoV, aortic valve; IVC, inferior vena cava; LA, left atrium; LV, left ventricle; MPA, main pulmonary artery; MV, mitral valve; PV, pulmonary valve; RA, right atrium; RV, right ventricle; SVC, superior vena cava; TV, tricuspid valve.
Source: Centers for Disease Control and Prevention, National Center on Birth Defects and Developmental Disabilities. https://www.cdc.gov/ncbddd/heartdefects/coarctationofaorta.html

Signs and Symptoms
- Blood pressure:
  - Hypertension in upper extremities
  - Hypotension, or lower blood pressures, in the lower extremities
- Pulses:
  - Bounding pulses in the arms
  - Weak or absent pulses in lower extremities
- Neonates
  - Absent or delayed femoral pulse
  - Cyanotic lower extremities
  - Diaphoresis
  - Heart failure

- Hepatomegaly
- Irritability
- Murmur
- Pale skin tone
- Preductal pulse ox saturation higher than postductal
- Poor pulses in extremities
- Older infants/children
  - Bounding pulses in upper extremities
  - Chest pain
  - Cold or cyanotic lower extremities
  - Headaches
  - Higher systolic pressures in upper extremities
  - Hypertension
  - Leg cramps
  - Lower systolic pressures in lower extremities
  - Nose bleeds

Diagnosis
Labs
There are no labs specific to diagnose coarctation of the aorta.

Diagnostic Testing
- Cardiac catheterization
- Cardiac MRI
- Chest x-ray
- Echocardiogram

Treatment
- Medication to palliate symptoms until the coarctation is corrected (see Table 6.2):
  - Furosemide to prevent fluid overload
  - Dopamine to improve cardiac contractility
  - Nifedipine for hypertension treatment
  - Prostaglandin E1
    - Administered to keep PDA open until surgery
    - Improves systemic blood flow supplying lower part of body
- Angioplasty or stent placement for mild cases
- Surgery: for removal or widening of narrowed part of the aorta

Nursing Interventions
- Administer hypertension medication if blood pressure remains high.
- Educate patient and family about symptoms of heart failure.
- Implement a high caloric, small volume, feeding regimen to maximize calories and minimize effort during feeds and educate families for home feeding management.
- Monitor four extremity blood pressures, assessing for higher systolic blood pressure in the upper extremities and lower systolic blood pressure in the lower extremities.
- Monitor upper and lower bilateral pulses, using Doppler if needed. Notify provider of absent pulses.
- Monitor strict I/O.
- Review the need for vaccination against respiratory syncytial virus.

 NURSING PEARL

Re-coarctation refers to stenosis after surgery or angioplasty. Symptoms include resting hypertension, headaches, and trouble walking or standing with pain and numbness.

Patient and Family Education

- Even with treatment, the coarctation can return. Recognize the signs and symptoms of a re-coarctation.
- Prevent prolonged crying after surgery.
- Regular follow-up appointments are important. There will be lifelong follow-up visits at least yearly with pediatrician or cardiologist and repeat imaging is necessary to monitor the repair.
- Watch for and notify the provider if there is increased respiratory effort, cyanosis/color change, or loss of consciousness.

 POP QUIZ 6.1

A laboring mother's prenatal ultrasound shows coarctation of the aorta in the fetus. What abnormal assessment findings should the nurse expect after delivery? What nursing interventions should be done to care for this baby after delivery?

HYPOPLASTIC LEFT HEART SYNDROME

Overview

- *HLHS* is a severe cardiac defect in which the left ventricle is underdeveloped or hypoplastic (too small) to support systemic circulation. This includes:
  - Hypoplasia of the atresia
  - Hypoplasia, or stenosis, of the aortic and/or mitral valves
  - Hypoplasia of the ascending aorta and arch
- This heart defect has a high mortality rate without intervention.
- HLHS results in a uni-ventricular circulatory system.
- Patients **must** have a PDA to maintain systemic circulation.
- The severity of the defect depends on the condition of the mitral and aortic valves.
- Due to it being a fatal condition without medical interventions, HLHS has raised many surgical, ethical, social, and economic issues. There is debate as to whether comfort care only should be presented as an option to family.

 COMPLICATIONS

Without treatment, HLHS is fatal. With treatment, complications include:

- Excessive fatigue
- Arrhythmias
- Edema in abdomen, legs, feet, lungs
- Growth retardation
- Blood clots causing emboli
- Development delays
- Additional surgery/transplantation in the future

Signs and Symptoms

- Acidosis
- Cool extremities
- Cyanosis
- Hepatomegaly
- Hypotension
- Poor feeding
- Respiratory distress
- Tachypnea

Diagnosis

Labs

There are no labs specific to diagnose HLHS.

Diagnostic Testing

- Diagnosis prenatally in 50% to 75% of cases
- Chest x-ray
- EKG
- Pulse oximetry

ALERT!

If diagnosed at a prenatal visit, choices that are given to the family are pursuant to additional testing, choice of delivery setting, termination of the pregnancy, and, where possible, prenatal intervention. Postnatal choices discussed are staged palliative surgery, heart transplant, or comfort care only.

Treatment

- PDA:
  - Prostaglandin E1 (see Table 6.2) to keep PDA open prior to initial surgery
  - Balloon PDA to keep open
- Three-stage palliative (not curative) surgical care:
  - Norwood
    - Completed in the first week of life
    - Creates a *neo-aorta*, or a single outflow tract from the heart, by fusing the aorta and the pulmonary artery
    - Establishes a source of pulmonary blood flow by placing a stent
    - Dissects atrial septum to allow for adequate mixing of oxygenated and deoxygenated blood
  - Glenn
    - Completed between 3 to 6 months of life
    - Original stent removed
    - Superior vena cava anastomosed to pulmonary artery
  - Fontan
    - Completed between 2 to 5 years of age
    - Creates a second pathway into the pulmonary artery using the inferior vena cava
    - Relieves cyanosis
- Medications beginning after Norwood (see Tables 6.2 and A.2)
  - Aspirin
  - Ace inhibitor
  - Digoxin
  - Diuretics

Nursing Interventions

- Administer cardiac medications as ordered and evaluate response.
- Auscultate heart sounds.
- Assess the family's coping mechanisms and continue to be supportive of family.
- Assess for infection at surgical site.
- Assess skin color, temperature, and moisture.
- Be mindful and supportive of the stress of coworkers and self when caring for these infants.
- Check peripheral pulses, including cap refill.
- Evaluate activity tolerance.
- Maintain chest tube(s) if present (Chapter 7).
  - Tubing and chamber should always be below chest level to maintain drainage.
  - Make sure all connections are secure and there are no kinks in the tubing.
  - Continuous bubbling my indicate a leak and should be investigated.
- Monitor pulse oximetry and CO_2.
- Promote breastfeeding during hospitalization, unless contraindicated.
- Provide resources for family, such as chaplain and palliative care team, if appropriate.
- Provide rest periods as needed. Disturb only if necessary. Do not allow a baby to cry for long periods.
- Monitor strict I/O.
- Supply oxygen as needed to maintain oxygen saturations within range for each stage of repair. Do not hyperoxygenate. These children will never have oxygen saturations of 100% due to the mixing of oxygenated and unoxygenated blood.
- Weigh patient every morning.

 NURSING PEARL

High oxygen saturations may be contraindicated in some cardiac patients due to the pulmonary vasodilation. Having high oxygen saturations could potentially be fatal to a patient with HLHS.

Patient and Family Education
- Avoid sick contacts and visitors.
- Express emotions and ask questions.
- Family should take time out for themselves.
- Higher calorie formula, fortified breast milk, or supplemental feeds may be recommended.
  - The coordinated suck, swallow, breathe burns a lot of calories.
  - The baby will need more calories because they are working harder to oxygenate their bodies.
  - They may need to be fed or supplemented via an NG tube.
- If surgery is not an option and the patient is not expected to survive, hold the baby and bond with them.
- Learn about the heart defect, treatment, medications, and management options.
- Learn to recognize signs and symptoms of infection.
- Seek support groups.

PULMONARY ATRESIA

Overview
- Pulmonary atresia is a congenital heart defect that is normally diagnosed soon after birth.
- *Pulmonary atresia* is a complete obstruction of the right ventricular outflow tract.
- The *pulmonary valve*, a heart valve that allows blood to flow out of the right ventricle to go to the lungs, does not completely form.
- Blood is unable to move from the right ventricle to the pulmonary artery and lungs.
- The ductus arteriosus must remain open, or patent, for the blood to flow to the lungs.
- There are two subcategories of pulmonary atresia:
  - Intact ventricular septum
  - VSD
- Pulmonary atresia with a VSD is very similar to TOF. Please refer to Tetralogy of Fallot section for more information.
- Left untreated, pulmonary atresia is fatal.

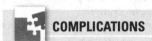 **COMPLICATIONS**

Pulmonary atresia can lead to complications such as arrhythmias, developmental delays, heart failure, narrowing of the atresia, and limited ability to perform activities.

Signs and Symptoms
- Cyanosis
- Decreased oxygen level
- Extreme sleepiness
- Murmur
- Poor feeding

Diagnosis
Diagnostic Testing
- Can be diagnosed prenatally, usually 18 to 22 weeks' gestation
- Cardiac catheterization
- Chest x-ray
- Echocardiogram
- EKG
- Prenatal ultrasound

Treatment

- Prostaglandin E1 to keep PDA open and maintain pulmonary circulation
- Probable cardiac catheterization to assess abnormalities and perform interventions
- Surgical repair with balloon or stent to keep the ductus arteriosus open
- Surgical repair to create or widen the pulmonary valve
- Surgical repair to patch the VSD if necessary

Nursing Interventions

- Educate families.
  - Encourage good dental care to minimize the risk of bacterial endocarditis.
  - Instruct family on home feeding regimen.
  - Monitor activity levels.
  - Review home medications, including anticoagulation requirements.
- Prepare patient and family emotionally for possible transplant.
- Provide emotional support to family as they adjust to their child's condition.
- Monitor strict I/O.

Patient and Family Education

- The child may need fortification of formula or breast milk for added calories.
- Long-term follow-up care will be needed.
- Patient will most likely require more surgeries as they get older.
- Prophylaxis antibiotics may be needed for certain procedures.
- Patients need to follow infection prevention instructions, such as proper hand hygiene, and avoid others who are sick to avoid risk of bacterial infections.
- The patient may need more rest periods than other children their age.
- Immunization schedule needs to be followed.

TETRALOGY OF FALLOT

Overview

- *TOF* is a heart defect with decreased pulmonary blood flow.
- There are four abnormalities that are, together, referred to as TOF (Figure 6.2):
  - *Ventricular septal defect*, or an opening between the left and right ventricles
  - *Pulmonary stenosis:* narrowing of the pulmonary valve and the pulmonary artery
  - *Overriding aorta:* aorta that overrides the ventricular septum, to the right above the VSD
  - *Right ventricular hypertrophy*, or thickening of the right ventricular wall
- The overriding aorta allows deoxygenated blood from the right ventricle to flow into the aorta and be mixed with the systemic blood flow.
- The right side of the heart develops hypertrophy because it works hard pushing against the obstruction at the pulmonary valve.
- TOF may present along with other deformities but typically presents with no other anomalies.
- Risk factors include:
  - Prematurity
  - Genetic predisposition
  - Environmental factors
  - A viral illness during pregnancy (e.g., rubella)
  - Alcoholism during pregnancy
  - Poor nutrition during pregnancy
  - A pregnant mother older than 40
  - A parent with TOF
  - The presence of trisomy 21 or DiGeorge syndrome
- A main sign of TOF is a tet spell, or a hypercyanotic episode, in which the child's skin, nails, and lips turn a dark blue. These episodes are caused by activities such as stooling or crying and caused by a decrease in blood flow to the lungs and decreased amount of oxygen in the blood.

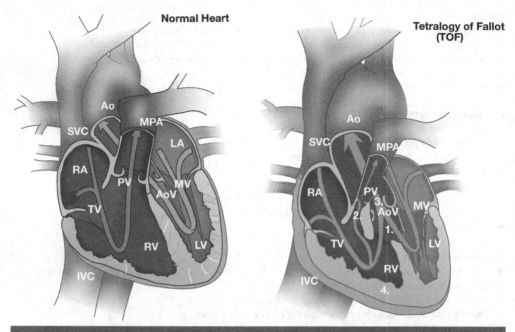

Figure 6.2 Normal heart and heart with TOF defects.

Ao, aorta; AoV, aortic valve; IVC, inferior vena cava; LA, left atrium; LV, left ventricle; MPA, main pulmonary artery; MV, mitral valve; PV, pulmonary valve; RA, right atrium; RV, right ventricle; SVC, superior vena cava; TV, tricuspid valve.
Source: Centers for Disease Control and Prevention, National Center on Birth Defects and Developmental Disabilities. Retrieved from https://www.cdc.gov/ncbddd/heartdefects/tetralogyoffallot.html

Signs and Symptoms
- Cyanosis
- Dyspnea
- Nail clubbing
- Poor appetite
- Polycythemia
- Systolic murmur
- Tet spells

Diagnosis
Diagnostic Testing
- Cardiac catheterization
- Chest x-ray
- Echocardiogram
- EKG
- Prenatal ultrasound

Treatment
- Medications:
    - Antibiotic prophylaxis prior to repair
    - Opioid for tet spells
    - Propranolol (see Table 6.2)

- Surgery:
  - Elective repair is usually done within the first year of life. This is dependent on the severity of cyanosis and the development of hypercyanotic spells.
  - Complete repair usually occurs between 6 and 12 months of life. Complete repair includes:
    - Closure of the VSD
    - Preserving right ventricle function
    - Relieving right ventricular outflow by removing obstruction
    - Procedure requires median sternotomy and the use of cardiopulmonary bypass

Nursing Interventions
- Unrepaired TOF:
  - Be prepared to treat tet spells.
    - Position child in a squat or knee-chest position.
    - Supply oxygen, although it does not always help oxygenation.
    - Administer an opioid.
    - Administer propranolol (see Table 6.2).
    - If interventions are not effective, emergency surgery is needed.
- Assess and medicate for pain as needed.
- Monitor for alterations in vital signs.
- Monitor for color changes (cyanosis).
- Monitor strict I/O.
- Provide emotional support to patient and family.
- Postoperative TOF care:
  - Assess and medicate for pain as needed.
  - Initiate sternal precautions.
    - Avoid lifting both arms overhead.
    - Avoid letting children reach behind their backs.
    - Do not allow children to push with their arms.
  - Monitor for postsurgical complications.
    - Chronic pulmonary regurgitation
    - Pulmonary valve dysfunction
    - Right ventricular enlargement and dysfunction
- Monitor strict I/O.

Patient and Family Education
- Activity may have to be limited as children with TOF may tire more easily.
- The child will need a yearly checkup with testing to monitor the surgical repair. The yearly visits will include:
  - Echocardiogram
  - Exercise testing
  - Other tests as needed
- Antibiotic prophylaxis will be needed before a dental visit.
- Learn about cardiac defect and signs of problems.
  - Tet spells
  - Cyanosis
  - Dizziness
  - Jugular vein distention
  - Palpitations
  - Syncope

 COMPLICATIONS

There are several possible complications from TOF repair, including the following:
- Altered cardiac rhythms
- Coagulation defects
- Infection
- Blood clots
- Heart failure
- Anemia
- Brain abscess
- Embolism
- Stroke
- Death

 ALERT!

Tet spells occur when the child becomes agitated and upset and can also occur if the child is in pain, has a fever, is anemic, or hypovolemic or after feeding, prolonged crying, or any activity or exercise. Tet spells present with fast, deep breathing, irritability, inconsolability, and progressively worsening cyanosis.

(continued)

Patient and Family Education *(continued)*

- Learn how to treat tet spells, such as knee-chest positioning. (See Nursing Interventions section.)
- Learn the "scoop lift," a technique to lift the patient under their bottom instead of under their arms. The "scoop lift" is used because the chest bone takes approximately 6 weeks to heal after surgery.
- The patient may need to have further heart surgery or interventional procedures as they age.

VENTRICULAR SEPTAL DEFECT

Overview

- *VSD* is a hole or, an opening, between the right and left ventricles of the heart, or the ventricular septum, which results in increased pulmonary blood flow.
- The VSD can vary in size from a small pinhole to absence of the septum. If the hole is small, the patient may be asymptomatic, and it may close spontaneously.
- Blood in the left ventricle (high pressure) will flow through the VSD into the right ventricle (lower pressure), creating a left-to-right shunt, which causes right ventricular hypertrophy.
- The effects and treatment depend on the size and pulmonary vascular resistance.

Signs and Symptoms

- Heart failure
- Hepatomegaly
- Increased work of breathing
  - Grunting
  - Rales
  - Retractions
- Murmur: loud, harsh at left sternal border
- Pallor
- Poor feeding
- Slow or no weight gain
- Tachycardia
- Tachypnea
- Thrill on auscultation

Diagnosis

Diagnostic Testing

- Can be detected in utero if moderate or large
- Chest x-ray
- Echocardiogram
- EKG
- Pulse oximeter

POP QUIZ 6.2

A toddler is brought into the ED crying. The patient is very cyanotic with an oxygen saturation level at 72%. They insist on squatting on the floor, their eyes are very red from crying, and their respirations are fast, at 80 per minute, and labored. The patient's mother states that this has been happening since they were a baby, but it is getting worse. The patient has not been eating well and has been more tired than usual. What do these signs and symptoms indicate? What can the nurse do to help this patient?

COMPLICATIONS

Complications associated with a VSD include pulmonary hypertension, heart failure, arrhythmias, stroke, endocarditis, aortic regurgitation, subaortic stenosis, left-to-right shunting at the atrial level, and right ventricle obstruction.

Treatment
- Mild or small: may close spontaneously
- Medications (see Table 6.2):
  - Inotropes for heart failure: dopamine
  - Furosemide for fluid overload
  - Spironolactone for fluid overload
- VSD closure:
  - Surgical closure: requires cardiopulmonary bypass
  - Transcatheter closure: reserved for patients who cannot tolerate bypass

Nursing Interventions
- Administer medications as ordered.
- Assess peripheral pulses and capillary refill.
- Evaluate nutritional status.
- Monitor vital signs, color, temperature, and heart sounds.
- Monitor EKG for changes.
- Monitor strict I/O.
- Weigh daily.

Patient and Family Education
- Family members should seek support groups to help face challenges and connect with other families going through similar experiences.
- Follow recommendations for the proper activity level for the patient.
- Learn about condition and when to call the doctor.
- Monitor child's weight and report a loss/failure to gain to physician.
- Recognize the importance of follow-up visits.
- Seek emotional support.
- Vaccinate the child.

INFLAMMATORY CARDIOVASCULAR CONDITIONS

ENDOCARDITIS, MYOCARDITIS, AND PERICARDITIS

Overview
Endocarditis, myocarditis, and pericarditis are inflammatory cardiovascular conditions (Table 6.1).

Signs and Symptoms
- Endocarditis
  - Abdominal pain
  - Bloody urine
  - Cough
  - Dyspnea
  - Enlarged spleen
  - Fever/chills
  - Heart murmur
  - Muscle, joint pain
  - Night sweats
  - Rashes, typically on hands and feet
  - Weight loss, poor appetite

 COMPLICATIONS

Complications with inflammation of the heart include:
- Endocarditis: embolus, arrhythmias, heart failure, sepsis
- Myocarditis: arrhythmias, cardiomyopathy, cardiogenic shock, pleural effusion, syncope
- Pericarditis: pericardial effusion, cardiac tamponade, constrictive pericarditis

- Myocarditis
  - Abdominal pain
  - Chest pain
  - Dyspnea
  - Edema, in the feet and legs
  - Fatigue
  - Fever
  - Palpitations
  - Syncope
  - Weakness
- Pericarditis
  - Chest pain
  - Dyspnea
  - Fever
  - Tachycardia

 ALERT!

MIS-C is a complication of COVID-19, the SARS-CoV-2 virus disease or exposure. MIS-C causes inflammation of many organs, and children may present with myocarditis or pericarditis. Care parameters are continually evolving. For current information on caring for patients with COVID-19, consult the National Institute of Health and the CDC.

Diagnosis
Labs
- Blood cultures
- CBC: monitor for increased WBC count
- CRP: monitor for increased level
- Kinase: monitor for increased level
- Troponin: monitor for increased level

Diagnostic Testing
- Cardiac CT or MRI
- Echocardiogram
- EKG
- Endomyocardial biopsy
- Pericardiocentesis

Nursing Interventions
- Administer medications as ordered or prior to procedures per protocol.
- Educate family on condition and provide support.
- Educate family about prophylaxis antibiotics and the importance of dental care.
- Monitor patient's vital signs, heart sounds, skin color, and weight.
- Monitor strict I/O.

Patient and Family Education
- Pericarditis can reoccur. Learn to recognize the symptoms of worsening condition, including chills/fever, dyspnea, excessive fatigue, and edema.
- Recognize the importance of dental hygiene and regular dental visits.
- There will be many follow-up appointments with lab work and testing.
- The provider may recommend limited physical activity.

Table 6.1 Inflammatory Cardiovascular Conditions

	Endocarditis	**Myocarditis**	**Pericarditis**
Description	• Inflammation of the inner lining of the heart including the chambers and the valves	• Inflammation of the actual heart muscle • Can be acute or chronic	• Infection of the fluid between the two layers of lining of the heart • Four types; acute, subacute, chronic, recurrent
Causes	• Bacteria • *Staph-aureus*: bacteria enter bloodstream during invasive procedure or IV drug use • *Strep* • Autoimmune disease; can also cause heart valve damage	• Viruses • Most commonly adenovirus, herpes, influenza, Sars-Cov-2, Zika virus • Autoimmune disease • Parasites: can cause Chagas disease; specific to Latin America • Side effects of medications[a] • Exposure to certain metals such as copper and lead • Radiation • Fungi	• Viruses • Autoimmune disease • Side effects of medications[a] • Fungi
Risk Factors	• Central venous catheters • Children with cyanotic heart disease • Rheumatic heart disease	• Exposure to virus	• Immunosuppression • Chest trauma • Thoracic surgery

[a]Medications include antidepressants, antibiotics, benzodiazepines, diuretics, cardiac medications, and vaccines.
Source: Data from National Heart, Lung, and Blood Institute. (2021). *Heart inflammation.* U.S. Department of Health and Human Services, National Heart, Lung, and Blood Institute. https://www.nhlbi.nih.gov/health-topics/heart-inflammation

RHEUMATIC FEVER

Overview

- *Rheumatic fever* is an inflammatory complication affecting the heart, joints, brain, and skin that can occur 2 to 4 weeks after group A *Streptococcus* pharyngitis.
- Rheumatic fever can cause the following:
  - Arthritis in major joints
  - Carditis
  - Chorea due to CNS involvement
  - *Erythema marginatum*, which is a pink, faint red rash that appears on the trunk and/or limbs
  - Subcutaneous painless nodules usually over bony prominences

 COMPLICATIONS

Rheumatic fever can cause long-term heart damage called rheumatic heart disease, which leads to atrial arrhythmias, weakened heart valves, cardiomyopathy, and pulmonary or systemic embolus. Rheumatic fever also may lead to death.

Signs and Symptoms

- Major symptoms:
  - Arthritis in large joints
  - Carditis and valvulitis
  - CNS (chorea)

- ○ Abrupt, nonrhythmic, involuntary movements
- ○ Emotional disturbance
- ○ Muscular weakness
- ○ Slurred speech
- Minor symptoms:
  - Arthralgia
  - Fever
  - Prolonged PR interval

Diagnosis
- Previous diagnosis of group A *Streptococcus* infection
- One of the following:
  - Two major symptoms
  - One major symptom and one minor symptom

Labs
- CRP, ESR: increased levels
- CBC: low Hgb and leukocytosis
- Throat culture: positive for group A *Streptococcus*

Diagnostic Testing
- Chest x-ray
- EKG
- Echocardiogram

Treatment
- Antibiotics for group A *Streptococcus* even if asymptomatic
- Symptom management:
  - Arthritis: NSAIDs (Table A.2)
- Carditis: treatment for heart failure
- Chorea:
  - Antibiotics (Table A.1)
  - Antidepressants (if severe and interfere with ADLs) (Table 16.2)
  - Rest

Nursing Interventions
- Assess neurologic status.
- Educate family on the condition and treatment plan.
- Educate the family that future sore throats must be treated promptly to avoid reoccurrence.
- Monitor labs daily, including CRP, ESR, CBC.
- Monitor vital signs, color, and temperature.
- Stress the importance of dental care.
- Stress the importance of finishing the antibiotics.
- Monitor strict I/O.

Patient and Family Education
- Activity level should be monitored to avoid overstimulation.
- Finishing antibiotics is important to completely eradicate bacteria.
- Seek emotional support as well as education.
- Understand the importance of treatment to prevent the heart from being damaged.

KAWASAKI DISEASE

Overview
- *Kawasaki disease* is an acute, self-limiting vasculitis.
- The cause is unknown, but it often develops after a respiratory or GI illness.
- Without treatment, approximately 20% to 25% of children develop cardiac involvement.
- Typical presentation includes fever and acute inflammation.
- The three phases are:
  - Acute: fever and irritability
  - Subacute: end of the fever until all clinical signs have resolved
  - Convalescent: from when clinical signs resolve until lab values resolve (6–8 weeks)

Signs and Symptoms
- Fever for 5 days or more
- Presence of at least four of the five symptoms:
  - Conjunctivitis:
    - Bilateral
    - Nonexudative
    - Photophobia
  - Oral mucus membrane changes:
    - Erythema and cracking of lips
    - Erythema of oral and pharyngeal mucosa
    - Strawberry tongue
  - Extremity changes:
    - Acute: erythema of the palms and soles
    - Edema of the hands and feet
    - Subacute: peeling, desquamation of the fingers and toes in second and third week
  - Cervical lymphadenopathy: at least one swollen lymph node
  - Rash:
    - Polymorphous exanthem
    - Trunk, extremities, and face

COMPLICATIONS

Kawasaki disease can result in:

- Shock syndrome
- Sustained systolic hypotension
- Clinical signs of poor perfusion
- Cardiac complications
- Noncoronary vascular involvement
- Urinary and renal disease
- GI abnormalities
- Central nervous system abnormalities
- Hearing loss

ALERT!

Signs and symptoms that may indicate coronary involvement include:

- Tachycardia out of proportion to the degree of fever
- Gallop rhythm
- Murmurs

Late signs include:

- Chest pain
- Abdominal pain
- Pallor
- Diaphoresis
- Inconsolable crying

Diagnosis
Labs
There are no labs specific to diagnose Kawasaki disease. However, the following may be helpful when determining severity and treatment:
- CBC
- CRP
- ESR
- Ferritin level
- Urinalysis

Diagnostic Testing
Echocardiogram to determine cardiac involvement.

Treatment
- Aspirin (Table A.2) as an anticoagulant to protect coronary arteries
- IVIG within first 10 days of diagnosis to reduce fever and chance of cardiac involvement

Nursing Interventions
- Educate family about condition.
- Encourage rest so that the body can heal and reduce the length of the illness.
- Ensure adequate hydration via either oral or intravenous fluids.
- Monitor and manage temperature.
- Monitor strict I/O.
- The more severe the involvement, the more involved the long-term treatment will be.

Patient and Family Education
- Attend all follow-up appointments for any cardiac involvement.
- Maintain rest and fluids at home to remain hydrated.
- Monitor symptoms and report any changes to the provider.
- Recovery time is typically 6 to 8 weeks.
- Patients who receive IVIG should not receive any vaccines for 1 year (Chapter 2).
- Review limitations on physical activity, if any.
- Take medications (aspirin) as prescribed (Table A.2).

 ALERT!

Children with Kawasaki disease are at risk for coronary artery abnormalities including MI, ischemia, and sudden death. This is more likely if the patient has not had IVIG early in the disease process. To prevent coronary thrombosis, low-dose aspirin is typically given for 4 to 6 weeks if there are no contraindications. Treatment depends on the size and persistence of coronary artery abnormalities.

 POP QUIZ 6.3

A 6-year-old child has been admitted with a diagnosis of Kawasaki disease. The patient has had a fever for 6 days, and their hands and feet are peeling. The parents are very upset and want to know what can be done to help their child. What anticipatory guidance should the nurse provide?

DEVICES AND PROCEDURES

CARDIAC CATHETERIZATION

Overview
- The main purpose of a cardiac catheterization is to collect hemodynamic data and/or to confirm a heart disease diagnosis.
- A cardiac catheterization can:
  - Detect heart defects
  - Measure pressures within the heart chambers and great vessels
  - Measure cardiac output
- It is an invasive procedure, usually performed in a cardiac catheterization lab, where a flexible catheter is inserted into an artery or vein, usually through either the femoral or radial arteries.
- During a cardiac catheterization, other procedures, such as closing heart defects (VSD, ASD, PDA), can also be performed by a cardiologist, interventional radiologist, or other qualified provider.

Nursing Interventions
- Assess affected extremity for color, temperature, and capillary refill.

 COMPLICATIONS

There are several major complications that can happen with cardiac catheterization:
- Arrhythmias
- Atrial thrombosis
- AV fistula
- Bleeding
- Death
- Embolism
- Infection
- Myocardial infarction
- Retroperitoneal extension
- Pseudoaneurysm
- Perforation of the heart or great vessels
- Radiation exposure
- Stroke
- Thrombosis at the catheter insertion site

- Assess patient and family's understanding of procedure.
- Assess pressure dressing according to protocol.
- Keep patient in bed in supine position for 6 hours following catheterization, keeping extremity straight.
- Monitor IV fluids; encourage PO as soon as appropriate.
- Monitor for bleeding at insertion site.
- Palpate distal pulses of extremity used.
- Provide warmth to opposite extremity.

Patient and Family Education
- Apply pressure to site if bleeding occurs.
- Learn what to look for in hands/feet of extremity used for procedure: temperature should be warm, color should be pink, and there should be good capillary refill.
- Notify provider of concerning changes, such as bleeding at the site, or pale or cool extremity.
- Patient should rest at home after procedure.
- Remove the pressure dressing after 24 hours or according to provider recommendation.

EKG MONITORING

Overview
- An *EKG* is a graphical representation of the electrical activity of the heart.
- Normal electrical activity of the heart
- The sinus node acts as the pacemaker in normal circumstances.
- Mediated by calcium currents, the node generates a slow action potential that activates the atrial myocardium.
- Sodium ions help to transmit the signal quickly.
- Once the atria are activated, the impulse reaches the AV node and then the bundle of His.
- From the bundle of His, the impulse is conducted to the right and left bundle branches.
- Through the bundles, it goes to the ventricular myocardium.
- EKGs are ordered on pediatric patients to:
  - Assess a baseline rhythm before any intervention.
  - Assess a change in rhythm or dysrhythmias seen on a monitor.
  - Assess the heart after procedure or surgery.
  - Diagnose structural or conductive heart abnormalities.
  - Evaluate the effectiveness of prescribed heart medications.
  - Monitor a patient with syncope.
- EKG strips have several components that are used to help interpret rhythms:
  - Small squares: 0.04 s
  - Large squares: 0.20 s
  - P wave: atrial depolarization
  - ST wave: atrial repolarization
  - PR interval: atrial depolarization and conduction through the AV node and Purkinje system
  - QRS: ventricular depolarization
  - T wave: ventricular repolarization
  - QT interval: ventricular repolarization

Normal Sinus Rhythm EKG Interpretation
- Normal sinus rhythm is a regular rhythm at the normal heart rate for age:
  - Infant: 100 to 180 beats/min
  - Toddler: 80 to 140 beats/min
  - Preschooler: 65 to 120 beats/min
  - School age: 70 to 110 beats/min
  - Adolescent: 60 to 100 beats/min

Normal Sinus Rhythm EKG Interpretation *(continued)*

- Normal sinus rhythm has a P wave before every QRS complex, and each PR interval is constant.
- Interpretation of normal sinus rhythm EKG strip:
  - Rhythm: Regular (slight variation of the R to R is normal in children)
  - Rate: 118 bpm (child is 19 months old)
  - P waves: Normal and upright
  - PRI: 122 ms
  - QRS: 76 ms
  - QT/QTc: 300/420 ms

Bradycardia

- *Sinus bradycardia* is a slower rate, or below the normal heart rate range for age.
- Bradycardia could be due to hypoxia, hypotension, cardiac post-op, anorexia, or medications such as opioids. Bradycardia can be a normal finding during sleep or adolescents with increased vagal tone.

Tachycardia

- *Sinus tachycardia* is a faster heart rate, or above the normal heart rate for age.
- Tachycardia can be due to fever, pain, anxiety, anemia, exercise, and dehydration.

Supraventricular Tachycardia

- SVT is a tachydysrhythmia characterized by a rapid regular heart rate of 200 to 300 beats/min.
- The onset of SVT is typically sudden.
- Treatment of SVT includes vagal maneuvers, applying ice to the face and Valsalva maneuver.

Ventricular Fibrillation

- *Ventricular fibrillation* is an irregular rhythm with no identifiable P waves, QRS complexes, or T waves.
- Ventricular fibrillation is a shockable rhythm.

Long QT Syndrome

- *Long QT syndrome* is a rhythm where the interval between the Q and the T is longer than expected.
- Long QT syndrome is commonly due to electrolyte imbalances or medications such as diuretics.
- A common sign or symptom of long QT syndrome is fainting or syncope.

First-Degree Heart Block

- *First-degree heart block* is a delay in conduction through the AV node causing a slower heart rate.
- First-degree heart block could be caused by beta-blockers or calcium channel blockers.

Second Degree Heart Block (Mobitz 1)

- Mobitz I is characterized by the electrical signals getting slower and skipping, or dropping, a beat.
- PR interval is longest before a dropped beat, and PR interval is shortest after a dropped beat.

Second-Degree Heart Block (Mobitz 2)

- Mobitz 2 is characterized by a dropped beat but there is no pattern of the signal getting slower.

Third-Degree Heart Block

- *Third-degree heart block* is when signals fail to conduct at all between the atria and ventricles.
- Third-degree heart block causes severe bradycardia and often results in needing a pacemaker.

VASCULAR ACCESS DEVICES

Overview
- Common venous access devices are peripheral catheters or IVs, central lines, and ports, while arterial lines provide vascular access via an artery.
- Peripheral access devices:
  - Venous access is obtained using an over-the-needle catheter.
  - Potential sites include extremities and the scalp.
  - Peripheral IVs are used for only a few days.
- Central venous access devices:
  - Types of central venous access devices include PICC lines, ports, and tunneled and nontunneled catheters.
  - Central venous access devices can be used over long periods of time for large volumes of fluid and/or irritating solutions and long-term medications.
  - Central access can be used for collection of blood for labs.
  - PICCs are used for short-term use, usually over weeks.
  - Central lines and ports are used over months or years.
  - Lines should be placed using ultrasound guidance, fluoroscopy, or in surgery under sterile procedure.
- Venous cutdown
- An emergency procedure in which the vein is surgically exposed, and an access device is placed by the surgeon under direct vision.
- Venous cutdown is only used when peripheral, central venous, and I/Os cannot be obtained.
- Saphenous is the best site in pediatrics, including infants.
- This is usually performed by an attending provider or surgeon.
- Arterial lines
  - An arterial line is placed into an artery by a provider for hemodynamic monitoring and for drawing atrial blood samples, such as for ABGs.
  - The radial artery, which is a peripheral artery, is the most reliable in pediatrics.
  - Femoral, posterior tibia, dorsal pedis, axillary, and brachial arteries can also be used if the radial is not available.
  - A child with an arterial line should be monitored in the ICU.

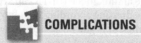

COMPLICATIONS

Possible complications of peripheral IVs include hematoma formation, infiltration, phlebitis, and thrombosis.

COMPLICATIONS

Complications of arterial lines include arterial vasospasm, emboli, sepsis, hemorrhage, and accidental drug injection.

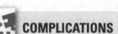

COMPLICATIONS

Complications of central venous access include CLABSIs, arterial punctures, malposition, hematomas, bleeding, and pneumothorax.

Nursing Interventions
- Explain the procedure at an appropriate developmental level to the patient.
- Provide emotional support throughout the process. Use child life specialist if available.
- Educate the patient and family about the vascular access device their child will be getting and ensure consent was obtained prior to PICC or central line placement.
- Prepare the patient for the central line placement procedure, whether it will be in the room, PICC suite, or in the operating room.
- Assess for infiltration and phlebitis.
- Maintain patency and flush line according to policy.
- Keep dressing clean, dry, and intact. Transparent dressings should be used to view the insertion site.
- Change dressing when visibly soiled, wet, or no longer intact. PICC or central line dressings should be changed in a sterile environment.

Nursing Interventions *(continued)*
- Prevent CLABSI in patients with PICCs or central lines:
  - Change antimicrobial barrier cap according to policy.
  - Change dressing according to policy and in sterile environment.
- Give chlorhexidine gluconate bath daily or according to policy.
  - Minimize number of times the line is accessed.
  - Use chlorhexidine to clean the insertion site when doing dressing changes.

Patient and Family Education
- Learn how to care for the CVC at home.
  - Prevent infection.
    - ○ Avoid having dental work done while the line is in place to prevent seeding of bacteria into the bloodstream from the mouth and gums.
    - ○ Keep the insertion site sterile to prevent infection.
    - ○ The dressing and antimicrobial cap must be changed every week.
  - Prevent line from getting wet.
    - ○ Cover the PICC line when showering to avoid getting wet.
    - ○ Do not swim while the line is in place.
  - Limit activity.
    - ○ Avoid strenuous activities while the line is in place.
    - ○ Do not participate in contact sports.
  - Flush the line properly.
  - Learn how to give medications through the line.
  - Never cut the dressing around the line with scissors.
  - Attach or tape the line to arm to prevent pulls or tears.
- Learn to care for a port at home.
  - Discomfort of insertion may last a week.
  - Report any redness, drainage, or warmness around the incision site.
  - Avoid lifting the arm on the same side as the port for 24 hours.
  - Flush with heparinized solution after medication administration (once per month if not in use).
  - Report any of the following to the provider:
    - ○ Blood backed up in the infusion tubing
    - ○ Fever or chills
    - ○ Insertion site that becomes hot, red, or tender
    - ○ Leaking from the med port site
    - ○ New or increased pain to site
    - ○ Resistance to flushing
    - ○ Purulent drainage or fluid coming from insertion site

Table 6.2 Cardiovascular Medications

Indications	Mechanism of Action	Contraindications, Precautions, and Adverse Effects
ACE inhibitor (enalapril)		
• Treat atrioventricular canal defect • Treat hypertension	• Inhibit angiotensin • Converting enzyme	• Medication is contraindicated in pediatric patients with a lowered GFR and contraindicated in patients with hypotension. • Use with caution in children under 6 years old. • Use with caution in patients with risk for hyperkalemia. • Adverse effects include hyperkalemia, myocardial infarction, renal failure, and hypotension.
Adrenergic agonist agent (dopamine)		
• Increase cardiac output • Increase blood pressure	• Stimulate adrenergic and dopaminergic receptors • Produce cardiac stimulation	• Medication is contraindicated in pheochromocytoma, tachyarrhythmias, and ventricular fibrillation. • Use extreme caution if patient is taking MAO inhibitors. • Precautions need to be taken in case of arrhythmias, extravasation, heart conditions, electrolyte imbalance, and shock. • Adverse effects include sloughing and necrosis of the IV site. Monitor closely. • Adverse effects also include anxiety, headache, cardiac rhythm changes, nausea, vomiting, dyspnea, polyuria, and increased intraocular pressure.
Anticoagulants (warfarin)		
• Anticoagulant	• Inactivate thrombin and prevent the conversion of fibrinogen to fibrin	• Contraindications include active bleeding, recent or planned surgery, major trauma, and acute intracranial hemorrhage. • Use precaution, as there is a risk of bleeding that must be weighed against not using the anticoagulant. • Adverse effects include thrombocytopenia, hemorrhage, pruritus, and skin necrosis.
Beta-blocker (propranolol)		
• Can be used to treat tet spells	• Reduce blood pressure, heart rate, cardiac output, and myocardial contractility	• Medication is contraindicated in patients with severe bradycardia. • Use with caution in patients with pulmonary disease. • Adverse effects include cardiac ischemia if discontinued suddenly, as well as acute MI, nausea/vomiting, and bronchitis.

(continued)

Table 6.2 Cardiovascular Medications *(continued)*

Indications	Mechanism of Action	Contraindications, Precautions, and Adverse Effects
Calcium channel blocker (nifedipine)		
• Treat hypertension	• Relax coronary vascular muscle and produce coronary vasodilation	• Caution must be used in patients with GI strictures, aortic stenosis, heart failure, and hepatic impairment. • Adverse effects include flushing, nausea, heartburn, dizziness, headache, Stevens–Johnson syndrome, and toxic epidermal necrolysis.
Diuretic (furosemide)		
• Remove excess fluid from the body	• Inhibit the reabsorption of sodium and chloride in the kidneys	• Contraindications include anuria. • Precautions should be used in patients with thyroid impairment, diabetes, urinary stricture, and lupus. • With chronic use, children can develop kidney stones. • Caution is needed if given before surgery, as patient may be volume depleted and blood pressure may be labile. • Adverse effects include necrotizing angiitis, Stevens–Johnson syndrome, and toxic epidermal necrolysis. • Medication can cause abdominal cramps, nausea/vomiting, constipation, and pancreatitis. • Medication can cause electrolyte imbalances, anemia, headache, vertigo, blurry vision, deafness, tinnitus, and dizziness.
Diuretic (spironolactone)		
• Treat heart failure • Treat hypertension	• Inhibit the action of aldosterone on the distal tubules • Increase NaCl and water excretion while conserving potassium and hydrogen ions	• Medication is contraindicated in patients with hyperkalemia, Addison's disease, and renal impairment. • Use with caution in patients with acid–base imbalance, metabolic acidosis, metabolic alkalosis, and respiratory acidosis. • Adverse effects include vasculitis, Stevens–Johnson syndrome, confusion, lethargy, headache, and dizziness.

Table 6.2 Cardiovascular Medications *(continued)*

Indications	Mechanism of Action	Contraindications, Precautions, and Adverse Effects
Inotropic agent (digoxin)		
• Treat HLHS and atrioventricular canal defect	• Increase force and velocity of myocardial contraction • Inhibit the Na-K-ATPase membrane pump	• Medication is contraindicated in patients with bradycardia, cardiomyopathy, thyroid disease, and myocarditis. • Use with caution in patients with renal impairment, hepatic impairment, and patients with electrolyte imbalances such as hypercalcemia, hyperkalemia, hypocalcemia, hypokalemia, and hypomagnesemia. • Monitor for symptoms of digoxin toxicity, including nausea, vomiting, and neurologic changes. • Adverse effects include bradycardia, tachycardia, palpitations, and electrolyte imbalances.
Prostaglandin E1		
• Maintain or reopen the patency of the ductus arteriosus • Used in an infant suspected of having a ductal-dependent congenital cardiac defect and ductal-dependent pulmonary blood flow to prevent hypoxia and metabolic acidosis	• Relax the smooth muscle of the ductus arteriosus	• Medication is contraindicated in neonates with respiratory distress syndrome. • Use caution in long-term use, as the medication can cause GI obstruction. • Adverse effects include inhibition of platelets, causing excessive bleeding. • Medication can cause flushing.

RESOURCES

Akamagwuna, U., & Badaly, D. (2019, May 7). Pediatric cardiac rehabilitation: A review. *Current Physical Medicine and Rehabilitation Reports, 7*, 67–80. https://link.springer.com/article/10.1007/s40141-019-00216-9#Sec13

American Heart Association. (2016, September 30). *Heart conduction disorders.* https://www.heart.org/en/health-to pics/arrhythmia/about-arrhythmia/conduction-disorders

American Heart Association. (2021). *Kawasaki disease.* https://www.heart.org/-/media/Files/Health-Topics/Answer s-by-Heart/What-is-Kawasaki-Disease.pdf

C.S. Mott Children's Hospital. (2020, August 31). *Congenital heart defect types.* https://www.mottchildren.org/health -library/tx4010

Carrozza, J. P. (2021). Complications of diagnostic cardiac catheterization. *UpToDate.* https://www.uptodate.com/ contents/complications-of-diagnostic-cardiac-catheterization?search=cardiac%20catheterization&source=searc h_result&selectedTitle=4~150&usage_type=default&display_rank=4

Centers for Disease Control and Prevention. (2018, November 1). *Rheumatic fever: All you need to know.* U.S. Department of Health and Human Services, Centers for Disease Control and Prevention. https://www.cdc.gov/ groupastrep/diseases-public/rheumatic-fever.html

Centers for Disease Control and Prevention. (2020a, November 17). *Facts about pulmonary atresia.* U.S. Department of Health and Human Services, Centers for Disease Control and Prevention. https://www.cdc.gov/ ncbddd/heartdefects/pulmonaryatresia.html

Centers for Disease Control and Prevention. (2020b, November 17). *Facts about ventricular septal defect.* U.S. Department of Health and Human Services, Centers for Disease Control and Prevention. https://www.cdc.gov/ ncbddd/heartdefects/ventricularseptaldefect.html

Centers for Disease Control and Prevention. (2020c). *Facts about tetralogy of Fallot*. U.S. Department of Health and Human Services, Centers for Disease Control and Prevention. https://www.cdc.gov/ncbddd/heartdefects/tetral ogyoffallot.html

Centers for Disease Control and Prevention. (2020d). *Facts about coarctation of the aorta*. U.S. Department of Health and Human Services, Centers for Disease Control and Prevention. https://www.cdc.gov/ncbddd/heartde fects/coarctationofaorta.html

Centers for Disease Control and Prevention. (2021, March 31). *Healthcare workers: Information on COVID-19*. U.S. Department of Health and Human Services, Centers for Disease Control and Prevention. https://www.cdc.gov/ coronavirus/2019-ncov/hcp/

Centers for Disease Control and Prevention. (n.d.). *Coronavirus disease 2019 (COVID-19) treatment guidelines*. U.S. Department of Health and Human Services, Centers for Disease Control and Prevention. www.covid19treatme ntguidelines.nih.gov

Fleishman, C. E., & Tugertimur, A. (2021). Clinical manifestations and diagnosis of atrioventricular (AV) canal defects. *UpToDate*. https://www.uptodate.com/contents/clinical-manifestations-and-diagnosis-of-atrioventricu lar-av-canal-defects?search=AVSD&source=search_result&selectedTitle=1~48&usage_type=default&display_ rank=1#H8312850

Fulton, D. R., & Saleeb, S. (2021). Management of isolated ventricular septal defects in infants and children. *UpToDate*. https://www.uptodate.com/contents/isolated-ventricular-septal-defects-in-infants-and-children-ana tomy-clinical-features-and-diagnosis?search=vsd&source=search_result&selectedTitle=1~150&usage_type=de fault&display_rank=1

Goldberger, A. L. (2021). Basic principles of electrographic interpretation. *UpToDate*. https://www.uptodate.com/ contents/ecg-tutorial-basic-principles-of-ecg-analysis?search=ecg%20interpretation&source=search_result& selectedTitle=1~150&usage_type=default&display_rank=1

Hockenberry, M., Wilson, D., & Rodgers, C. (2019). *Wong's nursing care of infants and children* (11th ed.). Elsevier.

Imazio, M. (2021). Purulent pericarditis. *UpToDate*. https://www.uptodate.com/contents/purulent-pericarditis?sear ch=pericarditis&source=search_result&selectedTitle=3~150&usage_type=default&display_rank=3#H3

Larkin, J., & Buttner, R. (2021, April 6). *AV block: 3rd degree*. Life in the Fastlane. https://litfl.com/av-block-3rd-de gree-complete-heart-block/

LeRoy, S. (2012). *Ventricular fibrillation*. C.S. Mott Children's Hospital Congenital Heart Center. https://www.mott children.org/conditions-treatments/ped-heart/conditions/ventricular-fibrillation

Lexicomp. (2021). Warfarin: Pediatric drug information [Drug Information]. *UpToDate*. https://www.uptodate.com /contents/warfarin-pediatric-drug-information?search=warfarin&source=panel_search_result&selectedTitle=2 ~148&usage_type=panel&kp_tab=drug_pediatric&display_rank=1

Lexicomp. (n.d.[a]). Alprostadil: Pediatric drug information [Drug Information]. *UpToDate*. https://www.uptodate. com/contents/alprostadil-pediatric-drug-information?search=alprostadil&source=panel_search_result&selecte dTitle=2~87&usage_type=panel&kp_tab=drug_pediatric&display_rank=1

Lexicomp. (n.d.[b]). Digoxin: Pediatric drug information [Drug Information]. *UpToDate*. https://www.uptodate.co m/contents/digoxin-pediatric-drug-information?search=digoxin&source=panel_search_result&selectedTitle=2 ~148&usage_type=panel&kp_tab=drug_pediatric&display_rank=1

Lexicomp. (n.d.[c]). Dopamine: Pediatric drug information [Drug Information]. *UpToDate*. https://www.uptodate. com/contents/search?search=dopamine&sp=0&searchType=PLAIN_TEXT&source=USER_INPUT&searchCo ntrol=TOP_PULLDOWN&searchOffset=1&autoComplete=false&language=en&max=10&index=&autoComp leteTerm=

Lexicomp. (n.d.[d]). Enalapril: Pediatric drug information [Drug Information]. *UpToDate*. https://www.uptodate .com/contents/enalapril-pediatric-drug-information?search=enalapril&selectedTitle=1~101&usage_type=panel& display_rank=1&kp_tab=drug_pediatric&source=panel_search_result

Lexicomp. (n.d.[e]). Nifedipine: pediatric drug information [Drug Information]. *UpToDate*. https://www.uptodate .com/contents/nifedipine-pediatric-drug-information?search=nifedipine&source=panel_search_result&selected Title=2~148&usage_type=panel&kp_tab=drug_pediatric&display_rank=1

Lexicomp. (n.d.[f]). Propranolol: Pediatric drug information [Drug Information]. *UpToDate*. https://www.uptodate. com/contents/propranolol-pediatric-drug-information?search=propranolol&source=panel_search_result&selec tedTitle=2~148&usage_type=panel&kp_tab=drug_pediatric&display_rank=1

Lexicomp. (n.d.[g]). Spironolactone: Pediatric drug information [Drug Information]. *UpToDate*. https://www.uptod ate.com/contents/spironolactone-pediatric-drug-information?search=spironolactone&source=panel_search_re sult&selectedTitle=2~148&usage_type=panel&kp_tab=drug_pediatric&display_rank=1

Machado, R. C., Gironés, P., Souza, A. R., Moreira, R. S., Jakitsch, C. B., & Branco, J. N. (2017). Nursing care protocol for patients with a ventricular assist device. *Revista Brasileira de Enfermagem, 70*(2), 335–341. https:// doi.org/10.1590/0034-7167-2016-0363

Myocarditis Foundation. (n.d.). *Discover myocarditis causes, symptoms, diagnosis and treatment*. https://www .myocarditisfoundation.org/about-myocarditis

National Center for Advancing Translational Sciences. (n.d.[a]). *Hypoplastic left heart syndrome*. U.S. Department of Health and Human Services, National Center for Advancing Translational Sciences. https://rarediseases.info .nih.gov/diseases/6739/hypoplastic-left-heart-syndrome/cases/31583

National Center for Advancing Translational Sciences. (n.d.[b]). *Rheumatic fever*. U.S. Department of Health and Human Services, National Center for Advancing Translational Sciences. https://rarediseases.info.nih.gov/diseases /5699/rheumatic-fever

National Down Syndrome Society. (n.d.). *The heart and Down syndrome*. https://www.ndss.org/resources/the-heart -down-syndrome/

National Heart, Lung, and Blood Institute. (2021). *Heart inflammation*. U.S. Department of Health and Human Services, National Heart, Lung, and Blood Institute. https://www.nhlbi.nih.gov/health-topics/heart-inflammation

National Organization for Rare Disorders. (n.d.). *Tetralogy of Fallot*. https://rarediseases.org/gard-rare-disease/tetra logy-of-fallot/

O'Brian, S. E. (2021). Infective endocarditis in children. *UpToDate*. https://www.uptodate.com/contents/infective -endocarditis-in-children?search=endocarditis&source=search_result&selectedTitle=1~150&usage_type= default&display_rank=1

O'Brien, P., & Marshall, A. C. (2015). Coarctation of the aorta. *Circulation, 131*, e363–365. https://www.ahajournals .org/doi/full/10.1161/circulationaha.114.008821

Prater, K. J., & Hubbard, J. E. (2017). *Normal to advanced rhythms. Pediatric arrhythmias and EKGs for the health care provider*. https://connect.springerpub.com/content/book/978-0-8261-9447-3/part/part03/chapter/ch06

Saenz, R. B., Beebe, D. K., & Triplett, L. C. (1999). Caring for infants with congenital heart disease and their families. *American Family Physician, 59*(7), 1857–1866. https://www.aafp.org/afp/1999/0401/p1857.html

Seattle Children's Hospital. (n.d.). *Tetralogy of Fallot*. https://www.seattlechildrens.org/conditions/tetralogy-of -fallot/

Tikkanen, A. U., Oyaga, A. R., Rlaño, O., Álvaro, E. M., & Rhodes, J. (2021, January 17). Paediatric cardiac rehabilitation in congenital heart disease: A systematic review. *Cardiology in the Young, 22*(3), 241–250. https:// www.cambridge.org/core/journals/cardiology-in-the-young/article/abs/paediatric-cardiac-rehabilitation-in -congenital-heart-disease-a-systematic-review/E04A0ACF723CC7A8D054F5B83B8C6AD4

University of California San Francisco Pediatric Cardiothoracic Surgery. (2021). *Atrial septal defect (ASD)*. https:// pedctsurgery.ucsf.edu/conditions--procedures/atrial-septal-defect.aspx

Vick, G. W., & Bezold, L. I. (2021). Isolated atrial septal defects in children: Management and outcome. *UpToDate*. https://www.uptodate.com/contents/isolated-atrial-septal-defects-in-children-management-and-outcome?search =asd&source=search_result&selectedTitle=2~150&usage_type=default&display_rank=2

RESPIRATORY SYSTEM

Overview

- Respiratory assessment
  - Airway and breathing are priority nursing assessments.
  - Normal respiratory rate varies by age.
    - Infant: 30 to 57 breaths/min
    - Toddler: 22 to 46 breaths/min
    - Preschooler: 20 to 29 breaths/min
    - School age: 16 to 24 breaths/min
    - Adolescent: 12 to 22 breaths/min
  - Normal pulse oximetry is 94% to 100%. However, the patient's baseline medical condition may alter the expected oxygen saturation level.
  - Inspection is an essential part of a physical assessment.
    - The shape of the chest wall should be symmetrical with a 1:2 ratio of anteroposterior diameter to transverse diameter.
    - Abnormal findings include cyanosis and pallor.
  - Observe respiration to provide critical information on the patient's status. Nurses need to note the following:
    - Rate: number of respirations per minute
    - Rhythm: regular, irregular, or periodic
    - Depth: deep or shallow
    - Quality: effortless or labored with retractions and accessory muscle use
  - Palpation and percussion provide additional information.
    - *Tactile fremitus*, or palpable vibrations of the chest wall caused by vocalization, is a normal finding when it is symmetric bilaterally.
    - Resonance is heard over healthy lung tissue.
    - Abnormal findings include dullness or hyperresonance.
  - Auscultation of breath sounds must be completed on every assessment.
    - Normal breath sounds are clear and equal bilaterally. Bronchial, bronchovesicular, and vesicular breath sounds are normal.
    - Abnormal findings include crackles, wheezes, stridor, and absent or diminished breath sounds.
- Blood gas interpretation
  - Arterial blood gases measure the acidity (pH), the partial pressure of carbon dioxide ($PaCO_2$), the bicarbonate level (HCO_3), and the partial pressure of oxygen (PaO_2).
    - Expected values (Table 7.1):
      - pH 7.35 to 7.45
      - $PaCO_2$ 35 to 45 mmHg
      - HCO_3, 21 to 28 mEq/L
  - Arterial blood gases are used to measure acid–base imbalances (Table 7.1).

Table 7.1 Arterial Blood Gas Acid–Base Imbalances Without Compensation

Imbalance	pH	PaCO$_2$ mmHg	HCO$_3$ mEq/L
Normal values	7.35–7.45	35–45	21–28
Metabolic acidosis	⬇	Normal	⬇
Metabolic alkalosis	⬆	Normal	⬆
Respiratory acidosis	⬇	⬆	Normal
Respiratory alkalosis	⬆	⬇	Normal

- End-tidal CO$_2$ monitoring
  - *End-tidal CO$_2$ monitoring* is a noninvasive measurement of the partial pressure of CO$_2$ in exhaled breath.
  - It is commonly used to assess ETT placement and adequacy of ventilation. It can also be used to monitor ventilation during sedation.
- Oxygen delivery
  - High-flow devices include a high flow nasal cannula, venturi mask, CPAP/BiPAP, and mechanical ventilation.
  - Low-flow devices include a nasal cannula, a simple face mask, and a nonrebreather mask.
  - Oxygen therapy increases the oxygen concentration the lungs are receiving, thereby increasing systemic oxygen delivery.
- Pulse oximetry
  - Pulse oximetry provides a measurement of oxygen saturation in the blood.
  - It is the saturation of the hemoglobin molecule with oxygen at the capillary bed using a light absorption sensor through a noninvasive probe that can be placed on the child's fingertip, toe, foot, or earlobe.
  - The expected levels are 94% to 100%.
- Suctioning
  - Suction is the primary intervention to clear secretions and mucus plugs from the nose, mouth, nasopharynx, or artificial airways such as ETT or tracheostomy tube.
  - Set suction pressure to 80 to 100 mmHg.
  - Use an appropriate size suction catheter for the age or size of an artificial airway.
  - Instill catheter to premeasured length, not until meeting resistance.
  - Do not apply suction on insertion.
  - Apply intermittent suction and gentle catheter rotation as the catheter is being removed.

NURSING PEARL

A mnemonic to help remember acid–base imbalances is ROME: **R**espiratory **O**pposite, **M**etabolic **E**qual. In respiratory imbalances, the affected values are inverse or the arrows are in opposite directions. In metabolic imbalances, the affected values are equal or in the same direction.

- Monitor pulse oximetry while suctioning.
- To help prevent hypoxia during suctioning, hyperventilate with oxygen or increase FiO_2 and limit suction passes.
- Tracheostomy care
  - *Tracheostomy* is a surgical opening in the trachea.
    - ○ Artificial airways are often used when there is a need for prolonged mechanical ventilation.
    - ○ Complications include obstruction, decannulation, and hemorrhage.
    - ○ Emergency supplies should always be nearby, including:
      - ■ An additional smaller-sized tracheostomy tube
      - ■ An extra same-sized tracheostomy tube
      - ■ Suction catheter
      - ■ Tracheostomy ties
    - ○ Maintain patent airway by suctioning secretions and performing tracheostomy care.
  - Tracheostomy care must be completed per shift.
    - ○ Assess the stoma and the surrounding skin.
    - ○ Change the tracheostomy tube weekly or according to policy.
    - ○ Keep the skin clean, dry, and free of infection.
    - ○ Use tracheostomy ties or securement device to hold the tracheostomy tube in place. Verify proper tension in the ties.
      - ■ Change ties according to facility policy or when soiled.
      - ■ Ties should be tight, allowing one finger width between ties and skin.

ASTHMA

Overview

- *Asthma* is a chronic disease of the lower respiratory tract and the lungs with acute flare ups or exacerbations. It is characterized by inflammation, increased mucus production, and bronchoconstriction.
- Asthma varies in symptom severity and frequency and can be classified as:
  - Intermittent
    - ○ Asthma symptoms occurring 2 or fewer days per week
    - ○ Use of SABA to relieve symptoms 2 or fewer days per week
    - ○ No interference with regular activities
  - Mild-persistent
    - ○ Asthma symptoms occurring more than 2 days per week
    - ○ Waking during sleep 3 to 4 times per month with symptoms
    - ○ Use of SABA to relieve symptoms more than 2 days per week
    - ○ Minor interference with regular activities
  - Moderate-persistent
    - ○ Asthma symptoms occurring daily
    - ○ Waking during sleep more than once a week with symptoms
    - ○ Use of SABA or bronchodilator daily for symptom relief
  - Severe-persistent
    - ○ Asthma symptoms occurring throughout day
    - ○ Waking from sleep often seven nights per week with symptoms
    - ○ Use of SABA several times per day to relieve symptoms
    - ○ Extremely limited in regular activities due to symptoms
- Risk factors include a family history of asthma, allergies, history of prematurity, and obesity.
- Triggers include allergens, irritants, exercise, environmental temperature changes, smoke exposure, and respiratory viruses.

 COMPLICATIONS

Status asthmaticus is a life-threatening, prolonged asthma attack characterized by wheezing, difficulty breathing, hypoxia, and tachycardia that does not improve with traditional treatments. Without appropriate medical care, it leads to respiratory failure.

Signs and Symptoms

- Chest tightness
- Coughing
- Difficulty speaking
- Dyspnea
- Eczema/atopic dermatitis
- Hypoxia
- Retractions
- Shortness of breath
- Tachycardia
- Tachypnea
- Wheezing (inspiratory and expiratory)

Diagnosis

Labs
- ABG for respiratory acidosis
- CBC for elevated WBC and elevated eosinophils

Diagnostic Testing
- Chest x-ray to rule out other respiratory conditions before asthma diagnosis
- PFT to measure lung volume, capacity, and flow rates

Treatment

- Medications (Table 7.2*):
  - Bronchodilators
  - Corticosteroids
  - LABA
  - Magnesium sulfate
  - SABA
  - Terbutaline
- Oxygen
- Heliox sometimes used for acute severe asthma

Nursing Interventions

- The goals of asthma management are to control symptoms and to prevent or reduce exacerbations.
- Administer inhaled medications as ordered.
- Administer oxygen therapy as ordered to maintain pulse oximetry above 90%.
- Assess airway, breathing, and vital signs.
  - Monitor for worsening work of breathing or dyspnea.
  - Monitor for increased agitation.
  - Monitor for increased respiratory rate.
  - Monitor for decreasing pulse oximetry reading.
  - Monitor for acute changes in heart rate and blood pressure.
- Assess for any barriers to care, such as access to a provider, transportation issues for follow-up appointments, or financial concerns.
- Assess the patient and family's understanding of the chronic disease and treatment plan.
- Auscultate breath sounds.
  - Monitor for worsening wheezing
  - Absent breath sounds are a medical emergency and indicate that air is not moving through the lungs because of inflammation, mucus, and/or bronchoconstriction.

---

* Table 7.2 is located at the end of this chapter.

- Involve case management to assist with obtaining prescriptions, spacers, peak flow meters, and referrals.
- Involve social work or school counselor to assist with school absences or hospitalizations.
- Notify the provider of any worsening symptoms; the patient may need escalation of management and treatment.

Patient and Family Education

- Adhere to the treatment plan.
  - Attend all follow-up appointments with pediatrician or pulmonologist. Appointments will be needed for:
    - ○ Annual visits and to discuss refills on inhalers
    - ○ Increased frequency of symptoms or asthma attacks
    - ○ Worsening peak flow meter measurements
  - Take controller medication every day, even when asymptomatic.
  - Take medications as prescribed.
- Avoid known triggers and allergens.
  - Allergens: dust mites, pollens, mold, pet dander, cockroaches
    - ○ Cover pillows and mattresses in allergen-proof cases.
    - ○ Vacuum weekly and use a damp cloth to dust.
    - ○ Limit outdoor activity when the pollen count is high. Change and wash clothing after being outdoors.
    - ○ To avoid mold, avoid damp areas such as basements or attics. Use a dehumidifier.
    - ○ Removing pets from home is the most effective way to prevent flare ups from pet dander.
    - ○ Wash hands after contact with an animal or pet.
    - ○ To avoid roaches, clean the kitchen area, keep food in sealed containers, and remove standing water.
  - Irritants: paint, exposure to chemicals, cleaning supplies, perfumes, strong odors, pollution
    - ○ Avoid exposure to irritants.
    - ○ Wear proper protective equipment around chemicals.
  - Respiratory viruses: flu, common cold, RSV
    - ○ Avoid sick contacts.
    - ○ Wash hands properly.
  - Smoke
    - ○ Do not smoke.
    - ○ Avoid secondhand smoke, especially in enclosed areas.
    - ○ Avoid smoke from fireplaces, firepits, or wood-burning stoves.
  - Weather: cold air, hot air, changes in temperatures
- Carry a rescue inhaler, especially if the child will be exposed to known triggers.
- Follow the personalized asthma action plan.
  - An action plan helps recognize the need for escalation in care and provides guidelines on when to call their provider and when to go to the ED.
  - Give action plan to family and school nurse(s).
- Recognize early symptoms of an asthma attack or exacerbation, such as cough, shortness of breath, or common cold or allergy symptoms.
- Remain up to date on immunizations, including the seasonal influenza vaccine.
- Rinse mouth out after using steroid inhalers to prevent thrush.
- Use peak flow meter for home monitoring.
  - Use a hand-held device to measure expiratory airflow.
  - Understand zones and when to escalate care
    - ○ Green = Go/Safe
      - ■ Breathing is normal with no cough or wheezing symptoms.
      - ■ Keep using preventative medications as prescribed.

ALERT!

Asthma is one of the most common childhood chronic diseases, a primary cause of school absences, and a leading cause of hospitalizations.

Patient and Family Education *(continued)*

- ○ Yellow = Caution
  - Mild symptoms are present (cough, mild wheeze, coughing at night) or exposed to known trigger.
  - Add quick-relief medication as prescribed and call provider.
- ○ Red = Danger/Emergency
  - Symptoms worsen (breathing fast, retractions, trouble speaking) and quick-relief medication is not improving symptoms.
  - Seek help from provider immediately or go to ED.
- Use a spacer with metered dose inhalers.
  - A spacer allows for slow inhale of medication, providing effective delivery to lungs.
  - Using a spacer helps to prevent thrush by delivering medication directly to lungs rather than the mouth or tongue.
- Utilize availability of support services and community resources such as counseling and social work.
  - Benefits children experiencing school absenteeism and frequent hospitalizations
  - Fosters communication in adolescents who are refusing or reluctant to adhere to treatment plan
  - Provides additional support to low-income families and households with limited access to care

POP QUIZ 7.1

What education should the nurse give to parents with a 6 year old newly diagnosed with asthma?

BRONCHIOLITIS

Overview

- *Bronchiolitis* is an acute inflammation of the lower respiratory tract and bronchioles.
- RSV is a viral respiratory illness that causes difficulty breathing. It is the most common cause of bronchiolitis.
- Bronchiolitis most often occurs from November to March and is typically preceded by common cold-like symptoms.
- Bronchiolitis, whether from RSV or other pathogens, most commonly affects children younger than 2 years old. It is usually a self-limiting viral illness but can cause respiratory distress, dehydration, and complications that require hospitalization.
- Risk factors for more severe illness include premature birth, chronic lung disease, and being immunocompromised.

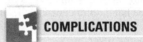

COMPLICATIONS

Infants and children under 2 years old may develop severe RSV bronchiolitis that progresses to pneumonia and requires hospitalization. It can cause complications such as apnea and dehydration.

Signs and Symptoms

- Cough
- Crackles
- Fever
- Nasal flaring
- Retractions
- Rhinorrhea
- Sneezing
- Tachypnea
- Upper airway congestion
- Vomiting
- Wheezing

Diagnosis

Labs
Viral PCR to identify RSV and rule out other respiratory viruses.

Diagnostic Testing
There are no diagnostic tests specific to diagnose bronchiolitis.

Treatment

- IV fluids for dehydration
- Nasal and nasopharyngeal suctioning
- Supplemental humidified oxygen

Nursing Interventions

- Assess pulse oximetry and vital signs.
  - Administer supplemental oxygen to keep SpO_2 greater than 90% to 92%.
  - Consider escalation of supplemental oxygen to high-flow nasal cannula or CPAP/BiPAP.
  - Notify provider of worsening pulse oximetry reading or increased work of breathing.
- Assess respiratory effort and auscultate breath sounds. Monitor for signs of increased work of breathing.
  - Abdominal breathing
  - Accessory muscle use
  - Nasal flaring
  - Retractions: subcostal, suprasternal, substernal, intercostal
- Monitor for tachypnea, fever, and decreasing pulse oximetry.
- Monitor intake, output, and hydration status.
- Stop oral intake for infants with tachypnea or increased work of breathing.
  - Obtain IV access for fluid administration.
  - Place NG tube for supplemental feedings if unable to PO feed.
- Suction nasal and nasopharyngeal secretions as necessary.

Patient and Family Education

- Call provider if respiratory symptoms worsen or if the child shows signs of dehydration.
- Prevent the spread of respiratory viral illness and RSV:
  - Avoid close contact with anyone with respiratory symptoms, viral illness, or RSV.
  - Clean and disinfect frequently touched surfaces.
  - If diagnosed with RSV, avoid spreading illness to others, especially infants.
  - Keep children home from school and day care when experiencing viral symptoms to prevent infecting others.
  - Place child on contact isolation if hospitalized.
  - Wash hands often and avoid touching eyes, nose, and mouth.
- Use bulb suction or oral nasal aspirator to clear secretions at home.
- Vaccinate high-risk infants with palivizumab.
  - Administered as one to five doses, monthly during first and second year of life.
  - Vaccination is recommended for at-risk infants:
    - Born before 29 weeks
    - Born prior to 32 weeks with chronic lung disease and an oxygen requirement for at least 28 days
    - With a congenital heart disease receiving medication to control congestive heart failure
    - With pulmonary hypertension

 ALERT!

Respiratory distress symptoms include:

- Color changes
- Grunting or wheezing
- Increased respiratory rate
- Increased work of breathing (i.e., retractions, abdominal breathing, accessory muscle use, nasal flaring, and head bobbing)
- Sweating

CARBON MONOXIDE POISONING

Overview

- *CO* is an odorless, colorless, tasteless gas produced when fossil fuel is burned, such as in cars, engines, stoves, fireplaces, and furnaces.
- CO replaces oxygen that is bound to hemoglobin because it has a greater affinity for hemoglobin than oxygen.
  - This causes inadequate oxygen transport and utilization as well as tissue damage.
  - Pulse oximetry is not considered a valid assessment for patients with CO poisoning. Since hemoglobin is fully saturated with CO, the patient may present with normal pulse oximetry measurements.
- Infants and toddlers may present with unspecific signs such as fussiness and feeding difficulties.
- Poisoning can happen when individuals breathe in CO that has built up in the air. Situations where individuals may breathe in CO from the air include breathing in exhaust from a vehicle or generator in an enclosed area such as a garage, using a charcoal grill indoors, or running a generator indoors.

> **COMPLICATIONS**
>
> Carbon monoxide poisoning can lead to neurologic issues such as loss of consciousness, seizures, syncope, coma, cardiac issues such as ischemia and arrhythmias, and even death.

Signs and Symptoms

- Chest pain
- Confusion
- Dizziness
- Feeding difficulty
- Fussiness
- Headache
- Nausea
- Shortness of breath
- Vomiting
- Weakness

Diagnosis

Labs
- ABG to evaluate for metabolic acidosis
- COHb elevated or greater than 10%

Diagnostic Testing
- Brain MRI to rule out other causes of neurologic dysfunction
- Chest x-ray in severe poisoning to monitor for pulmonary edema
- EKG to monitor for any cardiovascular involvement or arrhythmias

Treatment

- 100% oxygen via high-flow oxygen delivery device until symptoms have resolved
- Remove from CO source
- Hyperbaric oxygen for severe cases, indicated by loss of consciousness and severe metabolic acidosis

Nursing Interventions

- Administer oxygen as ordered.
- Allow family to stay with the child.

- Assess for any barriers to resources and consult social worker.
  - Access to an appropriate heating system in the home
  - Financial concerns
- Monitor CO and COHb level.
- Perform frequent neurologic assessments due to the possibility of delayed symptoms, including syncope and seizures.

Patient and Family Education

Prevent CO poisoning.
- Do not leave automobiles running inside a closed garage.
- Do not use a gas range or oven to heat the home.
- Do not use generators, gas, or charcoal grills inside or within 20 feet of the home.
- Ensure home furnaces, heating systems, and gas or oil-burning appliances are inspected each year.
- Install CO detectors with alarms in the home.

 NURSING PEARL

Educate families to ensure CO detectors with alarms are installed in the home. They should be near each bedroom and on each floor of the home.

CROUP

Overview

- *Croup* is a group of respiratory syndromes characterized by a hoarse, seal-like barky cough, inspiratory stridor, and respiratory distress due to subglottic swelling, narrowing, and obstruction of the larynx, trachea, or bronchi.
- *Laryngotracheobronchitis* is the medical terminology for croup due to inflammation extending to bronchi and involving the lower respiratory tract.
- Croup is most often secondary to viral infections such as parainfluenza, RSV, and adenoviruses.
  - Viral croup
    - Characterized by nasal congestion and fever
    - Self-limiting viral illness
  - Spasmodic croup
    - Abrupt onset
    - Occurs at night

 COMPLICATIONS

Croup is often a self-limiting viral illness, but the severe illness can lead to ear infections, pneumonia, and respiratory distress.

Signs and Symptoms

- Barky cough
- Hoarseness
- Nasal congestion
- Stridor

Diagnosis

Labs
There are no labs specific to diagnose croup.

Diagnostic Testing
There are no diagnostic tests specific to diagnose croup.

 NURSING PEARL

Remember the 3 Ss of croup symptoms:
- **S**tridor
- **S**ubglottic swelling
- **S**eal-like barky cough

Treatment

- Mild: symptomatic therapy including giving antipyretics and encouraging fluid intake
- Moderate to severe:
  - Dexamethasone (Table 7.2)
  - Nebulized racemic epinephrine (Table 7.2)
  - Oxygen

Nursing Interventions

- Administer supplemental oxygen as ordered.
- Help to keep the child calm and reduce anxiety to prevent airway obstruction.
- Monitor respiratory status and pulse oximetry.
  - Monitor for decreasing pulse oximetry reading.
  - Monitor for worsening stridor, hypoxia, and increased work of breathing.

Patient and Family Education

- Include home treatment supportive care, such as antipyretics and fluid intake.
- Notify provider or seek medical care if the child develops any of the following symptoms:
  - Difficulty breathing or increased work of breathing
  - Difficulty swallowing or drooling
  - Severe coughing episodes
  - Stridor at rest
- There is limited evidence about the benefits of exposing children to steam or cold air; both techniques may help briefly relieve symptoms.

CYSTIC FIBROSIS

Overview

- *CF* is an inherited autosomal recessive disease of the exocrine glands that affects the respiratory, digestive, and endocrine systems.
- Characteristics include persistent respiratory infections, elevated sweat chloride levels, and pancreatic insufficiency.
- Infants present with respiratory symptoms, meconium ileus, and failure to thrive.
- The primary clinical manifestation is thick, sticky mucus that obstructs the bronchioles, creates an ideal environment for infections, and prevents absorption of nutrients from the GI tract.

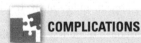

COMPLICATIONS

Gastrointestinal complications may occur from infancy through adolescents. Infants who present with a meconium ileus need to be evaluated for CF. Children and adolescents may have constipation from malabsorption, not taking prescribed pancreatic enzymes, decreased intestinal mobility, and increased intestinal secretions.

Signs and Symptoms

- Cough
- Difficulty breathing
- Diminished lung sounds
- Frequent and chronic infections
- Nasal polyps
- Poor growth or failure to thrive (due to malabsorption of fat and proteins)
- Salty tasting skin
- Shortness of breath
- Steatorrhea (frequent, greasy, foul-smelling stools)
- Wheezing

Diagnosis

Labs

- Newborn screening for CF
- Quantitative sweat chloride test to confirm CF
- Stool studies (fecal elastase) to evaluate fat in stool and evaluate GI function

Diagnostic Testing

- Chest x-ray to evaluate for changes over time in patients with CF or rule out respiratory infections
- PFT to evaluate for changes over time in patients with CF

Treatment

- Airway clearance
  - Chest PT
  - Exercise
  - Flutter mucus clearance device
  - High-frequency chest compressions
  - Percussion
  - Postural drainage
- Antibiotics for infections
- Bronchodilators
- Mucus thinners
  - Hypertonic saline
  - Recombinant human deoxyribonuclease (Table 7.2)
- Pancreatic enzymes
- Vitamins A, D, E, K
- Lung transplant if treatments fail progression

Nursing Interventions

- Administer pancreatic enzymes with every meal and snack.
- Assess lung sounds, respiratory status, cough, and congestion for worsening symptoms or overall disease progression. Recognize that patients with CF may be stable with baseline respiratory symptoms, but changes in clinical status require escalation in care.
- Assess the patient's understanding of chronic disease and management plan. Navigate and encourage adolescents' compliance with treatments.
- Assess stools and monitor for abdominal distention.
- Assist with airway clearance regimens.
- Monitor blood glucose levels.
  - Due to pancreas involvement, patients may become insulin deficient.
  - Use the point of care glucometer to monitor blood glucose levels.
  - Notify provider of either low or high abnormal results.

Patient and Family Education

- Adhere to the medication schedule.
- Call the provider if there are any changes in breathing, cough, or appetite.
- Continue airway clearance techniques.
- Eat a diet high in protein and calories.
- Maintain adequate hydration and exercise to prevent constipation.
- Take pancreatic enzymes before and within 30 minutes of eating meals and snacks.

 POP QUIZ 7.2

An infant presents with meconium ileus and minor respiratory issues. What disease do these conditions indicate, and what test does the nurse anticipate the provider will order to facilitate the diagnosis?

EPIGLOTTITIS

Overview

- *Epiglottitis* is a life-threatening obstructive, inflammatory illness of the epiglottis.
- Characteristics include an absence of cough, drooling, and restlessness.
- Its rapid onset leads to severe respiratory distress.
- Most often caused by Hib, the main risk factor is being unvaccinated.

COMPLICATIONS

Acute epiglottitis is a medical emergency due to its rapid progression. It leads to airway obstruction that can be fatal if not immediately treated.

Signs and Symptoms

- Cyanosis
- Distress, irritability, restlessness
- Drooling
- Dysphagia
- Fever
- Hypoxia
- Retractions
- Stridor
- Tripod, or sniffing, position: trunk leaning forward, neck hyperextended, and chin positioned up

NURSING PEARL

Remember the 3 Ds of epiglottitis symptoms:

- **D**rooling
- **D**ysphagia
- **D**istress

Diagnosis

Labs

There are no labs specific to diagnose epiglottitis.

Diagnostic Testing

Lateral neck x-ray to confirm thickening of the epiglottis and narrowing of the upper airway, which is diagnostic for epiglottitis

Treatment

- Antibiotic therapy (Table A.1)
- Corticosteroids (Table 7.2)
- IV hydration
- Supplemental oxygen or intubation

Nursing Interventions

- Administer supplemental oxygen and protect the airway.
  - Escalate to bag-valve-mask ventilation if status deteriorates.
  - Prepare for intubation.
- Help keep the patient calm.
- Monitor vital signs and pulse oximetry.
  - Assess for tachypnea and worsening oxygen saturation.
  - Assess for tachycardia.

ALERT!

Inspection of the throat with a tongue depressor should be avoided unless emergency intubation equipment and personnel are readily available.

Patient and Family Education

- Recognize the signs of respiratory distress.
- Remain up to date on immunizations, including Hib.

POP QUIZ 7.3

What symptoms indicate that a 4-year-old patient's respiration is worsening and the child's condition is becoming an emergency?

PERTUSSIS

Overview

- *Pertussis* is a highly contagious bacterial respiratory disease.
- Violent coughing episodes differentiate pertussis from other respiratory illnesses.
- Whooping cough is the colloquial term for pertussis. It describes the whooping sound patients make with inspiration as they gasp for air during uncontrolled coughing spells. Risk factors include infants who are not fully vaccinated, immunocompromised individuals, or older children and adolescents who are not vaccinated.

 COMPLICATIONS

Although more severe in infants and those who are unvaccinated, adolescents may have serious complications, include syncope, urinary incontinence, pneumonia, and rib fractures from severe coughing episodes.

Signs and Symptoms

- Apnea
- Low-grade fever
- Nasal congestion
- Vomiting, or poor intake
- Whooping cough spells

Diagnosis

Labs
- CBC to evaluate for elevated WBC
- Nasopharyngeal swab or aspirate culture

Diagnostic Testing
There are no diagnostic tests specific to diagnose pertussis.

Treatment

- Antibiotics: erythromycin (Table A.1)
- Supplemental oxygen and escalate to intubation if severe

Nursing Interventions

- Administer supplemental oxygen.
- Assess respiratory status and pulse oximetry.
  - Monitor for apnea and hypoxia.
  - Monitor severity of coughing spells.
- Monitor intake and output for signs of dehydration.
- Utilize standard and droplet precautions.

Patient and Family Education

- Adult family should receive pertussis boosters.
- Family members and close contacts may be treated prophylactically.
- Infected children should remain out of school and daycare for at least 5 days after the start of antibiotics or for 21 days after the onset of symptoms.
- Keep infants and unvaccinated children away from anyone with pertussis.
- Remain up to date on immunizations, specifically DtaP and Tdap.
- Stay hydrated by drinking fluids. Eat small meals to avoid vomiting with coughing spells.

PNEUMONIA

Overview

- *Pneumonia* is inflammation of the lungs secondary to a bacterial, viral, or fungal infection or an aspiration that may lead to alveolar consolidation.
  - Children less than 5 years old are most likely to have viral pneumonia.
  - Children older than 5 years old are most likely to have bacterial pneumonia.
- Pneumonia may either be the result of a primary disease process or a complication of another respiratory illness.
- Aspiration pneumonia is more likely to occur in children with neurologic diseases, reduced level of consciousness, dysphagia, or foreign body aspiration.

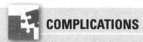 **COMPLICATIONS**

A symptomatic pneumothorax or a pleural effusion may develop when there is an accumulation of air or fluid in the pleural space, causing increased respiratory distress and the need for a chest tube to evacuate the air or fluid.

Signs and Symptoms

- Absent breath sounds (pneumothorax)
- Adventitious breath sounds
- Chest tightness
- Cough
- Fever
- Hypoxemia
- Lack of appetite
- Lethargy
- Tachypnea

Diagnosis

Labs

- CBC to evaluate for elevated WBC, and increased neutrophils
- Sputum culture to identify the pathogen

Diagnostic Testing

Chest x-ray to confirm pneumonia or as follow up from chest tube removal to monitor for reoccurrence of pneumothorax.

Treatment

- Antibiotics for bacterial pneumonia
- Antipyretics
- IV hydration
- Supplemental oxygen
- Chest tubes
  - Indications for a thoracostomy chest tube include:
    - *Hemothorax*: a collection of blood in the pleural space
    - *Pneumothorax*: accumulation of air between the visceral or the parietal space and the lung
      - The accumulation of air can cause the lung to collapse.
      - A *tension pneumothorax* is when air enters the pleural space on inhalation but cannot exit during expiration. It can be spontaneous or caused by trauma.
    - *Pleural effusion*: collection of fluid (serous fluid, or pus) in the pleural space

Nursing Interventions

- Administer supplemental oxygen to keep SpO_2 greater than 94%.
- Encourage oral intake or administer IV fluids to prevent dehydration.
- Encourage using incentive spirometer or blowing bubbles for younger children as deep breathing exercises.
- Manage secretions with chest PT and suctioning.
- Monitor respiratory status.
- Chest tube interventions:
  - Assisting with placement:
    - Administer pain or sedation medication as ordered.
    - Monitor vital signs, airway, breathing, and circulation.
  - Managing chest tubes:
    - There are two types of chest tube drainage systems.
      - Wet system allows suction up to 20 cm of water
      - Dry system allows suction up to 40 cm of water
    - Set up chest tube drainage system.
    - Attach to the level of suction, or gravity, as ordered.
  - Assess chest tube drainage and function.
    - If the chest tube is dislodged from the patient's chest, cover the site with sterile gauze, tape on three sides, and notify the provider.
    - If the chest tube drainage system has disconnected, place tubing from patient into a bottle of sterile water.
    - Monitor the water seal chamber for signs of an air leak or excessive bubbling.
    - Monitor for subcutaneous emphysema (air crackling around the chest tube insertion site).
    - Monitor drainage in the drainage collection chamber. Note the amount, color, and consistency.
    - Monitor dressing. Maintain clean, dry, and intact dressing at the insertion site.
  - Keep drainage system below the level of the patient's chest.
    - Avoid clamping tubing.
    - Do not attach the drainage system to a moveable part of the crib or bed, such as the side rails.
    - Do not milk or strip tubing.
    - Ensure tubing is free of dependent loops.
  - Assist with removal.
    - Administer pain or sedation medication as ordered.
    - Assist the patient in taking a deep exhale while the catheter is being removed.
    - Consider the age of the child and developmentally appropriate techniques for support. For example, asking a preschooler or school-aged child to "blow out a candle" to support exhaling.
    - Gather sterile occlusive dressing and apply according to policy.

Patient and Family Education

- Avoid others with respiratory illness and perform hand hygiene.
- For children with chest tubes:
  - Ask for help when getting out of bed or walking to the restroom.
  - Family members should be cautious not to tip over or move the drainage system.
- Prevent dehydration by drinking fluids.
- Take antibiotics as prescribed.

Table 7.2 Medications for Respiratory System

Indications	Mechanism of Action	Contraindications, Precautions, and Adverse Effects
Bronchodilators (magnesium sulfate)		
• Used parenterally or via oral inhalation for severe acute asthma exacerbation • Used when asthma symptoms are not resolved by first-line therapy	• Relax bronchial smooth muscle	• Adverse effects include hypotension, skin flushing, and dry mouth. • Use with caution in children less than 5 years old.
Corticosteroids (dexamethasone)		
• Used for moderate to severe asthma exacerbations or status asthmaticus	• Reduce swelling and inflammation in airways	• Adverse effects on growth. Use caution in immunosuppression and inhibition of bone growth; monitor for fractures.
Corticosteroids (methylprednisolone, prednisolone, prednisone)		
• Used for moderate to severe asthma exacerbations or status asthmaticus • Oral administration (prednisolone and prednisone) and IV or IM administration (methylprednisolone)	• Suppress inflammation	• Adverse effects include GI upset, weight gain, and mood changes. • Medication is contraindicated in patients with fungal, viral, and bacterial infections. • Prednisolone is contraindicated in patients with sulfite or tartrazine hypersensitivity. • Use with caution in patients with immunosuppression, growth inhibition, adrenal suppression, and increased intracranial pressure.
Inhaled corticosteroids (budesonide, fluticasone)		
• Anti-inflammatory used for long-term or maintenance control of asthma • Decrease airway inflammation and bronchoconstriction • Used in conjunction with SABA and LABA inhalers	• Reduce swelling in airways	• Adverse effects include thrush. Rinse mouth after each use. • Medication is contraindicated in acute asthma attacks. • Use with caution in immunocompromised patients. • Do not abruptly discontinue, and monitor for adrenal insufficiency.
Long-acting beta-2 agonists (formoterol, salmeterol)		
• Maintenance or preventative therapy for asthma • Must be used in conjunction with inhaled corticosteroids	• Relax bronchial smooth muscle	• Adverse effects include paradoxical bronchospasm, tachycardia, arrhythmias, palpitations, and tremors. • Medication is contraindicated for use in acute asthma attacks. • Use cautiously in patients under the age of 6 or patients taking MAOIs

Table 7.2 Medications for Respiratory System *(continued)*

Indications	Mechanism of Action	Contraindications, Precautions, and Adverse Effects
Mucolytic (recombinant human deoxyribonuclease)		
• Mucolytic agent • Improve lung function and decrease exacerbations in children with CF • Reduce sputum viscosity	• Select and hydrolyze extracellular DNA to reduce mucous viscosity	• Adverse effects include pharyngitis and hoarseness. • Use with caution in children under 5 years old.
Short-acting beta-2 agonists (albuterol, levalbuterol)		
• Short-acting rescue or quick-relief agent for asthma • Frequently used in conjunction with inhaled corticosteroids	• Relax bronchial smooth muscle	• Adverse effects include paradoxical bronchospasm, tachycardia, palpitations, and tremors. • Use caution in patients with hyperthyroidism, cardiovascular disorders, and diabetes mellitus.
Short-acting beta-2 agonists (racemic epinephrine)		
• Nebulized agent used to reduce airway edema, reduce bronchospasm, and improve stridor	• Relax bronchial smooth muscle • Reduce swelling in airways	• Adverse effects include tachycardia, headache, restlessness, tremor, and sweating. • Medication is contraindicated for patients taking MAO inhibitors. • Monitor for return of symptoms or rebound airway swelling, as multiple doses may be needed for severe symptoms. • Use caution in patients with heart disease, hypertension, diabetes, and thyroid disease.
Short-acting beta-2 agonists (terbutaline)		
• Treat and prevent acute bronchospasm and asthma exacerbation. Can be given orally, subcutaneously, or intravenously.	• Stimulate beta-2 receptors to relax bronchial smooth muscle	• Adverse effects include paradoxical bronchospasm, hypertension, tachycardia, headache, restlessness, and tremors. • Medication is contraindicated in patients taking MAOIs or tricyclic antidepressants. • Use caution in patients with cardiovascular disorders, hyperthyroidism, seizure disorders, and diabetes.

RESOURCES

American Heart Association. (2016). *Pediatric advanced life support provider manual*. https://www.uptodate.com/contents/pediatric-advanced-life-support-pals/print

Asthma and Allergy Foundation of America. (2021). *Asthma action plan*. https://www.aafa.org/asthma-treatment-action-plan/

Centers for Disease Control and Prevention. (2018, March 21). *Carbon monoxide*. U.S. Department of Health and Human Services, Centers for Disease Control and Prevention. https://www.cdc.gov/disasters/co-materials.html

Centers for Disease Control and Prevention. (2020a, December 18). *RSV in infants and young children*. U.S. Department of Health and Human Services, Centers for Disease Control and Prevention. https://www.cdc.gov/rsv/high-risk/infants-young-children.html

Centers for Disease Control and Prevention. (2020b, January 23). *Pertussis*. U.S. Department of Health and Human Services, Centers for Disease Control and Prevention. https://www.cdc.gov/pertussis/clinical/prevention.html

Centers for Disease Control and Prevention. (2021a, January 19). *Carbon monoxide poisoning*. U.S. Department of Health and Human Services, Centers for Disease Control and Prevention. https://www.cdc.gov/nceh/features/copoisoning/index.html#:~:text=The%20most%20common%20symptoms%20of,CO%20poisoning%20is%20entirely%20preventable

Centers for Disease Control and Prevention. (2021b, July 1). *Asthma*. U.S. Department of Health and Human Services, Centers for Disease Control and Prevention. https://www.cdc.gov/asthma/faqs.htm

Cystic Fibrosis Foundation. (n.d.). *About cystic fibrosis*. https://www.cff.org/What-is-CF/About-Cystic-Fibrosis/

Davalos Bichara, M., & Goldman, R. D. (2009). Magnesium for treatment of asthma in children. *Canadian Family Physician Medecin de Famille Canadien, 55*(9), 887–889. https://www.ncbi.nlm.nih.gov/pmc/articles/PMC2743582/

Fanta, C. (2021). Treatment of intermittent and mild persistent asthma in adolescents and adults. *UpToDate*. https://www.uptodate.com/contents/treatment-of-intermittent-and-mild-persistent-asthma-in-adolescents-and-adults?search=asthma%20classification%20children&sectionRank=2&usage_type=default&anchor=H2&source=machineLearning&selectedTitle=1~150&display_rank=1#H2

Hockenberry, M., Wilson, D., & Rodgers, C. (2017). *Wong's essentials of pediatric nursing*. Elsevier.

Lexicomp. (2021a). Albuterol (salbutamol): Pediatric drug information [Drug information]. *UpToDate*. https://www.uptodate.com/contents/albuterol-salbutamol-pediatric-drug-information?search=albuterol&source=panel_search_result&selectedTitle=2~148&usage_type=panel&kp_tab=drug_pediatric&display_rank=1

Lexicomp. (2021b). Budesonide (oral inhalation): Pediatric drug information [Drug information]. *UpToDate*. https://www.uptodate.com/contents/budesonide-oral-inhalation-drug-information?search=budesonide&source=panel_search_result&selectedTitle=1~140&usage_type=panel&display_rank=1

Lexicomp. (2021c). Dexamethasone: Pediatric drug information [Drug information]. *UpToDate*. https://www.uptodate.com/contents/dexamethasone-systemic-pediatric-drug-information?search=dexamethasone&source=panel_search_result&selectedTitle=2~145&usage_type=panel&display_rank=2#F8015706

Lexicomp. (2021d). Epinephrine (oral inhalation): Pediatric drug information [Drug information]. *UpToDate*. https://www.google.com/search?q=is+racemic+epinephrine+a+beta+2+agoniswt&rlz=1C5CHFA_enUS862US863&sxsrf=AOaemvJLJqQfStluy8Fm8jkBQkgWKRG0jQ%3A1634326614540&ei=VthpYY66ILOLytMP3-avGA&ved=0ahUKEwiOvbmKlc3zAhWzhXIEHV_zCwMQ4dUDCA4&uact=5&oq=is+racemic+epinephrine+a+beta+2+agoniswt&gs_lcp=Cgdnd3Mtd2l6EAMyBwghEAoQoAEyBQghEKsCOgYIABAHEB46BQgAEIAEOgYIABAWEB46BQgAEIYDOggIIRAWEB0QHjoFCCEQoAFKBAhBGABQlZcCWMnmAmCZ6AJoAHACeACAAbwBiAHmEZIBBTEwLjEwMAEAoAEBwAEB&sclient=gws-wiz

Lexicomp. (2021e). Fluticasone: Pediatric drug information [Drug information]. *UpToDate*. https://www.uptodate.com/contents/fluticasone-oral-inhalation-pediatric-drug-information?search=fluticasone&source=panel_search_result&selectedTitle=2~92&usage_type=panel&display_rank=2

Lexicomp. (2021f). Formoterol: Pediatric drug information [Drug information]. *UpToDate*. https://www.uptodate.com/contents/formoterol-pediatric-drug-information?search=formoterol&source=panel_search_result&selectedTitle=2~70&usage_type=panel&kp_tab=drug_pediatric&display_rank=1

Lexicomp. (2021g). Magnesium sulfate [Drug Information]. *UpToDate*. https://www.uptodate.com/contents/magnesium-sulfate-pediatric-drug-information?search=magnesium%20sulfate&source=panel_search_result&selectedTitle=2~148&usage_type=panel&kp_tab=drug_pediatric&display_rank=1#F191053

Lexicomp. (2021h). Terbutaline: Pediatric drug information [Drug information]. *UpToDate*. https://www.uptodate.com/contents/terbutaline-pediatric-drug-information?search=terbutaline&source=panel_search_result&selectedTitle=2~60&usage_type=panel&kp_tab=drug_pediatric&display_rank=1#F225646

Shefrin, A. E., & Goldman, R. D. (2009). Use of dexamethasone and prednisone in acute asthma exacerbations in pediatric patients. *Canadian Family Physician, 55*(7), 704–706. https://www.ncbi.nlm.nih.gov/pmc/articles/PMC2718595/

Theodore, A. (2020). Arterial blood gases. *UpToDate*. https://www.uptodate.com/contents/arterial-blood-gases?search=acid%20base%20imbalance&source=search_result&selectedTitle=3~150&usage_type=default&display_rank=3#H12

APPENDICITIS

Overview

- *Appendicitis* is inflammation or infection of the appendix.
- The *appendix* is a nonessential organ that lies in the RLQ of the abdomen. The appendix projects from the cecum and the large intestine.
- The appendix acts as a container for beneficial microbes, which aid in digestion.
- Appendicitis is usually caused by an obstruction of undigested food or stool that hardens and obstructs the appendix lumen.

Signs and Symptoms

- Anorexia
- Fever (late sign)
- Periumbilical pain
- Rebound tenderness
- Rigid abdomen
- RLQ tenderness
- Vomiting

Diagnosis

Labs

There are no labs specific to diagnose appendicitis. However, the following may be helpful when determining severity and treatment:

- ANC, CRP, and WBC to show if infection is present
- Urinalysis to rule out UTI or kidney stone
- PAS scoring system (Table 8.1):
  - Low risk: score of 3 or less
  - High risk: score of 7 or 8

Diagnostic Testing

- CT
- MRI
- Ultrasound

COMPLICATIONS

If the appendix is found to be perforated during surgery, the patient must be on IV antibiotics for several days after the surgery. If the WBC is still high after 5 to 7 days, diagnostic imaging should be done to rule out an abdominal or pelvic abscess. If an abscess is found, IV fluids and parenteral nutrition, if needed, will be started. Antibiotics and pain management will be prescribed. If necessary, a drain insertion under CT guidance will be done. Adhesions can form, which can cause a paralytic ileus or a mechanical bowel obstruction.

NURSING PEARL

The presentation of appendicitis may be different in young children. The most reliable clinical sign is local tenderness with rigidity at McBurney's point (one-third of the distance along a line from the anterior superior iliac crest to the umbilicus).

Table 8.1 The Pediatric Appendicitis Score	
Pediatric Appendicitis Symptom	**Score**
Anorexia	1
Nausea/vomiting	1
Migration of pain	1
Fever greater than 100.4 °F (38 °C)	1
Pain with cough, percussion, or hopping	2
RLQ tenderness	2
WBC greater than 10,000	1
Neutrophils plus band forms greater than 7,500 cells/uL	1
Total	10

Source: Data from Samuel, M. (2002, June). Pediatric appendicitis score. *Journal of Pediatric Surgery, 37*, 877–881. https://doi.org/10.1053/jpsu.2002.32893

Treatment

- Antibiotics (Tables A.1 and 8.6*) for all appendicitis patients:
  - Ceftriaxone: may be used as prophylaxis
  - Metronidazole: in cases of perforation
  - Piperacillin and tazobactam: in cases of perforation
- Pain medications: morphine, ketorolac, and acetaminophen postoperatively (Table A.2)
- Surgery
  - Laparoscopic or open abdominal
  - Appendectomy removes an inflamed or swollen appendix
  - Possible interval appendectomy after a 4- to 6-week course of IV antibiotics

Nursing Interventions

- Assess pain and vital signs after surgery.
  - Administer pain medications as ordered.
  - Monitor for fever or change in vital signs as sign of infection or complications. (See below.)
  - If any signs of complications, notify surgeon immediately.
- Administer antibiotics pre- and postoperatively.
- Administer IV fluids per order.
- Ensure patient is NPO status before surgery.
- Place an NG tube.
  - If the patient is vomiting or has abdominal distention, place the tube to intermittent suction.
  - The NG tube can also be used for feeds if the patient does not require GI suction.

 COMPLICATIONS

Complications that can occur after an appendectomy are:

- Paralytic ileus, bowel obstruction due to adhesions, constipation
- Infections include wound abscesses, abdominal or pelvic abscesses
- Symptoms: fever, anorexia, inability to tolerate a normal diet 3 to 5 days after surgery, weight loss, continued pain in the abdomen
- Inflammation of the tissue around the appendicular tissue; can happen months or years after appendectomy

---

* Table 8.6 is located at the end of this chapter.

- Post-op:
  - Start PO diet slowly to avoid nausea/vomiting.
  - Encourage early ambulation.

Patient and Family Education

- Call provider for any signs and symptoms of infection, fever, anorexia, fatigue, if concerned about an infection, or if the pain medication is inadequate.
- Do not engage in any vigorous activity for 2 weeks and rest to allow the abdomen to heal. Pain medications should relieve pain but may not eliminate it entirely.
- Learn how to splint with a pillow to reduce pain when coughing.
- Review the dose and schedule of pain medications at home.

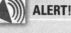

ALERT!

Never place heat on the lower right abdomen of patient with appendicitis before surgery because it can cause the appendix to rupture. After the appendectomy, heat can be administered for gas pain.

CELIAC DISEASE

Overview

- *Celiac disease* is an immune-mediated inflammatory disease of the small intestine due to exposure to dietary gluten that cannot be digested.
- *Gluten* is a protein found naturally in certain grains, including wheat, barley, and rye.
- Gluten is added to many foods and products.
- Nonceliac sensitivity:
  - These patients test negative for celiac disease.
  - Patients present with the same GI symptoms as celiac disease but lack the antibodies and intestinal damage seen in celiac.
  - Gluten sensitivity often produces non-GI symptoms after eating gluten, such as headache, foggy thinking, joint pain, and numbness.
  - A gluten-free diet is the only treatment for nonceliac sensitivity.
- Risk factors for developing celiac disease are:
  - Autoimmune thyroiditis
  - Down syndrome
  - Family history of celiac disease
  - Juvenile chronic arthritis
  - Turner syndrome
  - Type 1 diabetes
  - Williams syndrome
- There are two categories of celiac disease.
  - Classic:
    - ○ Patient has malabsorption symptoms such as weight loss, vitamin deficiencies, and steatorrhea which resolve with a gluten-free diet. In this case, eating gluten damages the lining of the small intestine.
  - Non-GI: There are no GI symptoms, but other body systems are involved.

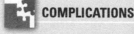

COMPLICATIONS

Complications of celiac disease include:
- Bone loss
- Cancer
- Irritability/depression
- Lactose intolerance
- Malnutrition

Signs and Symptoms

- Classic:
  - Abdominal distention and pain
  - Anemia
  - Anorexia

(continued)

Signs and Symptoms *(continued)*

- Chronic diarrhea
- Constipation
- Flatulence
- FTT
- Rash
- Weight loss
- Non-GI:
  - Arthritis
  - Bone disease
  - Delayed puberty
  - Dental enamel defects
  - Developmental delay
  - Epilepsy
  - Headache
  - Hypotonia
  - Vitamin and iron deficiency
  - Liver disease
  - Short stature

 ALERT!

Some patients with celiac disease also present with dermatitis herpetiformis. This is an itchy, blistering skin rash that appears on the elbows, knees, buttocks, back, or scalp. This may be the only symptom in some patients. It may take some time, but the rash will heal when gluten is no longer in the diet.

Diagnosis

Labs
IgA antibody testing that shows tissue transglutaminase

Diagnostic Testing
- Endoscopy with intestinal biopsy
- Stools for fecal fat

Treatment

- Gluten-free diet, avoiding wheat, barley, rye, and oats
- Food ingredient labels; packaged foods should read "gluten free"
- Total healing: may take months to years

Nursing Interventions

- Advise that follow-up visits will be necessary to determine response and the compliance of the family with the diet.
- Educate patient and family on diagnosis and need for diet and lifestyle changes.
- If steroids are prescribed, teach family how to give them.
- Provide emotional support and resources for support groups to patient and family.
  - There may be a need for a dietician for help in planning meals.
  - There are also books, apps, and online help for families to make the transition.

Patient and Family Education

- Before the initial antibody test, it is necessary to continue eating gluten. If patients have been gluten-free, they must have at least 3 g per day for 6 weeks before the test to ensure accurate results.
- Family may want to pack a lunch for school-aged child to ease concerns about cafeteria choices.
- Learn about the condition and ask questions.
- Learn which foods contain gluten to avoid them:
  - Wheat, barley, rye, durum, farina, graham flour, malt, and semolina
  - Processed foods such as canned soups, salad dressings, ice cream, candy bars, instant coffee, lunchmeats, condiments, yogurt, pasta, and pastries

- Learn which nonfood products may contain gluten, such as medications, supplements, cosmetics, toothpaste, skin and hair products, and vitamins.
- Recognize the importance of reading labels due to the high prevalence of hidden gluten. Labels should read "gluten free."
- Symptom improvement may occur as soon as a few weeks after starting a gluten-free diet.

ENTERAL TUBE PLACEMENT AND MAINTENANCE

Overview

- Enteral tubes provide nutrition for those unable to consume sufficient calories by mouth.
- Tubes can be placed in the mouth or nose and terminate in the stomach, duodenum, or jejunum (NG, OG, ND, NJ tubes).
- Surgically placed tubes include GT and JT or a combination of these listed (GJ tube). Surgically placed tubes are typically for feedings for long-term use.
- ND, NJ, and JTs are used to bypass the stomach and terminate in the duodenum or jejunum. They are commonly used in patients with severe reflex.
- Enteral tubes can used for the entire diet, supplementary feeds, and/or to give enteral medications.
- Indications for placement of an enteral tube include:
  - Eating disorders
  - Excessive metabolic demands
  - Impaired digestion and/or absorption
  - Inability to swallow
  - Oral aversion
  - Oral motor impairment
- Enteral feedings may be necessary for children with CF, short gut syndrome, Crohn's disease, renal disease, cardiac disease, biliary atresia, FTT, critical illness or injury, cancer, and stroke.

 COMPLICATIONS

Some of the possible complications from enteral tube feeding include:

- Aspiration
- Incorrectly positioned or dislodged tube
- Refeeding syndrome
- Medication-related complications
- Fluid imbalance
- Insertion-site infection
- Agitation

Tube placement can meet with resistance upon insertion and can cause gagging/vomiting, respiratory distress, and nasal bleeding.

Diagnosis

Labs
Point-of-care pH testing of gastric content for NG and OG tubes.

Diagnostic Testing
X-ray to confirm placement of NG, OG, and ND tubes when the tube will used for feedings or medications.

Nursing Interventions

Nasogastric Tube Placement
- Collect supplies:
  - Emesis basin
  - Gloves
  - Lubricant
  - NG tube
  - pH testing paper

 ALERT!

Testing the pH of gastric contents is a preferred method of tube placement confirmation. However, if the patient is on a proton pump inhibitor, the results will not be accurate, and it should not be used. When the tube is used for feeding, an x-ray **must** be done. If the tube is being used for stomach decompression, aspiration of contents is enough verification. If the tube is incorrectly placed and terminates in the lung, there will be no liquid returned, and the patient may cough and possibly turn blue. Auscultation of air inserted into the NGT is not a reliable method of confirming placement.

(continued)

Nursing Interventions (continued)

- Stethoscope
- Suction
- Syringe
- Tape
- Water or pacifier
- Explain procedure to patient at age-appropriate level.
- Wash hands and put on gloves.
- Position patient upright with neck flexed.
- Apply pulse oximeter and monitor patient status during insertion.
- Assess nares for possible deviation and patency.
- Determine NG tube length by measuring from the nose to the ear to the xiphoid process.
- Determine OG tube length by measuring from the mouth to the ear to the xiphoid process.
- Lubricate the tip of the tube.
- Insert tube and proceed slowly.
- When gagging starts, ask patient, if able, to sip water or suck on pacifier.
- When the measurement mark is reached, stop, aspirate, and check pH level. Point-of-care gastric pH: 4 or 5.
- If placement is correct, tape in place.
- If used for stomach decompression, aspirate contents.
- If used for feeding, obtain a chest x-ray to confirm placement.

Nasogastric Tube Management

- Place the tube as ordered.
- If used for decompression or drainage of stomach, monitor and record amount and description of contents.
- If used for feeding, check placement before all feeds.
- Monitor the nutritional and hydration status of patient.
- Reassess the need for the NG tube in patient's treatment.
- For patients on intermittent feeds that have enteral medications:
  - Administer the medication.
  - Flush the tube with water.
  - Clamp the tube for at least 30 minutes.
- There is no need to stop continuous feeding to administer medication.
- Provide arm immobilizers to young children to prevent them from dislodging the tube.

Surgically Placed Tube Management

- Educate patient and family about surgical procedure and ensure informed consent prior to surgery.
- Assess the patient and administer medications for pain relief postsurgery.
- Monitor surgical site for signs of infection or drainage.
- Visualize site, clean around tube, and change dressing according to facility policy.
- Ensure tube is clamped and access ports are closed when not in use.
- Educate patients and family about type and brand of tube, and how to manage it.

Patient and Family Education

- Do not pull the tube out.
- Learn how to replace the tube if it is pulled out and proper maintenance of the tube if being discharged home with tube.
- Obtain information on procedure and post-op care for surgically placed GT or JT.
- Pin the hanging part of the NG to clothing to help prevent accidental removal.
- Understand reasons for the NG.

 POP QUIZ 8.1

What are some indications for when an NG tube should be placed?

FAILURE TO THRIVE

Overview

- *FTT* is defined as failure to gain weight appropriately.
- Weight gain is much slower than that of other children of similar age and sex.

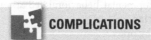

COMPLICATIONS

If the malnutrition is severe, linear growth and head circumference will be affected.

If left untreated, FTT can lead to:

- Brain damage
- CNS damage
- Short stature
- Immune deficiency

Signs and Symptoms

- Constipation
- Delayed physical, mental, and/or social skills
- Delayed secondary sexual characteristics
- Growth has stopped or slowed significantly
- Irritability
- Low height, weight, and head circumference
- Lethargy
- Weight is either:
  - In the 3rd percentile based on the standard growth charts
  - 20% lower than ideal weight

Diagnosis

Labs

There are no labs specific to diagnose FTT. However, the following may be helpful when determining severity and treatment:

- CBC
- Electrolytes
- Hemoglobin
- Thyroid studies
- Urinalysis

Diagnostic Testing

- Denver Developmental Screening Test to assess developmental disability
- Bone x-rays to check bone growth

Treatment

- Correction of mineral and vitamin deficiencies
- Identification and treatment of possible medical causes
- Calorie and fluid increase

Nursing Interventions

- To complete an evaluation, do medical, nutritional, developmental, and behavioral examinations.
- A thorough history must be obtained, including the following topics:
  - Access to resources
  - Necessity of home check for possible toxin exposure
  - Child neglect
  - Family education and skills, nutrition education
  - Poverty, food insecurity
  - Psychologic stressors for the family
  - Testing for possible physical causes such as anemia, chronic infection, inflammation, and malignancy

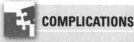

COMPLICATIONS

Refeeding syndrome can cause cardiac failure. To prevent this, a child's caloric and fluid intake should be increased slowly to prevent electrolyte imbalances.

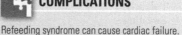

(continued)

Nursing Interventions *(continued)*

- Many professionals are involved in care, including:
  - Developmental, behavioral pediatrician
  - Dietician
  - Social worker
  - Occupational therapist
  - Speech therapist
- Monitor for refeeding syndrome.
- Review child's dietary history to identify any deficits.
- Use standardized growth charts at initial and subsequent assessments.

Patient and Family Education

- Follow proper diet for the patient's age.
- Many medical professionals will be involved; attend all follow-up appointments.
- Obtain information on food sources if food insecure.

FLUID AND ELECTROLYTE ADMINISTRATION

Overview

- Fluid therapy is designed to maintain normal volume and replace lost body fluids.
- Dehydration causes a compromise in tissue and organ perfusion due to volume depletion.
- The most common sites of extracellular fluid loss occur in the GI tract, the skin, and urine.
- Intravascular hypovolemia can result from third spacing due to edema, liver failure, malnutrition, heart failure, bleeding, and ascites.
- Children are at high risk for dehydration. Common causes of dehydration in pediatrics include:
  - Chronic medical conditions like CF or diabetes
  - Decreased intake related to inability to communicate
  - Diarrhea and vomiting due to gastroenteritis
  - Higher insensible losses
- Water loss is caused by:
  - Burns
  - Fever
  - GI illness
  - Polyuria
  - Sweating
- The clinical manifestations of dehydration are:
  - Dry mouth, lips, and skin
  - Hypernatremia
  - Dizziness
  - Lightheadedness
  - Somnolence
  - Tachycardia
  - Thirst
- The components of fluid replacement and maintenance therapy are:
  - Water
  - Electrolytes
  - Dextrose

 NURSING PEARL

To meet the needs of the ill pediatric patient, there are two formulas available to calculate a child's maintenance fluid requirements. The formulas, based on the Holliday-Segar nomogram, calculate milliliters per hour or day using a patient's weight in kilograms.

To calculate hourly fluid requirement, use the 4-2-1 rule. This is figured by giving 4 mL/kg/hr for the first 10 kg, 2 mL/kg/hr for the next 10 kg, and 1 mL/kg/hr for each kg after (Table 8.2).

To calculate daily fluid requirement, use the 100-50-20 rule. To use, figure 100 mL/kg for the first 10 kg, 50 mL/kg for the 2nd 10 kg, and 20 mL/kg for the remaining weight (Table 8.3).

- Common fluids used for IV replacement and management include:
  - LR
  - NS
  - D5/10
- The goal of treatment is to preserve volume and electrolytes.
- Pediatric maintenance fluid requirement is calculated based on patient weight in kilograms (Tables 8.2 and 8.3)
- When calculating fluid balance, consider the following:
  - Intake
  - Insensible losses
  - Sensible losses
  - Urine output
- Common electrolytes that are monitored include:
  - Ca++
  - Na+
  - Cl-
  - K+
- Fluid balance and electrolyte abnormalities are associated with:
  - Diarrhea
  - Renal failure

Diagnosis

Labs
- Bicarbonate
- BUN/creatinine
- Potassium
- Sodium
- Urine osmolality, specific gravity

Table 8.2 Hourly Fluid Calculations

WEIGHT (kg)	Amount
Up to 10	Weight (kg) × 4 mL/kg/hr
10–20	40 mL/hr + [weight (kg) × 2 mL/kg/hr] for any weight >10 kg
Greater than 20	60 mL/hr + [weight (kg) × 1 mL/kg/hr] for weight >20 kg

Source: Data from Somers, M. J. (2021b). Maintenance intravenous fluid therapy in children. *UpToDate.* https://www.uptodate.com/contents/maintenance-intravenous-fluid-therapy-in-children?search=iv%20 therapy&source=search_result&selectedTitle=1~150&usage_type=default&display_rank=1

Table 8.3 Daily Fluid Calculations

WEIGHT (kg)	Amount
Up to 10	Weight (kg) × 100 mL/kg
11–20	1,000 mL plus + [weight (kg) × 50 mL/kg] for every kilo over 10 kg
Greater than 20	1,500 mL + [weight (kg) × 20 mL/kg] for every kg over 20 kg (up to a maximum of 2,400 mL daily)

Source: Data from Somers, M. J. (2021b). Maintenance intravenous fluid therapy in children. *UpToDate.* https://www.uptodate.com/contents/maintenance-intravenous-fluid-therapy-in-children?search=iv%20 therapy&source=search_result&selectedTitle=1~150&usage_type=default&display_rank=1

Nursing Interventions

- Assess urine color, amount, and clarity.
- Assess for signs of dehydration.
- Assess for fluid overload.
  - Adventitious breath sounds
  - Bounding pulses
  - Edema
- Evaluate nutrition and control intake of electrolytes as needed.
- Give diuretics if needed.
- Maintain strict I/O.
- Monitor vital signs and weight.
- Obtain and assess IV access.

 ALERT!

Severe dehydration is a medical emergency and requires:

- An immediate IV
- A rapid infusion of 20 mL/kg of isotonic solution.

Patient and Family Education

- Monitor weight at home.
- Notify the physician if the following occurs:
  - Diarrhea lasts for more than 2 days
  - Vomiting continues for more than 1 day
  - Patient is unable to keep fluids down
- Oral rehydration therapy is an important way to restore hydration (Chapter 8).

GASTROENTERITIS

Overview

- *Gastroenteritis* is defined as three or more loose, watery stools in a 24-hour period.
- It may last less than 1 week, but not more than 2 weeks.
- Gastroenteritis can be viral or bacterial in origin. Common viral pathogens include rotavirus, enteric adenovirus, and norovirus.
- Viruses and bacteria can be spread through contaminated food or water or by touching a contaminated surface.
- Patients may or may not have fever, vomiting, and/or abdominal pain.
- Patients most likely to have severe cases are infants, young children, and those who are immunocompromised.

 COMPLICATIONS

Complications of acute viral gastroenteritis include dehydration, electrolyte imbalances, and skin irritation. If there is high fever, no/low urine output, or bloody diarrhea, the physician should be notified.

Signs and Symptoms

- Abdominal pain
- Anorexia
- Diarrhea
- Dysuria
- Fever
- Headache
- Myalgia
- Vomiting

Diagnosis

Labs
In severe cases, multiple labs:
- BMP: monitor for electrolyte imbalances and hypoglycemia
- CBC: screen for increased WBC indicating infection
- Stool studies: identify responsible organism
- Urinalysis: rule out UTI

Treatment

- ORT for dehydration in children
  - Advantages of ORT:
    - Lower cost than IV hydration
    - Easier to administer
    - May be continued at home
    - Fewer visits to the ED
  - Contraindications:
    - Altered mental status
    - Abdominal ileus
    - Short gut, carbohydrate malabsorption
    - Severe dehydration
- Phases of correcting dehydration:
  - Rehydration phase:
    - Fluid deficit replaced
    - Fluid given by spoon or syringe
    - Small amount given frequently in case of emesis
    - Breastfeeding to continue
  - Maintenance phase: age-appropriate diet
- Oral fluids:
  - Commercially prepared pediatric electrolyte fluids
  - Half-strength apple juice (equal parts apple juice and water)
  - ORT fluids by WHO
  - Not used: soft drinks, juices, sports drinks, tea, gelatin, and chicken soup
- IV fluids for severe cases:
  - Maintenance fluids
  - Bolus fluids

Nursing Interventions

- Administer medications to treat symptoms, such as acetaminophen and oral rehydration fluids.
- Administer IV fluids per order, typically NS, D5 fluids, and LR.
- Clean and treat skin irritation.
- Encourage rest.
- Monitor input/output and vital signs to monitor for signs of dehydration and/or hypovolemia.
- Provide oral fluids and nutrition.
- Place patient on contact precautions.
- Use antidiarrheal medications cautiously, as they may cause further issues.
- Wear gloves when changing all diapers, as most GI viruses are spread through the fecal-oral route.

Patient and Family Education

- Administer oral rehydration therapy as directed.
- Avoid fatty, greasy foods.
- Eat a bland diet, such as crackers and toast, and eat small meals.
- Family should consider the rotavirus vaccine if child is under age 1.

(continued)

Patient and Family Education *(continued)*

- Family should monitor fluid intake, urine output, and learn the signs of dehydration.
  - Children in diapers should have at least six wet diapers in 24 hours.
  - For infants, learn how to feel the fontanels for dehydration.
- Isolate patient from others in the household to prevent spreading to other household members.
- Keep kitchen surfaces clean, especially when cooking raw meat or eggs.
- Maintain oral fluid intake.
- Use proper handwashing technique.

GASTROESOPHAGEAL REFLUX DISEASE

Overview

- *GER* is the passage of gastric contents into the esophagus. This can happen periodically with no harm, or it can become serious.
- GERD includes complications such as esophagitis or poor weight gain.

Signs and Symptoms

- Infants
  - Most infants have GER, which resolves by age 1.
  - When infants have GERD, the symptoms include:
    - Arching of the back during or after eating
    - Anemia
    - Difficulty sleeping
    - FTT
    - Hematemesis
    - Irritability
    - Refusal to eat
    - Respiratory symptoms
    - Trouble swallowing
- Preschool-aged children
  - GERD symptoms include:
    - Decreased food intake
    - Food aversion
    - Intermittent regurgitation
    - Persistent wheezing
- School-aged children and adolescents
  - GERD symptoms are very similar to adult symptoms and include:
    - Chronic heartburn and regurgitation
    - Dysphagia
    - Epigastric pain
    - Nausea

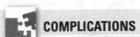 **COMPLICATIONS**

There can be serious complications from GERD. They include:

- Asthma
- Barrett's esophagus, permanent damage to the lining of the esophagus
- Dental erosion, gum disease
- Esophagitis
- Esophageal cancer
- Esophageal stricture

Diagnosis

Labs
There are no labs specific to diagnose GERD.

Diagnostic Testing
- Start 4- to 8-week course of a PPI (e.g., omeprazole) before ordering further testing (Table 8.2).
- Additional diagnostic tests for no positive results from PPI:
  - Endoscopy with histology
  - Esophageal pH probe monitoring
  - Swallowing study evaluation

Treatment

- Lifestyle changes
  - Avoid second-hand cigarette smoke, and do not smoke or vape (specifically for school-aged children and adolescents).
  - Avoid irritating foods.
    - Patients need to determine which foods are irritating to them by testing them.
    - Acidic foods, citrus, tomato sauce, carbonated beverages, and spicy foods are common irritants.
    - High-fat foods may not be limited in children depending on overall nutritional status.
  - Avoid eating meals 2 to 3 hours prior to bedtime. Elevate head of bed.
  - Feed infants in an upright position.
  - Maintain a healthy weight and avoid overeating.
  - Promote salivation by chewing gum.
- Formula change
  - Some infant formulas come with added rice. These can be used to help prevent GE reflux. It is important that the infant is not on any antacids if these formulas are used.
- Medications (see Table 8.6):
  - Antacids
  - Histamine type 2 receptor antagonists (famotidine)
  - PPIs (omeprazole)
- Surgery involves the following:
  - Surgical G-tubes for neurologically impaired children
  - Nissen fundoplication
  - G tube placement and fundoplication: A fundoplication is a surgical procedure where the stomach is wrapped around the esophagus to prevent regurgitation. This can be done in various degrees of tightness.

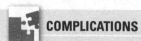

COMPLICATIONS

Complications after having a fundoplication include *dumping syndrome*: when gastric contents are emptied faster than normal into the duodenum (small intestine), which can cause glucose imbalances.

Controlling glucose levels will help prevent dumping syndrome; therefore, glucose levels must be checked and monitored after surgery.

Nursing Interventions

- Assess for aspiration.
- Encourage small, frequent meals high in calories.
- Patients should not lie down for 2 hours after eating.
- Keep infant upright 30 minutes after feeding.
- Monitor patient's weight and nutritional status.

Patient and Family Education

- Do not lie in a supine position after eating.
- Eat slowly and chew food thoroughly.
- Learn the signs of aspiration.
- Utilize a dietician to provide healthy meals.

HIRSCHSPRUNG DISEASE

Overview

- *Hirschsprung disease*, also known as aganglionic megacolon, is a congenital disease, present at birth and associated with genetic conditions.
- It is characterized by the lack of ganglion cells (which cause peristalsis) in the large intestine.
- Muscles in the intestine are unable to move stool, causing a functional obstruction as the colon enlarges (megacolon) prior to the segment of bowel that does not have ganglionic cells that cause peristalsis.

Signs and Symptoms

- Neonatal:
  - Failure to pass meconium or any stool within the first 48 hours of life
  - Development of bilious emesis and abdominal distention
  - Enterocolitis and/or sepsis
- Infants:
  - Chronic constipation
  - Ribbon-like stools (from stool passing through narrowed portion of colon)
  - FTT
  - Swelling of the abdomen
  - Unexplained fever
  - Vomiting

Diagnosis

Labs
There are no labs specific to diagnose Hirschsprung disease.

Diagnostic Testing
- Abdominal x-ray
- Barium enema
- Rectal biopsy
  - Gold standard
  - Positive if no ganglia present on mucosa
- Rectal manometry: test where pressure sensors are placed inside rectum to test muscle relaxation; Hirschsprung disease may prevent rectum muscle relaxation

Treatment

- Pull-through surgery: surgical resection of a ganglionic section
- Ostomy surgery
  - Connecting the normal tissue to an ostomy in the abdomen
  - Connecting the healthy colon back to the rectum

Nursing Interventions

- Administer antibiotics and IV hydration.
- Educate patient on condition and treatment goals.

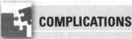

COMPLICATIONS

Hirschsprung-associated enterocolitis is a serious, life-threatening complication.

- It can happen before surgery, immediately after surgery, or years after surgery.
- Symptoms include:
  - Explosive, foul-smelling diarrhea
  - Fever, vomiting
  - Abdominal pain and distension
  - Can be mistakenly diagnosed as gastroenteritis
  - Bowel obstruction shown through radiology

COMPLICATIONS

Possible complications of surgery that will improve with time include:

- Bowel enterocolitis
- Constipation
- Delays in toilet training
- Diarrhea
- Fecal incontinence

Notify surgeon immediately if bleeding from the rectum, fever, swollen abdomen, or vomiting occurs.

- Ensure patient is NPO prior to surgery.
- Prior to surgery, place decompression tube or double-lumen NG tube to suction and either perform digital rectal exams or NS rectal irrigations three to four times per day per order.
- Postoperatively, give pain medications PRN and monitor skin integrity, especially if patient had a colostomy.
- Perform routine ostomy care, keeping the skin around the ostomy site clean and dry.

Patient and Family Education

- Address body image or self-esteem concerns for patients with a newly placed ostomy.
- Avoid constipation by slowly adding in a high-fiber diet. If not eating solid foods yet, provide information about formulas high in fiber.
- Discuss home medications including antibiotics and probiotics. Many pharmacies can flavor bad-tasting medicines to make it easier to administer.
- Drink more fluids after surgery to prevent dehydration.
- Learn about disease, treatment, and postoperative pain management.
- Learn how to care for colostomy at home and obtain supplies.
- Understand that there will be an adjustment to the child having a colostomy and learn care of the ostomy.

INFLAMMATORY BOWEL DISEASE

Overview

- GI disorders may present as chronic abdominal pain, change in bowel habits, and chronic intestinal inflammation.
- Under the broader category of IBD, there are two disorders: Crohn's disease and ulcerative colitis (Table 8.4).
  - *Crohn's disease* is a chronic disease that affects the digestive tract from mouth to anus, but most often affects the terminal ileum and involves all layers of the intestinal wall.
  - *Ulcerative colitis* affects only the colon and rectum and involves inflammation of the mucosal layer.
- Symptoms can be triggered by stress, anxiety, and fatigue.
- Disease processes include exacerbations and periods of remission.

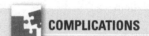 **COMPLICATIONS**

Complications of inflammatory bowel disease include:

- Fistulae
- Localized peritonitis
- Abdominal abscess
- Small bowel obstruction
- Perianal disease
- Oral lesions
- Esophageal and gastric disease

Signs and Symptoms

- Abdominal tenderness
- Anal skin tags
- Anorexia
- Cramping rectal pain
- Extra-intestinal symptoms
- Growth failure/delayed puberty
- Diarrhea/loose stools
- Fatigue
- Fever
- Joint pain
- Mass in RLQ

(continued)

Table 8.4 Comparing Crohn's Disease and Ulcerative Colitis

	Crohn's Disease	Ulcerative Colitis
Fistulas and anal fissures	Yes	No
Bloody stool	Minimal	Yes
Mucous or pus in stool	No	Yes
Colon obstruction	Yes	Rare
Small bowel disease	Yes	No
Small bowel obstruction	Yes	Rare
RLQ mass	Sometimes	Rare
Upper GI tract involvement	Yes	No

Source: Data from Higuchi, L. M., & Bousvaros, A. (2021). Clinical presentation and diagnosis of inflammatory bowel disease in children. *UpToDate.* http://uptodate/contents/clinical-presentation-and-diagnosis-of-inflammatory-bowel-disease-in-children

Signs and Symptoms *(continued)*

- Occult blood in stool
- Oral ulcerations
- Pain
- Perianal fissures
- Rash
- Weight loss

POP QUIZ 8.2

A child presents with diarrhea, fatigue, weight loss, and abdominal pain. What additional symptoms would be consistent with an ulcerative colitis presentation?

Diagnosis

Labs
- Albumin to check for malnutrition or inflammatory disease
- ALT and AST to measure liver function
- BUN/creatinine to check for dehydration
- Ca++, Mg to check for electrolyte imbalances
- CBC to check for infection
- CRP to check for inflammation
- ESR to measure inflammation
- Lipase to rule out other causes of diarrhea. Abnormal levels of lipase indicate other causes for diarrhea, such as celiac disease
- Stool testing to rule out other causes of diarrhea
  - Occult blood
  - Culture: *Clostridioides difficile* stool antigen and toxin

Diagnostic Testing
- Small bowel imaging
- Endoscopies with biopsies
- Colonoscopy

Treatment

- Crohn's disease
  - Medications (see Table 8.6):
    - ○ Amino salicylates (e.g., mesalamine)
    - ○ Anti-inflammatory drugs (e.g., sulfasalazine)
    - ○ Anti-TNF antibodies (e.g., infliximab)
    - ○ If severe, glucocorticoids (e.g., dexamethasone)
  - Reducing difficult-to-digest carbs from the diet
  - Using surgical resection of disease bowel
- Ulcerative colitis
  - Aminosalicylates, either oral or topical
  - Intravenous glucocorticoids
  - Sigmoidoscopy
  - Surgery
  - Anti-TNF and thiopurines (see Table 8.6)
- Nonpharmacologic treatments to treat IBD
  - Behavioral and psychological therapy
  - Body awareness therapy
  - Functional relaxation
  - Hypnotherapy
  - Meditation
  - Mindfulness therapy
  - Relaxation
  - Stress management
  - Yoga, tai chi

Nursing Interventions

- Administer medications, which may include antidiarrheal, laxatives, antibiotics, dietary supplements, and antispasmodics.
- Assess for signs of infection, typically fever, anorexia, abnormal vital signs, and labs.
- Interpret lab results, especially if labs get worse, indicating more bleeding, infection, or inflammation.
- Maintain adequate nutrition and monitor intake. If poor intake, an NG may be necessary.
- Monitor vital signs for possible infection and bleeding.
- Use PUCAI tool for monitoring ulcerative colitis disease activity (Table 8.5).
- Support family and patient as they adjust to a chronic disease and identify possible barriers to care.
- Teach family and patient about the condition and answer their questions.

Table 8.5 Pediatric Ulcerative Colitis Activity Index

Abdominal Activity	Points
Pain Level	
No pain	0
Pain can be ignored	5
Pain cannot be ignored	10

(continued)

Table 8.6 Pediatric Ulcerative Colitis Activity Index *(continued)*

Abdominal Activity	Points
Rectal Bleeding	
None	0
Small amount only, <50% of stools	10
Small amount with most stools	20
Large amount (more than 50% of stool content)	30
Consistency of Most Stools	
Formed	0
Partially formed	5
Completely unformed	10
Number of Stools per 24 Hours	
0–2	0
3–5	5
6–8	10
>8	15
Nocturnal Stools (any episode causing awakening)	
No	0
Yes	10
Activity Level	
No limitation of activity	0
Occasional limitation of activity	5
Severe limitation of activity	10
Total Points	

PUCAI interpretation
- 0–9 points: remission
- 10–34 points: mild disease
- 35–64 points: moderate disease
- 65–85 points: severe disease

Source: Data from Hyams, J. S., Ferry, G. D., Mandel, F. S., Gryboski, J. D., Kibort, P. M., Kirschner, B. S., Griffiths, A. M., Katz, A. J., Grand, R. J., Boyle, J. T., Michener, W. M., Levy, J. S., & Lesser, M. L. (1991). Development and validation of a pediatric Crohn's disease activity index. *Journal of Pediatric Gastroenterology and Nutrition, 12*, 439–447. https://doi.org/10.1097/00005176-199105000-00005

Patient and Family Education

- Diet should be adjusted to each individual patient.
  - Caffeine, dairy, beans, cabbage, and high fat and processed foods may make symptoms worse.
  - Gluten may also make symptoms worse in some people.
  - When not having an exacerbation, eat a diet high in soluble fiber from fruits, vegetables, and whole grains.
  - Keep a food diary to see which foods cause GI distress.
- Seek emotional support, including a mental health provider if needed.
- Some studies have shown that probiotics may help symptoms as well as exercise and hydration.
- Understand that in severe cases, the risk for colorectal cancer increases. Routine colonoscopies should start 8 to 10 years after diagnosis.

INTUSSUSCEPTION

Overview

- *Intussusception* is characterized by part of the intestine telescoping into another segment of the intestine, causing obstruction of blood flow that can lead to edema and ischemia.
- Most cases are idiopathic but can be preceded by a virus that swells the intestinal lining.
- A lead point in the intestine can also cause intussusception. A *lead point* is a lesion in the bowel that is trapped by peristalsis and dragged into the intestine, causing the intussusception. Multiple conditions can cause a lead point, including:
  - Meckel diverticulum
  - Polyp
  - Cyst
  - Tumor
  - Hematoma
  - Vascular malformation
- Typically, it presents between ages 6 and 36 months.
- Characterized by intermittent, painful episodes that occur every 15 to 20 minutes.

 COMPLICATIONS

If left untreated, an intussusception can lead to several complications:

- Bowel obstruction
- Dehydration
- Death of part of the intestine due to lack of blood flow
- Peritonitis
- Sepsis
- Shock

Signs and Symptoms

- Abdominal mass
- Abdominal pain episodes
  - Sudden and intermittent
  - Children will often pull their legs up to their abdomen.
- Bloody stool that looks like currant jelly
- Confusion
- Lethargy
- Vomiting: starts as nonbilious but becomes bilious

 NURSING PEARL

A classic sign of intussusception is a sausage-shaped mass felt at the right side of the abdomen.

Diagnosis

Diagnostic Testing
- Abdominal x-ray
- Fluoroscopy
- Ultrasound

Treatment

- Barium enema reduction under fluoroscopy
  - Air or water-soluble enema
  - Surgery not necessary; however, intussusception may reoccur
  - Possibly temporary and resolves without treatment
- Surgery if barium enema reduction is unsuccessful

Nursing Interventions

- Administer antibiotics prior to surgical repair (e.g., ceftriaxone; Table A.1).
- Determine NPO time.
- Give emotional support to caregivers. It may be the first time the child has had such severe pain and may need surgery.
- Insert an NG if ordered.
- Manage pain with medications as ordered.
- Monitor I/O.
- Monitor for possible recurrence or incarceration of the bowel.
- Start IV to hydrate patient in preparation for reduction and possible surgery.

Patient and Family Education

- Learn about the condition and ask questions.
- If reduction works, is possible that it can happen again.
- If patient has surgery, take pain medications as directed by provider.

PYLORIC STENOSIS

Overview

- The *pylorus* is a muscular sphincter at the end of the stomach where the stomach meets the small intestine.
- *Pyloric stenosis* is hypertrophy of the pyloric sphincter causing gastric outlet obstruction and projectile nonbilious vomiting.
- It is typically diagnosed in the newborn period, between the ages of 3 and 12 weeks.
- More common in Caucasians and first-born male infants.

Signs and Symptoms

- Changes in stools
- Failure to gain weight or weight loss
- Forceful projectile vomiting immediately after eating
- Irritability
- Ravenously hungry
- Wave-like motion in the abdomen right after eating

 NURSING PEARL

A classic sign of pyloric stenosis is projectile, nonbilious vomiting.

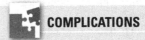 **COMPLICATIONS**

Complications of pyloric stenosis include:
- Duodenal perforation
- Post-op vomiting
- Incomplete pyloric stenosis
- Wound infection

Diagnosis

Labs

There are no labs specific to diagnose pyloric stenosis. However, the following may be helpful when determining severity and treatment:

- BMP—assessing for hypochloremia and hypokalemia, increased BUN and creatinine

Diagnostic Testing

- Abdominal ultrasound
- Upper GI

Treatment

- Surgery: pyloromyotomy

Nursing Interventions

- Keep the patient NPO preoperatively.
- Advance feeds as ordered postoperatively.
  - Feedings may start as little as 4 hours after surgery.
  - The feeds may or may not be graduated.
- Assess surgical site for drainage or signs of infection.
- Monitor infant 24 hours before discharge.
- Offer family emotional support. If breastfeeding, provide a breast pump so mother can continue to provide breast milk until the baby can eat.

Patient and Family Education

- Acetaminophen or ibuprofen should be adequate for pain control after surgery.
- Adhere to the postoperative feeding schedule.
- Breastfeeding may continue normally after surgery.
- Keep the incision site clean and dry. Sponge bath only for the first 2 days.
- Learn about the condition and ask questions.
- Learn signs of complications after surgery, including persistent projectile vomiting, wound infection, or intense pain.

NURSING PEARL

A classic sign of pyloric stenosis is the palpation of an olive-shaped mass in the RUQ. This is the enlarged pyloric sphincter.

POP QUIZ 8.3

A 6-week-old infant is brought into the ED by their parents. The mother states that her baby has not been able to keep anything down for 2 days. The patient vomits immediately after eating and she says, "It flies across the room." Based on this description, what other symptoms would be expected on further assessments?

ALERT!

Labs show metabolic alkalosis due to the loss of large amounts of hydrochloric acid due to emesis. Other labs can be normal.

Table 8.6 GI Medications

Indications	Mechanism of Action	Contraindications, Precautions, and Adverse Effects
5-aminosalicylic acid derivative (mesalamine)		
• Treat mild to moderate UC	• Block production of arachidonic acid metabolites in colon	• Precautions needed in those with renal impairment, pyloric stenosis, hepatic disease, and sodium restriction. • Also use caution in patients with pericarditis, myocarditis, preexisting skin conditions, renal impairment, and hepatic impairment. • Adverse effects include abdominal pain, constipation, headache, sore throat, hypertension, acne, chest pain and Stevens–Johnson syndrome, gout, and gastritis.

(continued)

Table 8.6 GI Medications *(continued)*

Indications	Mechanism of Action	Contraindications, Precautions, and Adverse Effects
5-aminosalicylic acid derivative (sulfasalazine)		
• Anti-inflammatory to treat ulcerative colitis and Crohn's disease	• Diminish the production of prostaglandins to reduce inflammation	• Medication is contraindicated in patients with porphyria and urinary or intestinal obstruction. • Medication is contraindicated in children under 6 years old. • Precaution needed in patients with renal impairment or failure and asthma. • Precautions needed in patients with blood dyscrasias, severe allergies, and G6PD deficiency. • Adverse effects include irreversible neuromuscular and CNS changes, severe skin reactions, fibrosing alveolitis, and GI discomfort. • Adverse effects also include sun sensitivity, skin rash, nausea/vomiting, anorexia, and headache.
Antiprotozoals (metronidazole)		
• Treatment of anaerobic bacteria infections	• Interact with DNA of susceptible organisms to inhibit protein synthesis, resulting in cell death	• Use with caution in renal, hepatic, and seizure disorder patients. • Medication may result in superinfection with prolonged use (*Clostridioides difficile*). • The intravenous formulation is high in sodium, so use cautiously in patients at risk for adverse effects from the additional sodium.
Histamine H$_2$ antagonist (famotidine)		
• Short-term relief of GERD if lifestyle changes not effective	• Block acid secretion by H$_2$ receptors	• Contraindications for OTC usage include: do not use if trouble or pain swallowing, vomiting blood, bloody or black stools, renal impairment, taking with other acid reducers. • Caution patients that tolerance can develop, which negates long-term therapy. • Precautions should be taken as medication increases risk of enteric infection, especially in *C. diff* and community-acquired pneumonia. • Adverse effects include: agitation, confusion, delirium, thrombocytopenia, severe skin conditions, and jaundice.

(continued)

Table 8.6 GI Medications *(continued)*

Indications	Mechanism of Action	Contraindications, Precautions, and Adverse Effects
Immunosuppressant (azathioprine)		
• Treatment of mild to moderate Crohn's disease	• Inhibit lymphocyte proliferation by impairing DNA synthesis	• Medication has contraindications in some patients with rheumatoid arthritis. • Use cautiously in patients with anemia, leukopenia, thrombocytopenia, hepatic disease, and renal disease. • Use caution, as it can cause GI toxicity, hematologic toxicity, hepatotoxicity, and increases risk of infection and malignancy. • Adverse effects include malaise, nausea/vomiting, diarrhea, leukopenia, and fever.
Immunosuppressant (infliximab)		
• Treat severe Crohn's disease, small bowel disease, ulcerating colonic disease	• Bind to TNF-α, which prevents it from interacting with its receptors on the cell	• Medication is contraindicated in some patients with heart failure. • Caution needed as medication may cause an increased risk for serious infection, antibody formation, autoimmune disorder, cardiovascular and cerebrovascular events, hematologic disorders, and hepatic reactions including hepatitis. • Lymphoma and other malignancies have been reported. • Medication may reactivate TB. • Adverse effects include abdominal pain, nausea, anemia, headache, cough, and vision disturbance.
Proton pump inhibitor (omeprazole)		
• Used for GERD occurring 2 or more times per week	• Suppress gastric acid secretion by inhibition of the proton pump excretion of H+	• Medication is contraindicated in OTC use if patient is having trouble/pain swallowing, bloody emesis, bloody/black stools, heartburn with lightheadedness, dizziness, diaphoresis, dyspnea, chest pain, or pain that spreads to arms, neck, or shoulders. • Use caution in patients with liver disease and lupus. • Use for the shortest time for desired effect. • Adverse effects include B12 deficiency and hypomagnesemia if taken long-term, bone fracture, abdominal pain, nausea/vomiting, muscle cramps, blurry vision, and tinnitus. • Discontinue gradually.

RESOURCES

Adamiak, T., & Francolla Plati, K. (2018). Pediatric esophageal disorders: Diagnosis and treatment of reflux and eosinophilic esophagitis. *Pediatrics in Review, 39*(8), 392–402. https://doi.org/10.1542/pir.2017-0266

Ambartsumyan, L., Smith, C., & Kapur, R. P. (2019). Diagnosis of Hirschsprung disease. *Pediatric and Developmental Pathology, 23*(1), 8–22. https://doi.org/10.1177/1093526619892351

Gotfried, J. (2021, September). *Overview of gastroenteritis.* Merck Manual Professional Version. https://www.merck manuals.com/professional/gastrointestinal-disorders/gastroenteritis/overview-of-gastroenteritis

Grossman, A. B., & Mamula, P. (2021, August 16). Pediatric Crohn disease. *Medscape.* https://emedicine.medscape .com/article/928288-overview

Higuchi, L. M., & Bousvaros, A. (2021). Clinical presentation and diagnosis of inflammatory bowel disease in children. *UpToDate.* http://uptodate/contents/clinical-presentation-and-diagnosis-of-inflammatory-bowel -disease-in-children

Houston, A., & Fuldauer, P. (2017, January 11). Enteral feeding: Indications, complications, and nursing care. *American Nurse.* https://www.myamericannurse.com/enteral-feeding-indications-complications-and-nursing -care/

Hyams, J. S., Ferry, G. D., Mandel, F. S., Gryboski, J. D., Kibort, P. M., Kirschner, B. S., Griffiths, A. M., Katz, A. J., Grand, R. J., Boyle, J. T., Michener, W. M., Levy, J. S., & Lesser, M. L. (1991). Development and validation of a pediatric Crohn's disease activity index. *Journal of Pediatric Gastroenterology and Nutrition, 12,* 439–447. https:// doi.org/10.1097/00005176-199105000-00005

Lexicomp. (2021a). Ceftriaxone: Pediatric drug information [Drug Information]. *UpToDate.* https://www.uptodate .com/contents/ceftriaxone-pediatric-drug-information?search=ceftriaxone&source=panel_search_result&select edTitle=2~148&usage_type=panel&kp_tab=drug_pediatric&display_rank=1

Lexicomp. (2021b). Dexamethasone: Pediatric drug information [Drug Information]. *UpToDate.* https://www.upto date.com/contents/dexamethasone-systemic-pediatric-drug-information?search=dexamethasone&source=pane l_search_result&selectedTitle=2~145&usage_type=panel&display_rank=2

Lexicomp. (2021c). Famotidine: Pediatric drug information [Drug Information]. *UpToDate.* https://www.uptodate .com/contents/famotidine-pediatric-drug-information?search=famotidine&source=panel_search_result&selecte dTitle=2~116&usage_type=panel&kp_tab=drug_pediatric&display_rank=1

Lexicomp. (2021d). Metoclopramide: Pediatric drug information [Drug Information]. *UpToDate.* https://www.upto date.com/contents/metoclopramide-pediatric-drug-information?search=metoclopramide&source=panel_search _result&selectedTitle=2~148&usage_type=panel&kp_tab=drug_pediatric&display_rank=1

Lexicomp. (2021e). Metronidazole: Pediatric drug information [Drug Information]. *UpToDate.* https://www.uptodate .com/contents/metronidazole-systemic-drug-information?search=metronidazole&source=panel_search_result& selectedTitle=2~145&usage_type=panel&display_rank=2

Lexicomp. (2021f). Omeprazole: Pediatric drug information [Drug Information]. *UpToDate.* https://www.uptodate. com/contents/omeprazole-pediatric-drug-information?search=omeprazole&source=panel_search_result&selec tedTitle=1~148&usage_type=panel&kp_tab=drug_pediatric&display_rank=1

Lexicomp. (2021g). Pentasa: Pediatric drug information [Drug Information]. *UpToDate.* https://www.uptodate.com /contents/mesalamine-mesalazine-pediatric-drug-information?search=pentasa&source=panel_search_result&s electedTitle=1~62&usage_type=panel&kp_tab=drug_pediatric&display_rank=1

Lexicomp. (2021h). Remicade: Pediatric drug information [Drug Information]. *UpToDate.* https://www.uptodate .com/contents/infliximab-including-biosimilars-of-infliximab-pediatric-drug-information?search=remicade&sour ce=panel_search_result&selectedTitle=1~148&usage_type=panel&kp_tab=drug_pediatric&display_rank=1

Lexicomp. (2021i). Simethicone: Pediatric drug information [Drug Information]. *UpToDate.* https://www.uptodate. com/contents/simethicone-pediatric-drug-information?search=simethicone&source=panel_search_result&sele ctedTitle=1~28&usage_type=panel&kp_tab=drug_pediatric&display_rank=1

Lexicomp. (2021j). Zosyn; Pediatric drug information [Drug Information]. *UpToDate.* https://www.uptodate.com/c ontents/piperacillin-and-tazobactam-pediatric-drug-information?search=zosyn&source=panel_search_result& selectedTitle=1~103&usage_type=panel&kp_tab=drug_pediatric&display_rank=1

MedlinePlus. (2021a). *Failure to thrive.* https://medlineplus.gov/ency/article/000991.htm

MedlinePlus. (2021b). *Pyloric stenosis in infants.* https://medlineplus.gov/ency/article/000970.htm

Mehanna, H. M., Moledina, J., & Travis, J. (2008, June 28). Refeeding syndrome: What it is, and how to prevent and treat it. *The BMJ, 336*(7659), 1495–1498. https://doi.org/10.1136/bmj.a301. https://www.ncbi.nlm.nih.gov/pmc/ articles/PMC2440847/

National Institute of Diabetes and Digestive and Kidney Diseases. (2017). *Symptoms and causes of Crohn's disease*. U.S. Department of Health and Human Services, National Institute of Diabetes and Digestive and Kidney Diseases. https://www.niddk.nih.gov/health-information/digestive-diseases/crohns-disease/symptoms-causes

National Institute of Diabetes and Digestive and Kidney Diseases. (2019). *Intussusception*. U.S. Department of Health and Human Services, National Institute of Diabetes and Digestive and Kidney Diseases. https://www.niddk.nih.gov/health-information/digestive-diseases/anatomic-problems-lower-gi-tract/intussusception

National Organization for Rare Diseases. (2019). *Pediatric Crohn's disease*. https://rarediseases.org/rare-diseases/pediatric-crohns-disease/

Ordas, I., Eckmann, L., Talamini, M., Baumgart, D. C., & Sandborn, W. J. (2012). Ulcerative colitis. *The Lancet, 380*(9853), 1606–1619. https://doi.org/10.1016/S0140-6736(12)60150-0. https://www.thelancet.com/journals/lancet/article/PIIS0140-6736(12)60150-0/fulltext#secd7051906e871

Philips, S. M., & Jensen, C. (2021). Laboratory and radiologic evaluation of nutritional status in children. *UpToDate*. http://uptodate.com/contents/laboratory-and-radiologic-evaluation-of-nutritional-status-in-children

Samuel, M. (2002, June). Pediatric appendicitis score. *Journal of Pediatric Surgery, 37*, 877–881. https://doi.org/10.1053/jpsu.2002.32893

Somers, M. J. (2021a). Clinical assessment and diagnosis of hypovolemia (dehydration) in children. *UpToDate*. https://www.uptodate.com/contents/clinical-assessment-and-diagnosis-of-hypovolemia-dehydration-in-children?search=hypovolemia&source=search_result&selectedTitle=1~150&usage_type=default&display_rank=1

Somers, M. J. (2021b). Maintenance intravenous fluid therapy in children. *UpToDate*. https://www.uptodate.com/contents/maintenance-intravenous-fluid-therapy-in-children?search=iv%20therapy&source=search_result&selectedTitle=1~150&usage_type=default&display_rank=1

Stewart, D. (2017). Surgical care of the pediatric Crohn's disease patient. *Seminars in Pediatric Surgery, 26*(6), 373–378. https://doi.org/10.1053/j.sempedsurg.2017.10.007. https://pubmed.ncbi.nlm.nih.gov/29126506/

Wesson, D. E., & Brandt, M. L. (2021). Acute appendicitis in children: Clinical manifestations and diagnosis. *UpToDate*. http://www.uptodate.com/contents/acute-appedicitis-in-children-clinical-manifestations-and-diagnosis

9

GENITOURINARY AND RENAL SYSTEM

ASSESSMENT AND MANAGEMENT OF DRAINS

Overview

- *Urinary catheterization* is the placement of a catheter through the urethra into the bladder.
- The procedure is done for the following reasons:
  - Accurately measure urine output
  - Assist in emptying the bladder
  - Obtain a sterile urine sample
  - Relieve urinary retention
- Types of urinary catheters include:
  - Indwelling (Foley catheter) for longer-term or postoperative use
  - Intermittent (straight catheter) for shorter-term use or for obtaining samples

 COMPLICATIONS

Prolonged urinary catheter usage is a major risk factor in developing CAUTI, which can lead to bloodstream infections, sepsis, increased morbidity, mortality, and prolonged hospital stays. Follow nursing guidelines for proper usage, insertion, and catheter care to help to minimize and prevent complications.

Nursing Interventions

- Provide privacy and developmentally appropriate explanation of procedure.
- Position patient appropriately for catheterization and perform peri-care.
- Insert appropriate size catheter for age, using sterile technique and sterile equipment.
- Secure closed-drainage system for indwelling catheters at a level lower than the bladder.
- Do not secure drainage system to movable crib or bedrail.
- Prevent dependent loops in tubing.
- To prevent infections while catheter is in place, clean the perineal area and around the insertion site routinely.
- Secure catheter to prevent tension or injury on urethra.
- Monitor for signs of infection:
  - Cloudy urine
  - Fever
  - Irritation at insertion site
  - Strong urine odor
- Ensure balloon is deflated prior to removal of indwelling catheter.

Urine Collection

- Catheterization sample
  - Obtain sample by using intermittent catheterization or accessing the sample port of an indwelling catheter.
  - Use this method to confirm a positive screen from a clean catch urine sample, with children unable to provide clean catch specimens, and/or to obtain a sterile urine culture.

(continued)

Urine Collection *(continued)*

- Clean catch
  - Give child specimen cup and antiseptic package.
  - Instruct females to clean by wiping from front to back and males to clean tip of the penis to prevent skin bacteria from getting into the sample.
  - Tell the patient to obtain a midstream sample by urinating into the toilet first, then into the specimen cup.
- Urine collection bags
  - Urine collection bags are appropriate for infants and toddlers who are unable to void on request, not toilet trained, or are wearing diapers.
  - Clean and dry the perineal area before applying the adhesive collection bag to skin.
  - Only use for collection of nonsterile specimens. Remove the collection bag once child has urinated and the specimen has been collected.
- Urine labs
  - UA
    - *Urinalysis* is a screening lab for urine. This can be done by sending urine sample to lab for testing or using a point-of-care dipstick for urinalysis.
    - Urinalysis lab notes the appearance and color of urine.
    - Urinalysis measures pH, protein, glucose, ketones, hemoglobin, bilirubin, urobilinogen, nitrites, leukocytes, and specific gravity.
    - Urine is examined for WBCs, RBCs, casts, crystals, bacteria, and yeast.
  - Urine culture
    - A *urine culture* is a diagnostic lab for infections.
    - It detects bacteria, yeast, and microorganisms in the urine.

 ALERT!

For infants and toddlers wearing diapers, to obtain a nonsterile urine sample that will not be used for cultures, place cotton balls in the diapers or inside the collection bag and then squeeze out the urine using a syringe into a specimen cup.

GLOMERULONEPHRITIS

Overview

- *Glomerulonephritis* is inflammation of the glomeruli in the kidneys.
- It may cause glomerular vascular damage, venous stasis, and intravascular coagulation.
- The inflammation can be acute or chronic. *Acute glomerulonephritis* is most common in preschool and school-age children. *Chronic glomerulonephritis* is a progressive disease that may result in kidney scaring or sclerosis, which can lead to renal failure.
- The primary risk factor for developing glomerulonephritis is a recent streptococcal skin or pharyngeal infection.

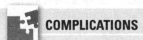 **COMPLICATIONS**

Post-streptococcal glomerulonephritis may resolve without treatment. However, if symptoms persist, treatment is needed to prevent severe complications such as acute renal failure, circulatory overload, hypertensive encephalopathy, and long-term kidney damage.

Signs and Symptoms

- Dark-colored urine
- Decreased urine output
- Edema in lower extremities and face
- Fatigue
- Hematuria
- Hypertension

- Irritability
- Lethargy
- Oliguria
- Proteinuria

Diagnosis

Labs

- Antistreptolysin to confirm recent streptococcal infection
- BMP to evaluate BUN and Cr (kidney function) and electrolyte levels
- CBC to assess for leukocytosis and underlying infection
- UA to assess for hematuria, proteinuria, and WBCs

Diagnostic Testing

- Renal biopsy

Treatment

- Antibiotics
- Antihypertensives
- Corticosteroids
- Diuretics
- Fluid restriction
- Sodium and potassium restriction

Nursing Interventions

- Assess patient for changes in neurologic status.
- Assess patient for edema and administer diuretics as ordered.
- Cluster nursing care.
- Educate on dietary changes, if necessary.
- Monitor BP at least every 4 hours.
- Monitor intake for fluid balance.
- Monitor urine output for blood, color, and amount.
- Notify provider of any changes in patient status, increased edema, or hypertension.
- Review labs for possible electrolyte imbalances and changes in renal function.
- Weigh patient daily.

 NURSING PEARL

Clustering care involves grouping together nursing interventions and treatments instead of spacing them throughout the shift. It provides for longer rest periods between care and interventions for the patient.

Patient and Family Education

- Ensure entire course of antibiotics is taken.
- Follow healthcare provider recommendations for dietary and fluid intake.
  - Most commonly, follow a regular diet with no added salt.
  - Restrict sodium and fluids if child is experiencing edema and hypertension.
  - Restrict potassium if child is experiencing oliguria.
- Monitor BP at home.
- Report if family notices an increase in child's swelling or edema.
- Treatment can be at home if BPs are normal and child has adequate urine output.
- Treatment will need to be in the hospital if child is experiencing more severe symptoms, such as hypertension, edema, hematuria, or oliguria.

 POP QUIZ 9.1

The parent of a 7-year-old states that the child's face looks swollen, and their urine is very dark in color. What labs should the nurse anticipate that the provider will order?

Overview

- *Nephrotic syndrome* is a condition in which the glomerular membrane is damaged, leading to edema, hyperlipidemia, hypoalbuminemia, and proteinuria.
- Nephrotic syndrome is characterized by increased glomerular permeability to plasma protein, resulting in urinary protein loss.
  - Proteins, such as albumin, can leak through the glomerular membrane and are lost in urine, resulting in hyperalbuminuria and reducing serum albumin level, leading to hypoalbuminemia.
- It can be primary, secondary, or congenital.
  - *Primary*, or idiopathic, which is also called *minimal-change nephrotic syndrome*, commonly affects children ages 2 to 3 years old.
  - *Secondary* occurs after glomerular damage from a known or presumed cause.
  - *Congenital* is inherited in an autosomal recessive pattern.
- Nephrotic syndrome typically presents in children between 2 and 7 years old.

 COMPLICATIONS

The first-line treatment, steroids, may cause several complications, including an increase in appetite, weight gain, mood swings, and increased risk for infection, which could lead to sepsis.

Signs and Symptoms

- Ascites
- BP is normal or slightly decreased
- Dark, foamy, frothy urine
- Decreased urine output
- Edema
  - Periorbital and facial
  - Lower extremities
  - Subsides throughout day
- Fatigue
- Hypoalbuminemia
- Hyperlipidemia
- Pallor
- Proteinuria
- Weight gain

 NURSING PEARL

Use the mnemonic PALE to remember the key signs and symptoms of nephrotic syndrome:

- **P** – Proteinuria
- **A** – Albumin low
- **L** – Lipids high
- **E** – Edema

Diagnosis

Labs

- Blood
  - Albumin, to monitor for decreased levels
  - BMP to monitor kidney function and electrolytes
  - Lipid panel to monitor elevated cholesterol levels
- Urine
  - 24-hour urine collection
  - First day void specimen for urine protein: creatine ratio
  - UA to measure increased urine protein levels

Diagnostic Testing

- Kidney biopsy
- Renal bladder ultrasound

Treatment

- Albumin replacement
- Limiting intake of sodium, potassium, and phosphorus
- Fluid restriction
- Medications (Tables 9.1* and A.3)
  - Corticosteroids (prednisone)
  - Diuretic (furosemide)
  - Immunosuppressant (cyclophosphamide)

Nursing Interventions

- Administer diuretics as ordered for edema and fluid balance.
- Assess diet and assist in implementing a low-salt diet to help control edema and sodium levels.
- Cluster care and provide rest periods.
- Monitor edema, assess degree of pitting, and elevate legs to relieve lower extremity edema.
- Monitor I/O and initiate fluid restriction if experiencing severe symptoms.
- Weigh patient daily.

Patient and Family Education

- Steroid treatment is typically for 6 to 8 weeks; understand the possible side effects of steroids.
- There is a possibility for relapse and repeated treatment.
  - Watch for early signs of relapse.
  - Use home urine monitoring by dipstick or watch for signs of puffiness, edema, swelling, or weight gain.
- Prevent infection when taking steroids or immunosuppressant medications, which increase infection risk, with hand hygiene and avoiding others who are sick.
- Remain up to date on immunizations, specifically the pneumococcal vaccine.
- Restrict sodium and cholesterol in diet.
  - Limit processed foods, red meat, and added salt.
  - Eat fresh fruits, vegetables, and whole grains.
  - Limit whole eggs and saturated fats.
- Watch for new weight gain and/or swelling.

PYELONEPHRITIS

Overview

- *Pyelonephritis* is a kidney infection that is typically severe and comes on suddenly.
- Usually, it begins as a UTI in the bladder, then ascends to the kidneys, resulting in inflammation of the upper urinary tract and kidneys.

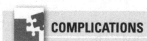

COMPLICATIONS

Pyelonephritis can cause renal scarring, which can lead to permanent kidney damage and chronic kidney disease.

Signs and Symptoms

- Chills
- Fever
- Lower back pain
- Nausea
- UTI symptoms
- Vomiting

---

* Table 9.1 is located at the end of this chapter.

Diagnosis

Labs
- UA
- Urine culture for bacteria detection

Diagnostic Testing
- Intravenous pyelogram
- Renal bladder ultrasound

Treatment

- Antibiotics (penicillins and cephalosporins) (Tables 9.1 and A.1)

Nursing Interventions

- Administer antibiotics and IV fluids as ordered.
- Encourage hydration.
- Monitor urine output, assessing urine for color and amount.
- Monitor vital signs, especially temperature for signs of fever improving or worsening.
- Perform sterile catheterization for urine culture collection.

Patient and Family Education

- Avoid urine retention.
  - Empty bladder completely.
  - Stay adequately hydrated.
  - Urinate frequently.
- Complete entire course of antibiotics.
- Maintain proper hydration by drinking fluids and staying adequately hydrated.
- Maintain proper peri-care and hygiene for diapered children.
- Perform proper perineal hygiene, wiping from front to back.
- Practice postcoital hygiene with sexually active adolescents.

URINARY TRACT INFECTION

Overview

- A *UTI* is an infection of the urinary tract that is caused by bacteria from the skin or rectum entering the urethra.
  - *Escherichia coli* is the most common bacterial pathogen of UTIs.
  - Most uropathogens originate in the GI tract.
- Females are at higher risk because their urethras are shorter and closer to the rectum.
- Risk factors include vesicoureteral reflux, urinary stasis, bubble baths, poor hygiene, onset of toilet training, and incomplete bladder emptying.

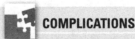 **COMPLICATIONS**

Untreated UTIs can progress to pyelonephritis and urosepsis, especially in infants who present with unspecific symptoms of irritability and fever or toddlers who may present with vomiting as the only symptom.

Signs and Symptoms

- Bloody urine
- Enuresis
- Feeling the need to urinate
- Fever
- Frequent urination
- Foul-smelling urine
- Irritability in infants
- Incontinence in a toilet-trained child
- Pain or cramping in the lower abdomen
- Painful urination
- Vomiting

Diagnosis

Labs
- UA for WBCs, leukocytes, nitrites, or blood
- Urine culture for detection of bacteria

Diagnostic Testing
- Renal bladder ultrasound

Treatment

- Antibiotics: cephalosporins (Table A.1)
- Prophylactic therapy for recurrent UTIs

Nursing Interventions

- Administer antibiotics as ordered.
- Educate patients and caregivers on proper hygiene and peri-care.
- Encourage hydration because increased fluid promotes flushing of the bladder.
- Monitor urine output.
- Monitor vital signs and temperature for signs of infection improving and notify provider if fever persists.

Patient and Family Education

- Identify contributing factors to reduce risk of another infection.
- Understand prophylactic therapy, if applicable for recurrent cases.
- Perform proper perineal hygiene, wiping from front to back.
- Maintain adequate fluid intake and dietary fiber to prevent constipation.
- Practice postcoital hygiene for sexually active adolescents.
- Stay adequately hydrated.
- Void as soon as there is an urge. Do not hold urine, and empty bladder completely.
- Wear cotton instead of nylon underwear.

POP QUIZ 9.2

Why are females at higher risk for UTIs, and what anticipatory education can be provided to prevent an infection?

VESICOURETERAL REFLUX

Overview

- *Vesicoureteral reflux* is a condition in which urine backflows from the bladder, through the ureters, and into the kidneys.
- It can be primary or secondary:
  - Primary: congenital malformation of the valves between the ureters and bladder
  - Secondary: result of blockage, narrowing, or nerve problems
- Vesicoureteral reflex increases risk of UTI.

> **COMPLICATIONS**
>
> Vesicoureteral reflux increases the risk of a child having recurrent, febrile, or symptomatic UTIs.

Signs and Symptoms

- Febrile UTIs
- Recurrent UTIs

Diagnosis

Labs
- There are no labs specific to diagnose vesicoureteral reflux.

Diagnostic Testing
- Renal bladder ultrasound
- Voiding cystourethrogram

Treatment

- Prophylactic antibiotics
- Surgical intervention
  - For patients at risk of renal scarring
  - For patients over 6 years old with significant degree of reflux

Nursing Interventions

- Monitor for signs and symptoms of UTIs (see Urinary Tract Infection topic).

Patient and Family Education

- Avoid holding urine.
  - Empty bladder completely.
  - Urinate frequently.
- Continue prophylactic antibiotics, even if asymptomatic.
- Perform proper perineal hygiene.
- Stay adequately hydrated.

> **POP QUIZ 9.3**
>
> A patient is diagnosed with primary vesicoureteral reflux and is awaiting the surgery date. What education is important to provide to prevent complications before and after surgery?

WILMS' TUMOR

Overview

- Wilms' tumor, or nephroblastoma, is the most common renal malignancy of childhood.
- It is most often categorized as a stage 1 cancer, limited to one kidney, and typically presents before the age of 5.

- In complicated cases, it may progress beyond stage 1 to include:
  - Both kidneys
  - Lymph node involvement
  - Metastasis to the lung, liver, and/or bone
- Risk factors include a family history of Wilms' tumor or congenital syndromes such as WAGR syndrome and Beckwith–Wiedemann syndrome.
  - *WAGR syndrome*, or 11p deletion syndrome, is a genetic disorder with characteristic associations being Wilms' tumor, *aniridia* or the absence of iris of the eye, genitourinary conditions, and intellectual disabilities.
  - *Beckwith–Wiedemann syndrome* is a growth disorder associated with being larger than normal as infants and children, larger abdominal organs, asymmetric growth, macroglossia, hypoglycemia, and increased risk for tumors, such as Wilms' tumor.
- The typical presenting symptom of Wilms' tumor is a painless abdominal mass.

> **COMPLICATIONS**
>
> The lungs are the most common secondary metastasis area for Wilms' tumor, leading to cough, chest tightness, dyspnea, and shortness of breath.

Signs and Symptoms

- Abdominal mass (nontender)
- Abdominal pain
- Anemia
- Constipation
- Fever
- Hematuria
- Hypertension

Diagnosis

Labs

- There are no labs specific to diagnose Wilms' tumor. However, the following may be helpful when determining severity and treatment:
- BMP to evaluate kidney function and electrolytes to determine if tumor has spread
- CBC to monitor for decreased hemoglobin levels
- Coagulation studies to screen for underlying diseases
- LFT to screen for liver involvement
- UA

Diagnostic Testing

- Abdominal ultrasound
- Chest x-ray
- Abdominal CT
- Abdominal MRI

Treatment

- Chemotherapy: when both kidneys are affected
- Surgery
  - Partial nephrectomy
  - Nephrectomy, which then requires dialysis and possible renal transplant

Nursing Interventions

- Do NOT palpate the abdomen.
- Encourage patients to wear loose clothing around abdomen.
- Monitor BP.

Nursing Interventions *(continued)*

- Prepare child for surgery by giving developmentally appropriate explanations and expectations.
  - Involve child life for therapeutic play.
  - Provide support for family; offer services such as social worker or chaplain.
- Postoperatively, monitor for intestinal obstruction by assessing for abdominal distension, vomiting, and auscultating for bowel sounds.

 ALERT!

Do not palpate abdomen because palpations may cause the tumor to rupture into the peritoneal cavity and allow cancer cells to spread.

Patient and Family Education

- Family members can join support groups or utilize community resources and friends and family to help with coping after learning diagnosis.
- Plan for radiation or chemotherapy.
- Understand and monitor for side effects of chemotherapy: nausea, vomiting, mouth sores, fatigue, hair loss, and weakened immune system.
- Understand the need for follow-up visits, postsurgery that will include lab work, and imaging to screen for reoccurrence or complications.

Table 9.1 Medications for GU and Renal Conditions

Indications	Mechanism of Action	Contraindications, Precautions, and Adverse Effects
Immunosuppressants (cyclophosphamide)		
• Used for management of nephrotic syndrome	• Immunosuppressant effects by selective suppression of B Lymphocyte activity	• Adverse effects include immunosuppression and serious infections that may require dose reduction or discontinuation. • Monitor for hemorrhagic cystitis after administration and ensure adequate hydration.
Diuretics (furosemide)		
• Reduce extra fluid and edema • Treat fluid imbalances and edema in patients with nephrotic syndrome and glomerulonephritis	• Inhibit sodium and chloride resorption and inhibit absorption of sodium and chloride in proximal and distal tubules	• Adverse effects include ototoxicity and acute kidney injury and hypovolemia due to fluid loss, hypokalemia, and electrolyte disturbances. • Do not administer intravenously too quickly, as this can cause ototoxicity.

RESOURCES

Centers for Disease Control and Prevention. (2015, November 5). *Catheter associated urinary tract infections*. U.S. Department of Health and Human Services, Centers for Disease Control and Prevention. https://www.cdc.gov/infectioncontrol/guidelines/cauti/background.html#:~:text=An%20estimated%2017%25%20to%2069,per%20year%20could%20be%20prevented

Centers for Disease Control and Prevention. (2018, November 1). *Post-streptococcal glomerulonephritis*. U.S. Department of Health and Human Services, Centers for Disease Control and Prevention. https://www.cdc.gov/groupastrep/diseases-hcp/post-streptococcal.html

Centers for Disease Control and Prevention. (2019, August 27). *Urinary tract infection*. U. S. Department of Health and Human Services, Centers for Disease Control and Prevention. https://www.cdc.gov/antibiotic-use/community/for-patients/common-illnesses/uti.html

Children's Hospital of Philadelphia. (2018, November). *Nephrotic syndrome in children*. https://www.chop.edu/conditions-diseases/nephrotic-syndrome-children?callsource=ctm&insitesid=1231&gclid=CjwKCAjw7J6EBhBDEiwA5UUM2ktOTZGcaxIrWTdIV0MKtSCJsPZ1Te8BBJt9SOiya6aVkTh_7W0DQxoCL_IQAvD_BwE

Chintagumpala, M. (2019). Presentation, diagnosis and staging of Wilms tumor. *UpToDate*. https://www.uptodate.com/contents/presentation-diagnosis-and-staging-of-wilms-tumor?search=wilms%20tumor%20children&source=search_result&selectedTitle=1~123&usage_type=default&display_rank=1

Hockenberry, M., Wilson, D., & Rodgers, C. (2017). *Wong's essentials of pediatric nursing*. Elsevier.

Lexicomp. (n.d.[a]). Cephalexin: Pediatric drug information. [Drug Information]. *UpToDate*. https://www.uptodate.com/contents/cephalexin-pediatric-drug-information?search=cephalexin&source=panel_search_result&selectedTitle=2~118&usage_type=panel&kp_tab=drug_pediatric&display_rank=1

Lexicomp. (n.d.[b]). Cyclophosphamide: Pediatric drug information. [Drug Information]. *UpToDate*. https://www.uptodate.com/contents/cephalexin-pediatric-drug-information?search=cephalexin&source=panel_search_result&selectedTitle=2~118&usage_type=panel&kp_tab=drug_pediatric&display_rank=1

Lexicomp. (n.d.[c]). Furosemide: Pediatric drug information. [Drug Information]. *UpToDate*. https://www.uptodate.com/contents/cyclophosphamide-pediatric-drug-information?search=Cyclophosphamide&source=panel_search_result&selectedTitle=2~148&usage_type=panel&kp_tab=drug_pediatric&display_rank=1

Lexicomp. (n.d.[d]). Prednisone: Pediatric drug information. [Drug Information]. *UpToDate*. https://www.uptodate.com/contents/prednisone-pediatric-drug-information?search=prednisone&source=panel_search_result&selectedTitle=2~148&usage_type=panel&kp_tab=drug_pediatric&display_rank=1

McGuire, M., & Pennathur, S. (2018). Nephrotic syndrome. In S. Saint & V. Chopra (Eds.), *The Saint-Chopra guide to inpatient medicine* (4th ed.). Oxford University Press. https://oxfordmedicine.com/view/10.1093/med/9780190862800.001.0001/med-9780190862800

National Institute of Diabetes and Digestive and Kidney Diseases. (2018, June). *Vesicoureteral reflux*. U.S. Department of Health and Human Services, National Institute of Diabetes and Digestive and Kidney Diseases. https://www.niddk.nih.gov/health-information/urologic-diseases/hydronephrosis-newborns/vesicoureteral-reflux

ENDOCRINE SYSTEM

DIABETES TYPE 1

Overview

- *Type 1 diabetes* is an insulin deficiency disorder characterized by the destruction of insulin-producing pancreatic beta cells.
- Risk factors for developing type 1 diabetes include:
  - Environmental factors: viruses that attack the beta cells of the pancreas
  - Ethnicity: highest prevalence in non-Hispanic whites
  - Genetic susceptibility
  - Many specialists will be involved in the care and treatment of a child with type 1 diabetes, such as:
    - Dentist
    - Diabetes educator
    - Dietician
    - Endocrinologist
    - Ophthalmologist
    - Pediatrician or primary care provider
- The common presenting symptoms are polyuria, polydipsia, and polyphagia.
- Type 1 diabetes can be a primary disorder or secondary to other diseases, including:
  - Addison's disease
  - Autoimmune thyroiditis
  - Celiac disease
  - Cystic fibrosis

 COMPLICATIONS

Diabetic ketoacidosis is a potentially life-threatening sequela of diabetes. When there is not enough insulin, the body breaks down fat and muscle for energy, resulting in ketone production. It is often the first sign that the child has type 1 diabetes. It can cause cerebral injury and death if left untreated. It includes the following characteristics:

- Acidosis
- Anorexia
- Confusion
- Drowsiness and lethargy
- Dry or flushed skin
- Fluid and electrolyte imbalances
- Frequent urination
- Fruity odor on the breath
- Hyperventilation or Kussmaul respirations
- Poor peripheral perfusion

Signs and Symptoms

Type 1 diabetes signs and symptoms include (Table 10.1):
- Flu-like symptoms
- Fruity smelling breath
- Hyperglycemia greater than 200 mg/dL
- Lethargy
- Metabolic acidosis pH less than 0.3
- Polydipsia
- Polyphagia
- Polyuria
- Slow-healing skin cuts/scrapes
- Visual disturbances
- Weight loss

Table 10.1 Type 1 vs. Type 2 Diabetes

Type 1	Type 2
• Recent weight loss	• Obesity
• 50% present before age 10	• Diagnosis usually after puberty
• Almost always symptomatic at the time of diagnosis	• 40% of patients are asymptomatic.
• Unusual to have clinical features of insulin resistance	Clinical features associated with insulin resistance: • Acanthosis nigricans • Dyslipidemia • Hypertension • PCOS
• 10% have a close family member with type 1 diabetes. • More common in non-Hispanic whites	• 75%–90% have 1st- or 2nd-degree relative with type 2 diabetes • More common among Hispanic, Black, Asian, Native American, and Pacific Islander patients

Source: Levitsky, L. L., & Misra, M. (2021). Insulin therapy for children and adolescents with type 1 diabetes mellitus. *UpToDate.* https://www.uptodate.com/contents/insulin-therapy-for-children-and-adolescents-with-type-1-diabetes-mellitus?search=kinds%20of%20insulin§ionRank=1&usage_type=default&anchor=H3940151930&source=machineLearning&selectedTitle=1~150&display_rank=1#H3940151930

Diagnosis

Labs
- ABG
- Beta-hydroxybutyrate
- BMP for electrolytes and glucose level
- HbA1C greater than 6.4: reflects the average blood sugar level for the past 2 to 3 months
- Plasma glucose greater than 200 mg/dL taken randomly in a patient that is symptomatic
- Plasma glucose greater than 200 mg/dL 2 hours after an oral glucose tolerance test
- Urine ketones

Diagnostic Testing
There are no diagnostic tests specific to diagnose diabetes type 1.

Treatment

- Goals:
  - Normal growth, development, self-care, and independence
  - Glycemic control with no hypo- or hyperglycemia (Table 10.2)
- Initial treatment:
  - Disease management basics
    - Blood glucose monitoring
    - Carbohydrate intake measurement
    - Hypoglycemia recognition and treatment
    - Insulin administration
    - Sick-day management
    - Urine ketone monitoring

 NURSING PEARL

Glucose in the urine is suggestive of diabetes but not diagnostic.

Table 10.2 Target Blood Sugar Levels by Age		
	Ages 6–12	**Ages 12–19**
Fasting	80–126	70–126
Glucose tolerance test	Above 200	Above 200
A1C	Less than 6.5%	Less than 7%

Source: Data from Centers for Disease Control and Prevention. (2021). *Preventing childhood obesity: 5 things you can do at home.* U.S. Department of Health and Human Services, Centers for Disease Control and Prevention. https://www.cdc.gov/nccdphp/dnpao/features/childhood-obesity/

- Insulin replacement for type 1 diabetes:
  - Insulin (Table 10.3*):
    - Intermediate-acting NPH
    - Long-acting glargine
    - Rapid-acting regular insulin
    - Short-acting lispro
- Ongoing treatment:
  - Dependent on the patient's communicative ability and developmental maturity
  - Infants:
    - Increased risk of severe hypoglycemia when compared to other age groups
    - Insulin management challenges because of frequent eating
    - Possible severe neurologic and developmental consequences for both hyper- and hypoglycemia
  - Toddlers:
    - Continued glucose monitoring preferred
    - Internal insulin pumps for toddlers' erratic eating and activity schedule
    - Temper tantrums: symptom of hypoglycemia
  - Preschool children:
    - Can start supervised self-care
    - Day or overnight diabetes camp: may provide a good support system
  - School-aged children:
    - Can administer injections and discuss routine care with family
    - If glucose monitoring, ensure back-up blood glucose monitor is at school
    - May affect school performance
    - Possible development of anxiety and depression related to illness
    - Significant caregiver involvement in all nonroutine decisions
  - Adolescents
    - Education on self-image promotion and effects of risk-taking behavior, like alcohol consumption, on disease management
    - Family-focused care: keeping the family working together as adolescents become more independent

 NURSING PEARL

Sick-day management includes a plan for when the patient is sick. It is important to have the sick-day management plan written out before the child gets sick. The child should continue taking prescribed medications, if possible. If they cannot, notify the provider. The dosages may need to be adjusted.

- Try to feed the child a regular diet with normal amounts and extra fluids.
- If the glucose level surpasses the limit recommended by the provider, give extra fluids.
- Check the child's blood sugar every 3 to 4 hours or more frequently if it rises quickly. Notify the provider to see if an additional dose of insulin is necessary.
- Check urine ketones.
- Check with the provider before giving any OTC medications. Some will affect blood sugar.
- Let the provider know if the child is vomiting or has diarrhea for more than 6 hours.

---

* Table 10.3 is located at the end of this chapter.

(continued)

Treatment *(continued)*

- ○ Insulin pumps and continuous blood glucose monitors
- ○ Key to transitioning to self-management; patient and family education
- ○ Eating disorders and under-dosing insulin for weight control

Nursing Interventions

- Check glucose on schedule and administer insulin per patient's parameters.
- Educate how to test for urine ketones, especially when the patient is ill.
- Educate on administering insulin and determining the amount needed based on the blood glucose test result.
- Educate the family to recognize the signs and symptoms of hypoglycemia. This can be difficult in a nonverbal patient or an infant. Family should check glucose in these situations.
- Educate the patient and family on the disease process, goals of management, and treatment options.
- Help the family make a plan for when the child is sick so they are prepared.
- Monitor for signs of hyperglycemia and hypoglycemia and intervene as needed.
- Observe for signs of depression or anxiety.
- Prevent skin breakdown and infections.
- Provide the patient with proper nutrition while considering glucose level, personal preferences, cultural customs, and lifestyle choices.
- Recommend that the child wear an emergency bracelet or necklace to inform possible emergency workers of the patient's condition.
- Recommend that the family consults and teaches the school nurse or other caregivers about the child's diabetes treatment plan.
- Reinforce points of education at subsequent visits especially if glycemic control is not ideal.
- Screen for vision changes.
- Suggest that the family/patient give the first dose and practice as many times as necessary to feel comfortable.
- Support family and patient emotionally and provide information on community resources.

Patient and Family Education

- A child should carry carbohydrate snacks as a precaution. Examples include fruit, peanut butter, and graham crackers.
- Keep all follow-up visits and appointments.
- Maintain exercise, personal hygiene, and health promotion.
- Obtain additional blood glucose supplies, insulin, emergency glucagon, tablets, and juice for a school setting and travel away from home.
- Older adolescents should prepare to transition to an adult diabetic management team.
- Older children and family should demonstrate performing glucose checks, preparing insulin, and injecting insulin.
- Stay up to date on immunizations, including the flu and the pneumococcal vaccines.

 NURSING PEARL

The diet for patients with diabetes type 1 is crucial, and the family and patient need to understand its importance. Carbohydrates are the food that has the greatest impact on blood sugar. Matching the carbohydrates eaten to the insulin given is the key to preventing long-term complications. Most type 1 diabetics are on long-term insulin, which lowers blood sugar over 24 hours. Low blood sugar will occur if no carbohydrates are ingested or if a meal is skipped or delayed. If a large amount of food is taken in, long-term insulin may not be enough, and short-term insulin will be added.

 ALERT!

Many family members have difficulty managing the illness when their child has diabetes. When they first receive the diagnosis, they can be in shock and very emotional. They should be given time to process the diagnosis before overwhelming them with a lot of information. Nurses can help family by:

- Assess the level of stress that the family is feeling. They may need professional help.
- Assure them they can call anytime with questions. Give the family a number they can use where someone will be available to help them.
- Encourage the family to join a support group.
- Listen to the family as they describe any problems following the diabetes plan.

- Family must help a child with or learn to use carbohydrate correction to determine the amount of insulin to take for a particular meal.
  - The provider determines the units of insulin per grams of carbohydrates.
  - If the ratio is 1 to 10, inject 1-unit insulin for 10 grams of carbohydrates.
  - If the meal has 60 grams of carbs, the dose is 6 units of insulin.
- Optimal nutrition for both type 1 and 2 diabetes:
  - Consume nonstarchy vegetables.
  - Limit added sugars, refined grains, and processed foods.
  - Try to eat approximately the same amount of carbs at each meal.
  - Portion control is very important. If eating out, portions are usually too big. Eat half and take the rest home.
  - Standard serving sizes include:
    - ○ 3 ounces of meat, fish, poultry (palm of hand)
    - ○ 1 cup or 1 medium fruit
    - ○ 1 to 2 ounces nuts or pretzels
    - ○ 1 ounce of cheese (tip of thumb)

POP QUIZ 10.1

An 8-year-old girl presents to her primary care physician's office for a well-child check, and the nurse notes weight loss since her last visit a year ago. The patient states she has been tired and thirsty. Her blood work shows blood glucose of 240 and hemoglobin A1C of 7.2%. What other questions would be appropriate to ask the patient and her caregiver on this visit?

DIABETES TYPE 2

Overview

- *Type 2 diabetes* is characterized by hyperglycemia, insulin resistance, and impaired insulin secretion.
- The incidence of diabetes type 2 has increased along with obesity since the 1990s, and it is considered preventable.
- Type 2 diabetes is a disease of insulin resistance.
- Type 1 and type 2 diabetes have similarities but also differences (Table 10.2).

Signs and Symptoms

- Blurry vision
- Darkened areas of skin, usually at the axilla and the neck
- Fatigue
- Nocturia
- Polydipsia
- Polyuria
- Vaginal candidiasis

Diagnosis

Labs

- Initial diagnosis:
  - Fasting plasma glucose greater than 126 mg/dL
  - HbA1C greater than 6.5 mg/dL
  - Nonfasting plasma glucose greater than 200 mg/dL
  - Oral glucose tolerance test greater than 200 mg/dL

COMPLICATIONS

Hyperosmolar hyperglycemic syndrome is a complication of type 2 diabetes. It presents as very high blood sugar glucose but little or no ketones present when measured using a ketone meter. Metabolic acidosis, dehydration, and decreased mental status are also present. It usually happens when the patient has not been diagnosed yet or has poor control of the disease. It can also happen when the patient has an infection.

NURSING PEARL

Point-of-care testing is done for many laboratory tests. The goal is to have better outcomes due to quicker results that allow treatment to begin sooner. Each test is more costly but has proven to be more cost-effective overall because it can shorten hospital stays and reduce complications. It is also associated with increased patient satisfaction and has been shown to increase adherence to treatment plans.

(continued)

Diagnosis *(continued)*

- Labs to differentiate between diabetes type 1 and type 2:
  - C-peptide levels (high levels suggest type 2; low levels, type 1)
  - Pancreatic antibodies (presence suggests type 1)
  - Serum insulin levels
  - Urine ketones (if present, more likely type 1)
  - Venous pH (if acidotic, more likely type 1)

Diagnostic Testing
There are no diagnostic tests specific to diagnose diabetes type 2.

Treatment

- Diet (see Diabetes Type 1 Patient and Family Education)
- Insulin replacement (Table 10.3):
  - Intermediate NPH
  - Long-acting glargine
  - Rapid-acting lispro
  - Short-acting regular insulin
- Oral medications: metformin (Table 10.3)
- Severe cases with ketosis/ketoacidosis referred to hospital
  - After acidosis resolves: metformin, with or without insulin
  - Initial management: high doses of insulin
- Treatment plan:
  - Appropriate weight-loss surgery referral if the patient is adhering to the plan but not progressing
  - Close blood glucose monitoring and medication adjustments as needed
  - HbA1C monitoring every 3 months
  - Increased physical activity
  - Weight loss encouraged

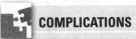

COMPLICATIONS

Type 2 diabetes affects almost every major organ in the body, including blood vessels, nerves, eyes, and kidneys. Long-term complications develop gradually over many years. Complications can be disabling and life-threatening and usually do not present until the patient is an adult. They include:

- Amputation due to severe nonhealing wounds or ulcers
- Fatty liver disease
- Heart and blood vessel disease
- High blood pressure
- High cholesterol
- Kidney disease
- Stroke
- Vision trouble

Nursing Interventions

- Educate patient and family about glucose monitoring.
- Ensure good nutrition.
- Identify children at risk and teach about healthy meals and increased activity.
- Monitor glucose and medicate when appropriate.
- Prevent skin breakdown and infection.
- Provide emotional support and actively listen to concerns.
- Provide hyper- and hypoglycemia education.
- Review adherence to a medication plan.
- Work with the patient and family if the patient struggles with the plan.
  - Ask the patient what specifically is hard for them.
  - Find resources to help (e.g., more practice time, games, books, internet).

Patient and Family Education

- Adhere to the follow-up visit regimen for success.
- Educate on the following:
  - Administering medications, including preparing and injecting insulin
  - Monitoring blood glucose levels and urine ketone levels
- Ensure good nutrition, exercise, and wound care.
- See Diabetes Type 1 Patient and Family Education.
- Use support groups.

 POP QUIZ 10.2

The family of a middle school-aged child brings the nurse's attention to the fact that they have to wait several days for testing each time their diabetes medications are adjusted, resulting in a hospital stay (due to fluctuating glucose levels) and frustration for the child. What could the nurse recommend and why?

DIABETES INSIPIDUS

Overview

- *DI* is a hormonal abnormality in which the patient's production of or response to antidiuretic hormone (vasopressin) is impaired, resulting in excess production of dilute urine.
- In children, it is divided into two subcategories.
  - Central
    - ○ Central DI is caused by damage to the hypothalamus or the pituitary gland, disrupting the production, storage, and release of vasopressin.
    - ○ Causes include:
      - ▪ Brain tumor that damages the hypothalamus or pituitary gland
      - ▪ Severe head injury that damages these glands
      - ▪ Complications of hypothalamus or pituitary surgery
      - ▪ Inflammation or infection of the brain
  - Nephrogenic
    - ○ Kidneys are unresponsive to vasopressin and produce dilute urine.
    - ○ Causes include:
      - ▪ Blockage of the urinary tract
      - ▪ Chronic kidney disease
      - ▪ High calcium levels in the blood
      - ▪ Idiopathic
      - ▪ Inherited
      - ▪ Low potassium levels in the blood
      - ▪ Medications (e.g., lithium)

COMPLICATIONS

Patients with DI may develop hypovolemic shock. Signs of hypovolemic shock include:

- Altered mental status
- Decreased peripheral perfusion
- Hypotension (late sign)
- Tachycardia
- Tachypnea

Signs and Symptoms

- Irritability and other neurologic symptoms
- Nocturia
- Polydipsia
- Polyuria: 3 to 20 quarts of urine per day

Diagnosis

Labs
- BMP
- Serum and urine osmolality
- Serum and urine sodium level
- Water deprivation test: urine, electrolytes, and weight check after 12 hours with no liquid intake

Diagnostic Testing

MRI of hypothalamus or pituitary gland.

Treatment

- Central: synthetic vasopressin, desmopressin (Table 10.3)
- Nephrogenic:
  - Anti-inflammatories: aspirin or ibuprofen to reduce urine volume
  - Calcium or potassium supplements to correct abnormalities
  - Low-solute diet: low salt and low protein
  - Thiazide diuretics (Table 10.3)

Nursing Interventions

- Administer IV fluids if the patient is unable to maintain adequate oral fluid intake.
- Educate patient and family about the disease process.
- Monitor I/O and urine output.
- Monitor labs.
  - Serum and urine osmolality
  - Serum and urine sodium levels
  - Serum potassium
  - Urine specific gravity
- Provide ice chips for comfort.
- Weigh daily.

Patient and Family Education

- Learn about the disease.
- Follow a low-solute diet.
- Devise a "sick-day" plan to adjust medication dosages when sick (see Diabetes Type 1 topic).
- Learn when to seek further medical attention.
- Weigh at the same time of the day.

HYPERTHYROIDISM

Overview

- *Hyperthyroidism* is a hormonal imbalance caused by the overproduction of thyroid hormone that affects growth and puberty.
- An insidious onset is characteristic of hyperthyroidism.
- Graves' disease is the primary cause of hyperthyroidism. With Graves' disease, autoantibodies bind to the thyrotropin receptor, stimulating the growth of the thyroid gland and the overproduction of thyroid hormone.

Signs and Symptoms

- Accelerated height
- Agitation
- Developmental delay
- Increased appetite, HR, and sweating
- Low HDL level
- Mood swings

 COMPLICATIONS

Thyroid storm is an acute, life-threatening event that presents with exaggerated hyperthyroidism symptoms: tachycardia, atrial fibrillation, agitation, fever, jaundice, delirium, nausea/vomiting, and anxiety. It can be caused by untreated hyperthyroidism, thyroid surgery, trauma, infection, or iodine overload. Labs show a low TSH and high T4/T3.

 NURSING PEARL

On physical exam, patients with hyperthyroidism may stare and have lid lag when closing their eyes.

- Neurologic tremor
- Poor sleep
- Weight loss

Diagnosis

Labs (normal)
- Serum thyroid antibody test
- Total T4 (normal: 5.0–12 mcg/dL): will be high
- Free T4 (normal: 0.7–1.8 ng/dL)
- Total T3 l (normal: 80–220 ng/dL)
- Free T3 (normal: 260–480 pg/dL)
- TSH l (normal: 0.5–5.0 mU/L): will be low

Diagnostic Testing
Radionuclide uptake and scan.

NURSING PEARL

High doses of biotin may cause false high levels of T4 and T3 or false low levels of TSH.

Treatment

- Beta-blockers to treat symptoms until a definitive solution
- Medications: anti-thyroid medications (Table 10.3)
- Definitive treatment; the destruction of abnormally functioning gland tissue:
  - Anti-thyroid medications (Table 10.3)
  - Radioactive iodine therapy (Table 10.3)
  - Subtotal thyroidectomy

ALERT!

Children are more sensitive to radiation than adults. Regardless of the source, both external and internal radiation from radioactive iodine therapy may cause sequela that may not be realized for years. One possible side effect is thyroid nodules, which are normally benign but should be investigated. Another possibility is thyroid cancer, but the prognosis is good if detected early. Lifelong follow-up is recommended.

Nursing Interventions

- Identify and manage symptoms.
- Monitor vital signs, including postural changes to blood pressure.
- Post-thyroidectomy, monitor for laryngospasm/airway swelling.
- Prepare family and school settings for emotional lability and irritability, which can interfere with studies and relationships.
- Provide a quiet, nonstimulating environment.

Patient and Family Education

- Recognize signs of thyroid storm and call the provider after the following symptoms:
  - Anxiety
  - Delirium
  - Fast HR
  - Fever
  - Nausea/vomiting
  - Yellow skin
- Provide information on the disease process and its effects on development, school performance, and behavior.
- Recognize the importance of:
  - Adhering to a medication schedule
  - Drinking fluids
  - Keeping follow-up visits
  - Monitoring diet, exercise, and weight
  - Providing a quiet environment that allows for rest and sleep

POP QUIZ 10.3

An 11-year-old patient is in for a checkup. They were diagnosed a month earlier with hypothyroidism and state they do not feel much better with her new medication, levothyroxine. When asked, the patients notes they take their medicine whenever they remember, usually around lunchtime along with their vitamin. What education should be provided to this patient about the medication?

HYPOTHYROIDISM

Overview

- There are two kinds of hypothyroidism that affect children.
  - Acquired:
    - ○ *Acquired hypothyroidism* is most often caused by autoimmune thyroiditis (Hashimoto thyroiditis).
    - ○ It can also be caused by thyroid disease and hypothalamus–pituitary disease.
  - Congenital:
    - ○ *Congenital hypothyroidism* is most often caused by an embryologic defect in the thyroid gland during development.
    - ○ It can also be caused by iodine deficiency. Taking iodine during pregnancy prevents this.

Signs and Symptoms

- Cold sensitivity
- Constipation
- Delayed permanent teeth
- Delayed puberty
- Depression
- Difficulty learning
- Dry skin
- Fatigue
- Menstrual disturbances
- Muscle weakness
- Poor growth and development
- Puffy face
- Thin hair
- Voice hoarseness
- Weight gain

Diagnosis

Labs
- T3 (normal: 80–220 ng/dL): will be elevated
- Free T4 (normal: 5–12 mcg/dL): will be low
- Newborn screening
- TSH (normal: 0.5–5.0 mU/L): will be high

Diagnostic Testing
- Thyroid radionuclide uptake and scan
- Thyroid ultrasound

Treatment

Levothyroxine (Table 10.3)
- Ideal dose: normal TSH levels and improved symptoms; monitor every 6 to 12 months as needed
- Monitor closely for 6 to 8 weeks
- Titrate upward slowly

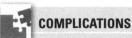

COMPLICATIONS

Prolonged, severe hypothyroidism can cause a myxedema coma, which is an endocrine emergency. Some of the symptoms include:

- Bradycardia
- Decrease in mental status
- Decrease in responsiveness
- Deposits of albumin and mucin on the skin
- Enlarged tongue
- History of thyroidectomy
- Hypoglycemia
- Hyponatremia
- Hypothermia
- Nonpitting edema
- Puffy face and hands
- Seizures
- Swollen lips, nose

Nursing Interventions

- Assess the thyroid by palpation to determine if firm, tender, or enlarged.
- Assess the thyroid from the front and side.
- Monitor for headaches or vision changes after initiation of levothyroxine.
- Monitor for hyperactivity.
- Monitor temperature.
- Promote rest.
- Protect against coldness and excessive heat.

Patient and Family Education

- Adhere to frequent follow-up visits.
- Avoid certain foods if low iodine levels cause hypothyroidism.
  - Cabbage, broccoli, kale, cauliflower, spinach
  - Highly processed foods
  - Iodine or selenium supplements unless otherwise directed by the physician
  - Millet
  - Nuts and seeds
  - Soy products including tofu, tempeh, edamame
  - Sweet potatoes, peaches, strawberries
- Common supplements, medications, or formulas may decrease the effectiveness of levothyroxine. Take alone.
  - Calcium
  - Concentrated iron
  - Fiber supplements
  - Soy protein formulas
  - Sucralfate
- Follow weight-loss plan when needed.
- Learn through self-awareness training why TSH levels fluctuate.
  - Medication dosage errors
  - Possible food interactions
  - Possible supplement interactions
  - The dose needs adjustment by the physician
- Take levothyroxine at the same time every day on an empty stomach.

OBESITY

Overview

- *Obesity* is one of the most important public health issues in the United States today and needs to be addressed early to prevent comorbidities.
  - An obese child is more likely to become an obese adult.
  - Behavior and genetics predispose a child to become overweight.
  - Communities can be involved in promoting healthy lifestyles by offering healthy food options and exercise opportunities in childcare centers, schools, and community activities.

COMPLICATIONS

Complications of obesity in childhood and adolescence include higher risk for inflammatory diseases, type 2 diabetes, and cardiovascular disease.

Psychosocial issues include poor self-esteem, anxiety, troubled relationships with peers, depression, and distorted body image.

- Economic factors come into play as children in low-income families have a higher rate of obesity than those in higher income families, possibly because of the availability of lower quality, cheaper food.
- Endocrinologists specialize in metabolic and hormone disorders and may be used to treat the patient if the obesity is caused by a physical problem.
- For severe cases, children's hospitals perform bariatric surgeries on teenagers.

(continued)

Overview *(continued)*

- BMI-for-age percentiles are used to measure obesity in children over 2 years of age.
  - Normal weight: between 5th and the 85th percentile for age and sex
  - Underweight: less than 5th percentile for age and sex
  - Overweight: between 85th and 95th percentile for age and sex
  - Obesity: greater than 95th percentile for age and sex
- Obesity is associated with many other health issues (comorbidities):
  - Asthma, sleep apnea, bone and joint problems, dyslipidemia (noted elevated concentrations of LDL cholesterol and a decreased concentration of HDL). It can also cause nonalcoholic fatty liver disease and gallstones. Impaired renal function is also more likely in obese children.
  - Endocrine concerns of obesity in children include glucose intolerance, diabetes mellitus, hyperandrogenism in females and onset of PCOS, and resulting abnormalities in growth and puberty.
  - Orthopedic complications include slipped capital femoral epiphysis, bowed legs, knock-knees, knee instability, knee pain, and tibial torsion. Obese children are also at higher risk for fractured bones.

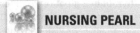 **NURSING PEARL**

In adolescents, the weight increase related to growth in height is accounted for in BMI. Therefore, a reduction in BMI is a better indicator.

Diagnosis

Labs

There are no labs specific to diagnose obesity. However, the following may be helpful when determining severity and treatment:

- ALT, AST
- Fasting glucose, HbA1C
- Fasting lipid profile
- Iron
- Vitamin D (low amounts may increase inflammation and impede weight loss)
- With high BP: electrolytes, BUN, creatinine, CBC, urinalysis

Diagnostic Testing

- Abdominal ultrasound
- X-rays of lower extremities

Treatment

- Counseling to establish goals and provide education for diet and activity
- Initial measurement of BMI and plotting on a chart to follow trends
- Medications for underlying conditions that may contribute to obesity (Table 10.3):
  - Diabetes: metformin
  - Diabetes, weight loss: liraglutide
  - Weight loss: orlistat
  - Hypothyroidism: levothyroxine
- Motivational counseling
- Referrals, if necessary:
  - Dietician
  - Mental health
  - Comprehensive weight management program
  - Comorbidities, as needed
  - Weight-loss surgery (adolescents only)

- Routine monitoring of BMI, assessment of obesity-related risk factors
- Structured weight-loss program

Nursing Interventions

- Explain medication side effects.
- Formulate an eating plan with family and patient.
- Identify realistic weekly goals for weight loss.
- Monitor blood pressure and blood glucose at well-child visits.
  - Obtain dietary and activity diaries as part of obesity evaluation.
  - Refer to a dietician to help educate patient and family.
  - Review medical, family, and psychosocial histories during physical exams.
  - There can also be psychologic problems such as anxiety and depression. Low self-esteem and issues with bullying can affect the obese child.
- Provide emotional support to family and patient.
- Provide information to family and patient on healthy diets and exercise options.
- Weigh periodically as indicated.

Patient and Family Education

- Learn about fad diets and why they do not work.
  - How to recognize a fad diet:
    - ○ Fad diets claim that a person can lose a great amount of weight very quickly.
    - ○ If it sounds too good to be true, it probably is.
    - ○ It limits entire food groups.
    - ○ Usually, they are costly (prepackaged meals or memberships)
  - They do not work because it takes time to lose weight and keep it off. Exercise is usually necessary. It is not healthy to ban entire groups of foods.
- Learn and practice behavior modification techniques.
  - Eat only while sitting down.
  - Do not watch television or talk on the phone while eating.
  - Keep tempting foods out of the house.
  - Stay out of the kitchen unless cooking.
  - Keep healthy snacks.
  - Do not skip meals.
  - Use small plates and bowls.
- Learn and practice strategies for dealing with cravings and temptations.
  - Go for a walk instead of snacking.
  - Drink water instead.
  - When tempted with a high-calorie treat, try to wait 20 minutes, and distract oneself with a physical activity.
  - Avoid grocery shopping when hungry or tired.

SYNDROME OF INAPPROPRIATE ANTIDIURETIC HORMONE SECRETION

Overview

- *SIADH* is characterized by excessive production of antidiuretic hormone in relation to the patient's fluid balance and electrolyte status.
- SIADH can be acute, where sodium levels drop rapidly, or chronic, where the symptoms gradually present over 48 hours or longer.
  - *Acute SIADH* is a medical emergency where the risk of complications is high.

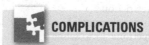

COMPLICATIONS

If not treated, SIADH can cause cerebral edema manifesting as confusion, hallucinations, seizures, and coma.

(continued)

Overview *(continued)*

- *Chronic SIADH* has less risk involved, and symptoms and complications are more manageable.
- Patients develop symptomatic hyponatremia if the serum sodium level drops to 125 mEq/L or lower.
- If the intake of water exceeds urine output, the ensuing water retention leads to hyponatremia.
- Causes of SIADH include:
  - Brain abscesses
  - Certain medications
  - Encephalitis
  - Genetics
  - Guillain-Barrè syndrome
  - Hemorrhage
  - Infection
  - Surgery, interventional procedures
  - Trauma

Signs and Symptoms

- Anorexia
- Irritability
- Malaise
- Nausea
- Obtundation (a reduced level of consciousness)
- Personality changes
- Vomiting

Diagnosis

Labs
- BUN
- Creatinine
- Glucose
- Plasma and serum potassium
- Sodium
  - 135 to 145 mEq/L: normal
  - 130 to 134 mEq/L: usually asymptomatic
  - 120 to 129 mEq/L: mild
  - Less than 120 mEq/L: severe
- Urine specific gravity

Diagnostic Testing
There are no diagnostic tests specific to diagnose SIADH.

Treatment

- Dependent on symptom severity and whether acute or chronic
- Two primary mechanisms to manage hyponatremia:
  - Fluid restriction
  - Sodium supplements
    - Hypertonic (3%) saline
    - Oral sodium supplement
- Must avoid correcting sodium levels too quickly

Nursing Interventions

- Administer medications as ordered.
- Assess muscular strength and neurologic status.
- Encourage foods with salt.
- Implement seizure precautions.
- Monitor fluid balance:
  - Daily weight
  - I/O monitoring
  - Mucous membranes
  - Skin turgor
- Monitor labs.
  - Serum and urine osmolality
  - Serum electrolytes

Patient and Family Education

- Family must also learn about the condition, the reason for fluid restriction, and the importance of daily weights.
- Listen to the body when rehydrating, but do not overhydrate; if athletic, sports drinks may be an option during vigorous activities.
- Take medications as ordered.
- Urine color is a good indicator of hydration status.

Table 10.3 Medications for Endocrine System		
Indications	**Mechanism of Action**	**Contraindications, Precautions, and Adverse Effects**
Antidiuretic hormone analog (vasopressin)		
• Treat central DI	• Antidiuretic effect by increasing water resorption at the renal collecting ducts	• There are no contraindications for antidiuretic hormone analog. • Use caution when discontinuing vasopressin, as it may cause DI. Monitor electrolytes, fluid status, and urine output after discontinuation. • Precautions include proper needle placement, as it can cause extravasation. It may also cause water intoxication. • Use caution in patients with migraines, renal disease, and vascular disease. • Adverse effects include atrial fibrillation, bradycardia, hyponatremia, renal insufficiency, decrease in platelets, and increased bilirubin.

(continued)

Table 10.3 Medications for Endocrine System *(continued)*

Indications	Mechanism of Action	Contraindications, Precautions, and Adverse Effects
Biguanide (metformin)		
• Treat diabetes type 2	• Decrease hepatic gluconeogenesis production • Decrease intestinal absorption • Improve insulin sensitivity	• Medication is contraindicated in type 1 diabetes, in the presence of diabetic ketoacidosis, or in patients with renal impairment. • Use caution in patients with heart failure, cardiac disease, and hepatic impairment. • Use caution and withhold if the patient experiences dehydration, fever, infection, trauma, surgery, or sepsis. • Adverse effects include GI symptoms at the beginning of therapy. • Adverse effects include chest discomfort, flushing, chills, dizziness, headache, dyspnea, and decreases in the absorption of B12 and folic acid.
Diuretics (hydrochlorothiazide)		
• Removes excess fluid from the body	• Inhibit reabsorption of sodium in the kidney, causing increased excretion of sodium, water, potassium, and hydrogen ions	• Medication can cause acute angle-closure glaucoma, acute myopia, hypercalcemia, hyperglycemia, hyperuricemia, hypokalemia, hyponatremia, hypotension, alopecia, rash, and toxic epidermal necrolysis. • Medication may cause abdominal cramps, anorexia, constipation, nausea/vomiting, gastritis, aplastic anemia, dizziness, restlessness, headache, vertigo, acute kidney injury, fever, and interstitial nephritis.
Glucagon-like peptide-1 receptor agonist (liraglutide)		
• Treat diabetes mellitus • Adjunct to diet and exercise for weight loss	• Increase glucose-dependent insulin secretion • Decrease glucagon secretion • Slow gastric emptying • Decrease food intake	• Medication is contraindicated in patients with history or family history of medullary thyroid cancer and in patients with multiple neoplasia syndrome type 2. • Use caution if an increased resting HR occurs. If sustained, manufacturer recommends discontinuation. • Use caution if patient has any psychiatric history. Medication can cause depression, suicidal thoughts, and mood changes. • Use caution in patients with renal or hepatic impairment. • Adverse effects include acute kidney injury, gallbladder disease, nausea, vomiting, diarrhea, abdominal pain, medullary thyroid cancer, and pancreatitis.

Table 10.3 Medications for Endocrine System *(continued)*

Indications	Mechanism of Action	Contraindications, Precautions, and Adverse Effects
Insulin: intermediate-acting (NPH)		
• Intermediate-acting insulin	• Lower glucose concentration by facilitation glucose uptake in muscle and adipose tissue • Regulate fat metabolism by enhancing fat storage • Increase protein synthesis • Inhibit protein breakdown in the muscle	• Medication is contraindicated in periods of hypoglycemia. • Ensure accurate dose and administration to maintain glycemic control and prevent hyper- and hypoglycemia. • Monitor potassium levels, as hypokalemia can result. • Use caution in patients with renal and hepatic impairment. • Adverse effects include hypoglycemia, hypokalemia, peripheral edema, injection site pruritus, swelling of extremities, and visual disturbance.
Insulin: long-acting (glargine)		
• Long-acting insulin to treat type 1 and 2 diabetes	• Regulate the metabolism of carbohydrates, proteins, and fats	• Medication is contraindicated in hypoglycemia. • Ensure accurate dose administration to maintain glycemic control and prevent hypoglycemia. • Monitor potassium levels, as hypokalemia can result. • Adverse effects include hypertension, peripheral edema, diarrhea, URI, depression, back and limb pain, and cataracts. • Administer as subcutaneous injection only. Medication is not for IV or IM administration. • Take at the same time each day. • Use only if clear and colorless.
Insulin: rapid-acting (lispro)		
• Rapid-acting insulin to treat type 1 and 2 diabetes	• Lower glucose concentration by facilitating glucose uptake in muscle and adipose tissue • Regulate fat metabolism by enhancing fat storage • Increase protein synthesis • Inhibit protein breakdown in the muscle	• Medication is contraindicated during episodes of hypoglycemia. • Use caution in patients with hepatic and renal impairment. It can cause hypoglycemia and hypokalemia. • Ensure accurate dose and administration to maintain glycemic control and prevent hyper- and hypoglycemia. • Monitor potassium levels as hypokalemia can result. • Adverse effects include erythema at injection site, headache, pain, cough, flu-like symptoms, and nasopharyngitis. • Do not mix with another insulin.

(continued)

Table 10.3 Medications for Endocrine System *(continued)*

Indications	Mechanism of Action	Contraindications, Precautions, and Adverse Effects
Insulin: regular/short-acting		
• Short-acting insulin formulation for use in diabetes type 1 and 2	• Lower glucose concentration by facilitating glucose uptake in muscle and adipose tissue • Regulate fat metabolism by enhancing fat storage • Increase protein synthesis • Inhibit protein breakdown in the muscle	• Medication is contraindicated during episodes of hypoglycemia. • Use caution in patients with renal and hepatic impairment. • Monitor potassium levels, as hypokalemia can result. • Caution is needed in maintaining glycemic control and preventing hyper- and hypoglycemia. • Adverse effects include peripheral edema, weight gain, and pruritus at injection site.
Lipase inhibitor (orlistat)		
• Obesity management	• Inhibit gastric and pancreatic lipases, which inhibits the absorption of dietary fats by 30%	• Medication is contraindicated in patients with malabsorption syndrome and cholestasis. • Use caution in patients with hepatic impairments, as the medication can cause severe liver injury. • Closely monitor patients with diabetes, as weight loss may affect glycemic control. • Adverse effects include gastrointestinal distress including oily rectal leakage, pedal edema, headache, fatigue, anxiety, and hypoglycemia.
Thyroid hormone (levothyroxine)		
• Treat hypothyroidism	• Act as endogenous thyroid hormone • Influence growth and maturation of tissues • Increase energy expenditure	• Contraindications include uncorrected adrenal insufficiency. • Caution is needed in patients with adrenal insufficiency. Treat with glucocorticoids before levothyroxine treatment. • Caution is needed in patients with benign thyroid nodules, CV disease, and diabetes. • Adverse effects include abdominal cramps, goiter, weight loss, alopecia, diaphoresis, cardiac arrhythmia, flushing, tachycardia, hypertension, increased liver enzymes, anxiety, fatigue, and dyspnea. • Take on an empty stomach 30–60 minutes before breakfast or 4 hours after evening meal. • Do not take within 4 hours of calcium or iron-containing products. • Do not give as a weight-reduction medication.

RESOURCES

Atkinson, M. A. (2016). Type 1 diabetes mellitus. In H. M. Kronenberg, P. R. Larsen, S. Melmed, & K. S. Polonsky (Eds.), *Williams textbook of endocrinology* (13th ed., pp. 1451–1483). Elsevier. https://www.sciencedirect.com/sd fe/pdf/download/eid/3-s2.0-B9780323297387000320/first-page-pdf

Bichet, D. G. (2021). Clinical manifestations and causes of central diabetes mellitus. *UpToDate*. https://www.uptoda te.com/contents/clinical-manifestations-and-causes-of-central-diabetes-insipidus?search=diabetes%20insipidus &source=search_result&selectedTitle=1~150&usage_type=default&display_rank=1

Bull, M. J., & Committee on Genetics. (2011). Health supervision for children with Down syndrome. *Pediatrics*, *128*(2). https://doi.org/10.1542/peds.2011-1605

Centers for Disease Control and Prevention. (2021). *Preventing childhood obesity: 5 things you can do at home*. U.S. Department of Health and Human Services, Centers for Disease Control and Prevention. https://www.cdc.gov/ nccdphp/dnpao/features/childhood-obesity/

Cheetham, T., & Boal, R. (2019). Graves' disease. *Paediatrics and Child Health*, *29*(7), 316–320. https://doi.org/10.10 16/j.paed.2019.04.006 https://www.paediatricsandchildhealthjournal.co.uk/article/S1751-7222(19)30092-7/ fulltext

Christ-Crain, M., Bichet, D. G., Fenske, W. K., Goldman, M. B., Rittig, S., Verbalis, J. G., & Verkman, A. S. (2019). Diabetes insipidus. *Nature Reviews Disease Primers*, *5*. https://doi.org/10.1038/s41572-019-0103-2

Counts, D., & Varma, S. K. (2009). Hypothyroidism in children. *Pediatrics in Review*, *30*(7), 251–258. https://doi.org /10.1542/pir.30.7.251

Deeb, A. (2017). Challenges of diabetes management in toddlers. *Diabetes Technology & Therapeutics*, *19*(7), 383–390. https://doi.org/10.1089/dia.2017.0130

Glaser, N. (2021, July). Diabetic ketoacidosis in children: Clinical features and diagnosis. *UpToDate*. https://www.up todate.com/contents/diabetic-ketoacidosis-in-children-clinical-features-and-diagnosis?search=hhs&source=sea rch_result&selectedTitle=4~150&usage_type=default&display_rank=4

LaFranchi, S. (2021a). Acquired hypothyroidism in childhood and adolescents. *UpToDate*. https://www.uptodate.co m/contents/acquired-hypothyroidism-in-childhood-and-adolescence?search=hypothyroidism&source=search_ result&selectedTitle=1~150&usage_type=default&display_rank=1

LaFranchi, S. (2021b). Treatment and prognosis of Graves disease in children and adolescents. *UpToDate*. https:// www.uptodate.com/contents/treatment-and-prognosis-of-graves-disease-in-children-and-adolescents?search=hy perthyroidism&source=search_result&selectedTitle=5~150&usage_type=default&display_rank=5

Levitsky, L. L., & Misra, M. (2021). Insulin therapy for children and adolescents with type 1 diabetes mellitus. *UpToDate*. https://www.uptodate.com/contents/insulin-therapy-for-children-and-adolescents-with-type-1-diab etes-mellitus?search=kinds%20of%20insulin&sectionRank=1&usage_type=default&anchor=H3940151930&so urce=machineLearning&selectedTitle=1~150&display_rank=1#H3940151930

Lexicomp. (2021a). Desmopressin: Pediatric drug information [Drug Information]. *UpToDate*. https://www.uptoda te.com/contents/desmopressin-pediatric-drug-information?search=desmopressin&source=panel_search_result &selectedTitle=1~117&usage_type=panel&kp_tab=drug_pediatric&display_rank=1

Lexicomp. (2021b). Insulin (Glargine): Pediatric drug information [Drug Information]. *UpToDate*. https://www.upt odate.com/contents/insulin-glargine-pediatric-drug-information?search=insulin&selectedTitle=1~150&usage_ type=panel&display_rank=1&kp_tab=drug_pediatric&source=panel_search_result

Lexicomp. (2021c). Insulin (Lispro): Pediatric drug information [Drug Information]. *UpToDate*. https://www.uptod ate.com/contents/insulin-lispro-conventional-and-faster-acting-pediatric-drug-information?search=insulin&se lectedTitle=1~150&usage_type=panel&display_rank=1&kp_tab=drug_pediatric&source=panel_search_result

Lexicomp. (2021d). Levothyroxine: Pediatric drug information [Drug Information]. *UpToDate*. https://www.uptoda te.com/contents/levothyroxine-pediatric-drug-information?search=levothyroxine&source=panel_search_result &selectedTitle=1~127&usage_type=panel&kp_tab=drug_pediatric&display_rank=1

Lexicomp. (2021e). Liraglutide: Pediatric drug information [Drug Information]. *UpToDate*. https://www.uptodate .com/contents/liraglutide-pediatric-drug-information?search=liraglutide&source=panel_search_result&selected Title=2~44&usage_type=panel&kp_tab=drug_pediatric&display_rank=1

Lexicomp. (2021f). Metformin: Pediatric drug information [Drug Information]. *UpToDate*. https://www.uptodate .com/contents/metformin-pediatric-drug-information?search=metformin&source=panel_search_result&selecte dTitle=1~148&usage_type=panel&kp_tab=drug_pediatric&display_rank=1

Lexicomp. (2021g). Orlistat: Pediatric drug information [Drug Information]. *UpToDate*. https://www.uptodate.com /contents/orlistat-pediatric-drug-information?search=orlistat&source=panel_search_result&selectedTitle=2~3 0&usage_type=panel&kp_tab=drug_pediatric&display_rank=1

Lexicomp. (2021h). Vasopressin: Pediatric drug information [Drug Information]. *UpToDate*. https://www.uptodate .com/contents/vasopressin-pediatric-drug-information?search=vasopressin&source=panel_search_result&selec tedTitle=1~148&usage_type=panel&kp_tab=drug_pediatric&display_rank=1

MedlinePlus. (2021a). *Diabetes*. https://medlineplus.gov/ency/article/001214.htm

MedlinePlus. (2021b). *Graves disease*. https://medlineplus.gov/ency/imagepages/17067.htm

National Institute of Child Health and Human Development. (2021). *Diabetes*. U.S. Department of Health and Human Services, National Institute of Child Health and Human Development. https://www.nichd.nih.gov/heal th/topics/diabetes

National Institute of Diabetes and Digestive and Kidney Diseases. (2015, October). *Diabetes insipidus*. U.S. Department of Health and Human Services, National Institute of Diabetes and Digestive and Kidney Diseases. https://www.niddk.nih.gov/health-information/kidney-disease/diabetes-insipidus

Physiopedia. (n.d). Grave's disease. *Physiopedia*. https://www.physio-pedia.com/Grave%27s_Disease

Ross, D. S., Burch, H. B., Cooper, D. S., Greenlee, M. C., Laurberg, P., Maia, A. L., Rivkees, S. A., Samuels, M., Sosa, J. A., Stan, M. N., & Walter, M. A. (2016). American thyroid association guidelines for diagnosis and management of hyperthyroidism and other causes of thyrotoxicosis. *Thyroid, 26*, 1343–1421. https://doi.org/10 .1089/thy.2016.0229

Somers, M. J., & Traum, A. Z. (2021). Hyponatremia in children: Evaluation and management. *UpToDate*. https:// www.uptodate.com/contents/hyponatremia-in-children-evaluation-and-management?search=hyponatremia&sou rce=search_result&selectedTitle=1~150&usage_type=default&display_rank=1

Sterns, R. (2021). Pathophysiology and etiology of the syndrome of inappropriate diuretic hormone (SIADH). *UpToDate*. https://www.uptodate.com/contents/pathophysiology-and-etiology-of-the-syndrome-of-inappropria te-antidiuretic-hormone-secretion-siadh?search=siadh&source=search_result&selectedTitle=1~150&usage_typ e=default&display_rank=1

HEMATOLOGY AND ONCOLOGY

IRON DEFICIENCY ANEMIA

Overview

- *Anemia* is a reduction in RBC count and/or hemoglobin concentrations.
- *Iron-deficiency anemia* is the most common type of anemia and is characterized by decreased hemoglobin production due to low iron levels. It can be acute or chronic.
- Possible causes include:
  - Blood loss
  - Decreased absorption of iron from the GI tract
  - Diets low in iron
  - Increased iron demand during growth spurts
- Risk factors include:
  - Cow's or goat's milk consumption before age 1
  - Low birth weight
  - Obesity
  - Premature birth
  - Restrictive diets
- Adolescents are at higher risk for iron deficiency due to:
  - Decreased body weight
  - Endurance training (athletes)
  - Heavy periods (school-age or adolescent females)
  - History of blood donation
  - Increased needs
  - Obesity
  - Vegetarian/vegan diet choice

Signs and Symptoms

- Brittle nails
- Chest pain or tachycardia
- Decrease in mental function
- Fatigue
- Hair loss
- Headache, dizziness, and lightheadedness
- Pallor
- Pica or pagophagia
- Restless leg syndrome

COMPLICATIONS

Patients with untreated iron-deficiency anemia can develop tachycardia and low oxygen levels, leading to heart failure and delayed growth and development.

ALERT!

Unmodified goat's milk and cow's milk is not suitable for infants. It is too high in protein and minerals and goat's milk in particular is too low in folate.

NURSING PEARL

LOW IRON Mnemonic

- **L** – Lethargy
- **O** – Overexerted easily
- **W** – Weird cravings
- **I** – Increased heart rate
- **R** – Reduced hemoglobin level
- **O** – Observed changes in RBCs
- **N** – Nail changes

(continued)

Signs and Symptoms *(continued)*

- Shortness of breath
- Tongue inflammation
- Weakness

Diagnosis

Labs

- CBC
  - Hematocrit less than 11 g/dL
  - Hemoglobin (two standard deviations below the mean for age)
- Ferritin less than 15 mcg/L
- Reticulocyte count
- Serum iron
- Total iron-binding capacity

Treatment

- Blood transfusion for clinically significant hematocrit or hemoglobin levels
- Iron-rich diet
- Iron supplementation to increase hemoglobin production and transportation of oxygen (see Table 11.2*)
- Treatment for any underlying occult bleeding

 ALERT!

Iron supplements may cause constipation and black, tarry stools.

Nursing Interventions

- Assess patient's diet and educate on iron-rich foods.
- Educate patient and family on iron supplementation.
- Monitor the patient for signs of occult bleeding.
- Prepare patient for administration of blood transfusion for severe anemia.

Patient and Family Education

- Include iron-rich foods.
  - Dark green leafy vegetables
  - Dried fruit
  - Iron-fortified cereals, bread, and pasta
  - Legumes
  - Red meat, pork, or poultry
  - Seafood
- Include foods containing vitamin C to enhance iron absorption.
  - Broccoli
  - Grapefruit
  - Kiwi
  - Leafy green vegetables
  - Melons and oranges

---

* Table 11.2 is located at the end of this chapter.

- Prevent iron-deficiency anemia in infants.
  - Do not give cow's milk or goat's milk to children under 1 year of age.
  - For exclusively breastfed infants, start an iron supplement at 4 months of age.
  - For exclusively formula-fed infants, additional iron supplementation is unneeded.
  - For infants over 6 months old, iron needs can be met through iron-rich foods/cereals.
  - Give breast milk or iron-fortified formula for the first year of life.
  - Monitor for anemia at well-child visits.

POP QUIZ 11.1

At a 4-month-old well-baby visit, the family tells the nurse that they are exclusively breastfeeding. What education should the nurse provide to help them prevent iron-deficiency anemia in their baby?

BLOOD PRODUCT ADMINISTRATION

Overview

- Blood products are used as replacement fluids for bleeding, volume depletion, deficiency syndromes, and surgery.
- Types of blood products are cryoprecipitate, FFP, PRBC, and platelets.
- Types of transfusion reactions include:
  - Acute hemolysis
  - Anaphylaxis
  - Delayed hemolytic transfusion reaction
  - Febrile nonhemolytic reaction
  - Sepsis
  - Transfusion-associated circulatory overload
  - Transfusion-related acute lung injury
  - Urticaria

Types of Blood Products

- Cryoprecipitate
  - Cryoprecipitate is prepared from plasma and contains fibrinogen, factor VIII, Van Willebrand factor, factor XIII, and fibronectin.
  - It is used to treat low fibrinogen levels.
- FFP
  - Administer appropriate volume: 12 to 15 mL/kg.
  - Ensure the product is compatible with the patient's blood type (Table 11.1).
    - It does not need to be Rh compatible.
    - It must be ABO compatible.
  - FFP is used to treat coagulation deficiencies or for loss of clotting factors.
    - Active bleeding
    - Disseminated intravascular coagulation
    - Surgery
- PRBC
  - Administer appropriate volume: 10 to 15 mL/kg.
  - Administer at room temperature within 4 hours of receipt from controlled storage to prevent bacterial contamination. If PRBCs are out of controlled storage for more than 30 minutes, they cannot be reused.

COMPLICATIONS

Blood administration complications may include:

- Febrile reactions
- Allergic reactions/anaphylaxis
- Circulatory overload
- Bacterial contamination; donors may have occult contamination
- Graft vs. host disease
  - Prevent by using irradiated products.
  - This is most likely to occur in high-risk patients, such as premature, low-birth-weight infants, chemotherapy patients, and patients with immunodeficiencies.
- Infection
  - Although extensively screened, it does happen. Products are screened for HIV, hepatitis B and C, human T cell leukemia, West Nile virus, and Zika virus.
- Iron overload
  - Patients getting chronic infusions may have iron overload; use chelation therapy to correct.
  - Use exchange transfusions in sickle cell patients to reduce this risk.
- Metabolic toxicity
  - Hyperkalemia may occur during exchange transfusion or massive transfusion.
  - Patients may develop hypocalcemia and hypoglycemia from the citrate in the preservative solution.

(continued)

Table 11.1 Compatibility of Recipient Blood With Donor Blood Components

Patient ABO Group	Whole Blood	Red Blood Cells	Platelets	FFP	Cryoprecipitate	Rh Factor Positive	Rh Factor Negative
O	O	O	Any	O, A, B, AB	N/A	O positive, O negative	O negative only
A	A	A or O	Any	A or AB	N/A	A positive, A negative	A negative only
B	B	B or O	Any	B or AB	N/A	B positive, B negative	B negative only
AB	AB	AB, B, O	Any	AB	N/A	AB positive, AB negative	AB negative only

Types of Blood Products (continued)

- Blood warmers are used in the following circumstances:
  - Cold agglutinin disease
  - Exchange transfusions
  - Massive transfusion
  - Rapid transfusion
  - Unstable infants
- Ensure the product is ABO and Rh compatible.
- PRBC are used to treat patients with anemia, bleeding, or as ordered before a surgical procedure.
- Platelets
  - Administer appropriate volume: 10 to 20 mL/kg.
  - Consider using an aphaeresis catheter for donation, which separates blood from platelets and returns blood to the donor.
  - Remember that the first choice is an ABO-compatible product, but any ABO and Rh could be transfused in urgent situations.
  - Platelets are used to treat thrombocytopenia or platelet dysfunction.

 NURSING PEARL

Because infants have higher blood volume per kilogram, they may need a volume at the high end of the range. Patients may be ordered a one-time dose of furosemide at the end of the transfusion if symptoms of fluid overload occur.

Signs and Symptoms

- Blood transfusion reaction symptoms include:
  - Anxiety
  - Bleeding
  - Chest pain
  - Dyspnea
  - Fever
  - Headache
  - Hematuria
  - Hypotension
  - Nausea
  - Pain
  - Pruritus
  - Rash
- Signs of needing a transfusion:
  - Bleeding or trauma
  - Hypotension
  - Low fibrinogen level

 COMPLICATIONS

Iron overload is a possible complication of multiple red blood cell infusions. If left untreated, it can cause organ damage. Symptoms are nonspecific, and develop gradually.

- Low hemoglobin
- Low platelets
- Tachycardia
- Volume depletion

Diagnosis

Labs
- CBC
- Type and screen

Nursing Interventions

- Prior to blood product administration:
  - Determine permissible level of hematologic support given patient's religious and spiritual beliefs.
  - Assess for any reactions to prior transfusions to determine if premedication is necessary.
  - Ensure type and screen have resulted.
  - Explain the procedure to the patient and the family.
  - Verify the provider has obtained signed consent.
- Steps during blood product administration:
  - Verify the correct patient and blood product.
  - Identify the patient using two-factor identification and verification of the armband.
  - Confirm ABO and Rh type compatibility of the product to the patient.
  - Use sodium chloride with blood products.
  - Use a dedicated vascular access device.
  - Obtain vital baseline signs.
  - Infuse blood product over ordered time, within 4 hours, due to risk of bacterial contamination at room temperature.
  - Record vital signs at the start of the infusion, 15 minutes after transfusion starts, and at the end of the transfusion.
  - Assess for change in vital signs, auscultate lung sounds for fluid overload, and assess skin for rashes during administration.
  - Obtain vital signs at the end of the transfusion.
- Steps to take if the patient has transfusion reaction:
  - Stop the infusion.
  - Start 0.9% sodium chloride.
  - Administer O_2 if the patient is short of breath.
  - Contact provider.
  - Administer antihistamine for mild reactions.
  - Monitor symptoms and treat as needed.

 ALERT!

Most Jehovah's Witnesses believe that voluntarily accepting a blood transfusion will affect their eternal salvation and object to autologous blood donation ahead of surgery as well. For some, blood products including immunoglobins, albumin, and coagulation factors are permitted, and apheresis, cardiopulmonary bypass, and other interoperative blood salvage systems may be acceptable. While this is the church's belief, not all church members will follow these rules. Check with each patient and family on their individual beliefs and inform them of any risks associated with refusing transfusions.

 ALERT!

If the only reaction or response is a change in temperature of less than 1 degree during a transfusion, the infusion may continue when symptoms subside.

(continued)

Nursing Interventions *(continued)*

- Provide emotional support to patient and family.
- Send the remaining blood product, the blood container, tubing, label, and transfusion record back to the lab.

Patient and Family Education

- Report any possible symptoms of a reaction to provider, as a delayed reaction may occur.
- Understand the procedure and reasons for blood transfusion.

POP QUIZ 11.2

Fifteen minutes after starting a blood transfusion, the patient tells the nurse that they feel "funny." The nurse asks for clarification, and the patient notes they feel like someone is standing on their chest. What is the most appropriate nursing intervention?

IMMUNE THROMBOCYTOPENIC PURPURA

Overview

- Formerly referred to as idiopathic thrombocytopenia purpura, *ITP* is an immune-mediated bleeding disorder in which autoantibodies destroy platelets.
  - Platelets form blood clots to prevent or stop bleeding.
  - With ITP, if platelets are destroyed, the patient is at risk for bleeding.
- Common viral illnesses that precede ITP by approximately 1 month include:
  - Epstein-Barr
  - HIV
  - Influenza
  - Varicella zoster virus
- It is considered primary ITP if there is no apparent cause.
- It is considered secondary ITP if thrombocytopenia occurs with an underlying cause.
- Reoccurrence after treatment is common.
- Secondary ITP can be caused by medications (rare in children), vaccines (MMR), or viral illness.
- Thrombocytopenia can be an incidental finding.

Signs and Symptoms

- Bleeding
- Ecchymoses
- Purpura
- Sudden appearance of petechial rash

Diagnosis

Labs
There are no labs specific to diagnose ITP. However, the following may be helpful when determining severity and treatment:
- CBC: platelets less than 100,000

Treatment

- Depends on bleeding severity, thrombocytopenia degree, and family's preferences
- No treatment required for asymptomatic patients or those with mild episodes
- Treatment options:
  - Glucocorticoid steroids (Table 11.2)
  - Intravenous anti-D to help increase platelets
  - Intravenous immune globulin, in addition to glucocorticoids to help increase platelets
  - Platelet transfusion

Nursing Interventions

- Monitor labs for decreased platelet levels.
- Prevent bleeding and injury. Watch for signs of bleeding.
- Prevent infections with appropriate hand hygiene.

Patient and Family Education

- Avoid aspirin and other NSAIDs.
- Delay live vaccines for up to 11 months after receiving intravenous immune globulin.
- Prevent infection, especially if taking steroids, by washing hands.
- Stress the importance of preventing injury to avoid creating a source of bleeding.
- Use stool softeners to prevent bleeding at the anus.

LEUKEMIA

Overview

- *Leukemia* is a cancer of the bone marrow that is responsible for producing blood cell lines.
  - Typically, leukemia is cancer of the white blood cells.
  - Patients with leukemia mass-produce immature WBCs called blasts.
  - The hyper-production of blasts suppresses the bone marrow from producing RBCs and platelets.
- There are two subcategories of leukemia most often seen in children.
  - *Acute lymphocytic leukemia* involves lymphocytes, immature B or T cells.
    - Acute lymphocytic leukemia is the most common pediatric cancer.
    - Almost 30% of children or teens with cancer have some form of leukemia.
  - *Acute myeloid leukemia* involves immature myeloid cells or blast cells.

COMPLICATIONS

Tumor lysis syndrome is an oncologic life-threatening emergency caused by massive tumor cell lysis and release of intracellular contents. It is characterized by electrolyte abnormalities from cell lysis releasing potassium, phosphate, and nucleic acid into the bloodstream. The increase in uric acid and phosphate causes acute kidney injury. Common symptoms include cardiac arrhythmias, diarrhea and vomiting, lethargy, and muscle cramps.

Signs and Symptoms

- Anemia
- Bleeding
- Bruising, petechiae
- Fever
- Headache
- Lethargy
- Pallor
- Palpable liver
- Recurrent infections
- Respiratory distress

Diagnosis

Labs
- Bone marrow aspiration and biopsy: cell types and sizes
- CBC with diff: very high WBC 100,000 to 400,000
- Cell morphology: blastocytes
- Cytochemistry
- Flow cytometry

Diagnostic Testing
- Chest x-ray
- CT of chest
- MRI
- PET scan

Treatment

- Chemotherapy (Table 11.2):
  - Induction phase
    - Goal: complete remission
    - Bone marrow examination for therapy response
    - Corticosteroids: daily
    - Chemotherapy during the first month (IV, oral, or intrathecal administration)
    - Radiation if needed for killing cancer cells or stopping their growth
  - Consolidation phase
    - Goal: Maximizing synergy and minimizing drug resistance
      - Combination of medications
      - Intensity depends on risk-group classification
    - Lasts 4 to 8 months
  - Maintenance phase
    - Less intense treatment regimen
    - Oral medications only
  - Prophylactic antibiotics for prolonged risk of infection
- Targeted therapy (Table 11.2)
  - Tyrosine kinase inhibitors
  - Immunotherapy drugs (blinatumomab)
- Radiation: used for treatment of leukemia that has spread to the brain, spinal cord, or testicles
- Stem cell transplant: infusion of stem cells to restore bone marrow, typically after higher doses of chemotherapy and radiation.

 ALERT!

Radiation treatment has advanced so much that some patients do not have any side effects. Others may have some side effects including skin problems like blistering, dryness, and peeling. Fatigue is another common side effect of radiation. Other side effects depend on the location of the therapy.

Nursing Interventions

- Administer chemotherapy, if certified to do so.
- Administer IV hydration to improve renal perfusion and to increase urine output.
- Assess and document patient's current height and weight. Chemotherapy dosing is based on body surface area.
- Assess the patient's emotional and social needs.
- Encourage fluids and maintain adequate hydration.
- Maintain a low level of activity.
- Maintain skin integrity and prevent further trauma from radiation.
- Manage central venous catheter.
- Monitor fluid balance and electrolyte levels.
- Monitor for complications:
  - Bleeding
  - Infection
    - Neutrophil count nadir is lowest 7 to 10 days after chemotherapy induction.
    - Septic shock or severe infection is most likely at or near the neutrophil nadir.

 ALERT!

Side effects of chemotherapy include alopecia, anemia, bruising easily, infection, appetite changes/weight loss, constipation, diarrhea, nausea, vomiting, infection, mouth, tongue, and throat issues such as metallic taste, pain, sores, stomatitis, mental fog, mood changes, peripheral neuropathy, and urine and bladder changes.

- Perform mouth care.
- Promote healthy nutrition and identify if the child cannot take in sufficient calories by monitoring weight and doing calorie counts.
- Provide emotional support for family and patient.
- Provide education regarding the side effects of chemotherapy (Table 11.2).
- Relieve pain as needed.
- Promote a healthy diet for the patient. It may be hard for the patient to maintain a healthy weight.
- Support side effects of chemotherapy with appropriate medications, as needed.
- Weight loss is common. Encourage healthy foods that patients enjoy. Weigh patients often.

Patient and Family Education

- Attend all follow-up visits and adhere to medication regimens.
- Contact provider with questions and report any concerns.
- Discuss any body image issues.
- Learn about the disease and treatment plans.
- Learn signs of infection and other complications.
- Seek out support for the side effects of treatment and how they affect daily life.
- Seek out support groups to help with possible socialization issues.
- Seek out resources for emotional support, if needed.

 ALERT!

High-risk patients may fail conventional therapy and require allogenic hematopoietic transplantation or a bone marrow transplant. Prepare patients and families for this possibility.

RETINOBLASTOMA

Overview

- *Retinoblastoma* is a highly curable cancer caused by a genetic mutation that forms in the retina of the eye.
- Types of retinoblastomas include:
  - *Heritable:* inherited gene mutation from parent, and retinoblastoma present at birth; can affect both eyes
  - *Sporadic:* gene mutation occurs after child is 1 year old
- Retinoblastomas typically occur in children less than 5 years old and affect either one eye or both eyes.
- A characteristic sign of retinoblastoma is *leukocoria*, known as the cat's eye reflex, which is a cloudy, white appearance of the pupil of the eye.

 COMPLICATIONS

Children with retinoblastomas are at higher risk for developing secondary cancers, commonly soft tissue sarcomas, such as osteosarcoma, even after the retinoblastoma has been treated or cured.

Signs and Symptoms

- Abnormal red-light reflex
- Blindness or poor vision
- Crossed eyes
- Glaucoma
- Heterochromia (different color of the iris)
- Pain
- Strabismus

 ALERT!

The *red reflex* is the reflection of light off the retina as it passes through the pupil. An abnormal red reflex, or whitening of the red reflex, is a sign of retinoblastoma and requires immediate examination by an ophthalmologist.

Diagnosis

Labs
Genetic testing for RB1 gene mutation

Diagnostic Testing
- Ophthalmoscopy exam
- CT or MRI

Treatment

- Chemotherapy: to decrease tumor size
- Photocoagulation: laser therapy to inhibit ability of tumor to receive nutrients
- Cryotherapy: freezing of the tumor
- Enucleation: removal of eye for severe cases

Nursing Interventions

- Educate family on retinoblastoma.
- Recommend genetic counseling.
- Provide support and resources such as social worker and chaplain during diagnosis and treatment.

Patient and Family Education

- Enucleation education
  - Prepare for procedure and expectations of prosthesis.
  - Learn about the need for eye patch after surgery.
  - Be prepared for facial appearance after surgery, with eye patch and some swelling or bruising.
  - Properly apply dressing changes and applying antibiotic ointment.
  - Clean prosthesis by soaking in hot water for several minutes.
- Adhere to follow-up appointment plan made by ophthalmologist.
- Ensure any younger siblings have eye exams in early infancy.

SICKLE CELL ANEMIA

Overview

- *Sickle cell anemia* is a genetic disease that causes decreased oxygen delivery and complications related to hypercoagulability.
- It causes the production of abnormal red blood cells that are sickle or crescent shaped.
- The sickle cells form clots or obstructions to blood flow more easily than healthy red blood cells, resulting in vaso-occlusive crisis complications such as hemolysis of red blood cells, damage to organs such as the liver and spleen, deep vein thrombosis, and pulmonary embolism.
- Risk factors include having a family history of sickle cell disease.
- Sickle cell anemia is inherited in an autosomal recessive pattern. It requires two affected genes; if only one gene is inherited, the individual is a carrier with sickle cell trait.
- Sickle cell anemia is more common in people of African, Asian, Indian, Mediterranean, and Middle Eastern descent and people from Central and South America.
- Sickle cells only live for about 10 to 20 days, and there are not enough healthy red blood cells to carry oxygen, which leads to anemia. Normal RBCs last for 120 days.

Signs and Symptoms

- Anemia
- Dactylitis (swelling of hands and feet)
- Delayed growth
- Dyspnea
- Infections and fevers
- Pain episodes and chronic pain
- Priapism (prolonged erection of the penis)
- Vision problems

DIAGNOSIS

Labs

- Blood smear for presence of sickle-shaped RBCs
- CBC to monitor for hemoglobin level
  - Hgb between 6 and 11 g/dL
- High-performance liquid chromatography
- Iron studies
- Newborn screening

Diagnostic Testing

There are no diagnostic tests specific to diagnose sickle cell anemia.

Treatment

- Primary goals for sickle cell anemia patients:
  - Decrease pain episodes and treat chronic pain
  - Decrease number of abnormal or sickle cells; increase healthy red blood cells
  - Prevent infections that may lead to sepsis
- Blood transfusions
- IV hydration
- Medications
  - Hydroxyurea (Table 11.2)
  - Opioids (Table A.2)
  - Prophylactic antibiotics (Table A.1)
- Oxygen therapy
- Stem cell/bone marrow transplant

Nursing Interventions

- Administer blood products or an exchange transfusion as ordered for severe anemia.
- Advocate for pain control.
  - Administer opioids.
  - Apply warm compresses.
  - Promote rest.
  - Remove restrictive clothing for perfusion.
- Assess for signs of infection and administer antibiotics as ordered.
- Keep extremities elevated to prevent swelling.
- Monitor perfusion and administer IV hydration.

COMPLICATIONS

Patients with sickle cell anemia may develop sickle cell crisis or an acute exacerbation that causes moderate to severe pain. Sickle cell crises are a direct result of hypercoagulation in the microvasculature, and complications include:

- Anemia
  - May be a result of splenic sequestration
    - Can lead to hypovolemic shock and death
    - Often reoccurs
    - Prevention: splenectomy
    - Splenic sequestration crisis: potentially life-threatening acute drop in hemoglobin
  - Will have compensated chronic anemia but can acutely get worse
- Cardiac: cardiomyopathy, heart failure
- Neurologic: stroke (ischemic and hemorrhagic), transient ischemic attack, seizures, encephalopathy
- Pulmonary
  - *Acute chest syndrome:* a syndrome caused by a new pulmonary infiltrate causing fever, chest pain, hypoxemia, wheezing, cough, respiratory distress; prevent with prophylactic antibiotics and immunizations
  - Asthma
  - Pulmonary hypertension
- Renal
  - Diabetes insipidus
  - Hematuria
  - Hypertension
  - Medication toxicities
  - Proteinuria
  - Renal infarct
  - Renal medullary carcinoma
- Skeletal
  - Avascular necrosis and osteomyelitis
  - Dactylitis
  - Osteoporosis

ALERT!

Rarely, individuals with sickle cell trait can experience pain crises, dehydration, low oxygen levels, or muscle breakdown related to exercise, extreme temperatures, or changes in altitude.

(continued)

Nursing Interventions *(continued)*

- Monitor respiratory status and administer oxygen as needed.
- Suggest nonpharmacologic ways to help alleviate pain, such as:
  - Acupuncture
  - Aquatic rehabilitation
  - Biofeedback
  - Cognitive behavioral therapy
  - Guided imagery
  - Hypnosis
  - Massage
  - Peer support groups
- Support family and patient by advocating for social worker, chaplain, and school assistance during hospital admissions.

Patient and Family Education

- Avoid extreme temperatures and changes in altitudes that could cause a vaso-occlusive crisis.
- Avoid smoking. Nicotine attaches to the hemoglobin and causes decreased oxygen delivery.
- Discuss self-esteem and social well-being.
- Prepare a list of triggers that precipitate pain, such as cold, low humidity, dehydration, stress, and menses.
- Remember that a compromised spleen causes an increased risk of infection, and it is important to follow infection prevention techniques:
  - Handwashing
  - Staying up to date on vaccinations
  - Taking prophylactic antibiotics as prescribed

 POP QUIZ 11.3

The nurse admits a patient with a history of sickle cell anemia for pain and shortness of breath. What should the nurse anticipate that the provider will order to treat this patient's pain and promote comfort?

Table 11.2 Medications for Hematology and Oncology

Indications	Mechanism of Action	Contraindications, Precautions, and Adverse Effects
Antimetabolites (hydroxyurea)		
• Treatment of abnormally shaped hemoglobin	• Increase hemoglobin F or fetal hemoglobin, which is larger and more flexible than other forms of hemoglobin • Decrease propensity of sickle cells to form clots	• Women who are pregnant or who may become pregnant should not handle the medication. • Individuals touching the medication should wear disposable gloves. • Do not administer live vaccines while taking hydroxyurea, as this can cause a life-threatening infection. • Medication is a carcinogenic agent to skin. Wear sun protection. • Medication can cause skin depigmentation and gastritis.

Table 11.2 Medications for Hematology and Oncology *(continued)*

Indications	Mechanism of Action	Contraindications, Precautions, and Adverse Effects
Iron (ferrous sulfate)		
• Correct low hemoglobin • Restore iron reserves	• Increase hemoglobin production • Allow for transportation of oxygen via hemoglobin	• Administer on an empty stomach or with orange juice to increase absorption. • Medication may cause constipation and black, tarry stools. • To prevent tooth staining, rinse the mouth with water or brush teeth after taking in liquid form. • Administer iron 2 hours before or 4 hours after calcium or antacids for optimal iron absorption. • Iron may decrease the concentration of levothyroxine. Administer iron 4 hours after levothyroxine. • Avoid in patients with ulcerative colitis or patients who received frequent blood transfusions.
Monoclonal antibodies (blinatumomab)		
• Treatment of ALL	• Bind to CD19 on B cells and CD3 cells on T cells	• Adverse effects include neurotoxicity, neutropenia, infection, and hepatotoxicity. • Monitor for fever, hypertension, anemia, thrombocytopenia, leukopenia, and weight gain, which have been reported more in children. • Medication is contraindicated in children less than 1 month old.
Tyrosine kinase inhibitors (imatinib)		
• Used for treatment of ALL and AML in patients positive for Philadelphia chromosome	• Inhibit tyrosine kinase which inhibits proliferation in leukemic cells from Philadelphia chromosome positive leukemia	• Adverse effects include nephrotoxicity, congestive heart failure, bleeding, and bone marrow suppression. • Medication may inhibit growth; take precautions against pregnancy in appropriate population. • Medication is contraindicated with vaccinations and should be avoided 2 weeks prior to administration of chemotherapy.

(continued)

Table 11.2 Medications for Hematology and Oncology *(continued)*

Indications	Mechanism of Action	Contraindications, Precautions, and Adverse Effects
Vinca alkaloids (vincristine)		
• Chemotherapy treatment for ALL and other cancers	• Exert cytotoxic effects on cell by interfering with microtubules	• Adverse effects include SIADH, ileus, seizures, alopecia, paresthesias, GI issues, dizziness, hearing loss, vertigo, rash, anemia, bone marrow suppression, and infection. • Use caution in patients with any neurologic problems and monitor for neurotoxicity. • Monitor for electrolyte abnormalities such as hyperkalemia, hyperphosphatemia, and hypocalcemia, which can be signs of tumor lysis syndrome. • Vaccinations should be avoided 2 weeks prior to administration of chemotherapy.

RESOURCES

American Association for Pediatric Ophthalmology and Strabismus. (2020). *Retinoblastoma*. https://aapos.org/glossary/retinoblastoma

American Cancer Society. (n.d.). *Treating acute lymphocytic leukemia (ALL)*. https://www.cancer.org/cancer/acute-lymphocytic-leukemia/treating.html

American Cancer Society. (2020, October 8). *Osteosarcoma risk factors*. https://www.cancer.org/cancer/osteosarcoma/causes-risks-prevention/risk-factors.html#:~:text=Some%20children%20have%20the%20inherited,soft%20tissue%20sarcomas%2C%20including%20osteosarcoma

Bussel, J. B. (2020, June). Immune thrombocytopenia in children: Clinical features and diagnosis. *UpToDate*. https://www.uptodate.com/contents/immune-thrombocytopenia-itp-in-children-clinical-features-and-diagnosis?search=thrombocytopenia&source=search_result&selectedTitle=8~150&usage_type=default&display_rank=8

Desmond, R., & Klein, H. (2021). *Blood transfusion*. https://oncohemakey.com/blood-transfusion/

Hockenberry, M., Wilson, D., & Rodgers, C. (2019). *Wong's nursing care of infants and children* (11th ed.). Elsevier.

Horton, T. M., Steuber, C. P., & Aster, J. C. (2021). Overview of the clinical presentation and diagnosis of acute lymphoblastic leukemia/lymphoma in children. *UpToDate*. https://www.uptodate.com/contents/overview-of-the-clinical-presentation-and-diagnosis-of-acute-lymphoblastic-leukemia-lymphoma-in-children?search=Overview%20of%20the%20clinical%20presentation%20and%20diagnosis%20of%20acute%20lymphoblastic%20leukemia%2Flymphoma%20in%20children&source=search_result&selectedTitle=1~150&usage_type=default&display_rank=1

Larson, R. A., & Pui, C.-H. (July, 2021a). Tumor lysis syndrome: Definition, pathogenesis, clinical manifestations, etiology, and risk factors. *UpToDate*. https://www.uptodate.com/contents/tumor-lysis-syndrome-definition-pathogenesis-clinical-manifestations-etiology-and-risk-factors?search=tumor%20lysis%20syndrome&source=search_result&selectedTitle=2~150&usage_type=default&display_rank=2

Larson, R. A., & Pui, C.-H. (July, 2021b). Tumor lysis syndrome: Prevention and treatment. *UpToDate*. https://www.uptodate.com/contents/tumor-lysis-syndrome-prevention-and-treatment?search=tumor%20lysis%20syndrome&source=search_result&selectedTitle=1~150&usage_type=default&display_rank=1

Lexicomp. (n.d.[a]). Blinatumomab: Pediatric drug information [Drug Information]. *UpToDate*. https://www.uptodate.com/contents/blinatumomab-pediatric-drug-information?search=blincyto&source=panel_search_result&selectedTitle=1~21&usage_type=panel&kp_tab=drug_pediatric&display_rank=1

Lexicomp. (n.d.[b]). Hydroxyurea: Pediatric drug information [Drug Information]. *UpToDate*. https://www.uptodate.com/contents/hydroxyurea-hydroxycarbamide-pediatric-drug-information?search=hydroxyurea&source=panel_search_result&selectedTitle=1~148&usage_type=panel&kp_tab=drug_pediatric&display_rank=1

Lexicomp. (n.d.[c]). Imatinib: Pediatric drug information [Drug Information]. *UpToDate*. https://www.uptodate.co
m/contents/imatinib-drug-information?source=auto_suggest&selectedTitle=1~1---1~4---gleevec&search=gle
evec

Lexicomp. (n.d.[d]). Iron: Pediatric drug information [Drug Information]. *UpToDate*. https://www.uptodate.com/c
ontents/ferrous-sulfate-pediatric-drug-information?search=ferrous%20sulfate&source=panel_search_result&se
lectedTitle=1~34&usage_type=panel&kp_tab=drug_pediatric&display_rank=1

Lexicomp. (n.d.[e]). Vincristine: Pediatric drug information [Drug Information]. *UpToDate*. https://www.uptodate.
com/contents/vincristine-conventional-drug-information?source=auto_suggest&selectedTitle=1~2---1~2---vin
cristine&search=vincristine

National Heart Lung and Blood Institute. (n.d.). *Iron deficiency anemia*. U.S. Department of Health and Human
Services, National Heart. https://www.nhlbi.nih.gov/health-topics/iron-deficiency-anemia

National Heart Lung and Blood Institute. (2020, September 1). *Sickle cell disease*. U.S. Department of Health and
Human Services, National Heart, Lung and Blood Institute. https://www.nhlbi.nih.gov/health-topics/sickle-cell
-disease

Powers, J. (2020). Iron deficiency in infants and children <12 years: Screening, prevention, clinical manifestations,
and diagnosis. *UpToDate*. https://www.uptodate.com/contents/iron-deficiency-in-infants-and-children-less-tha
n12-years-screening-prevention-clinical-manifestations-and-diagnosis

Powers, J. M. (2021). Approach to the child with anemia. *UpToDate*. https://www.uptodate.com/contents/approach
-to-the-child-with-anemia?search=anemia&source=search_result&selectedTitle=1~150&usage_type=default&
display_rank=1

Rodgers, G., George, A., & Strouse, J. (2020). Hydroxyurea use in sickle cell disease. *UpToDate*. https://www.uptoda
te.com/contents/hydroxyurea-use-in-sickle-cell-disease?search=hydroxyurea%20sickle%20cell&source=search_
result&selectedTitle=1~150&usage_type=default&display_rank=1#H4245273999

Tarlock, K., & Cooper, T. M. (2021). Acute myeloid leukemia in children and adolescents. *UpToDate*. https://www.u
ptodate.com/contents/acute-myeloid-leukemia-in-children-and-adolescents?search=AML&source=search_resu
lt&selectedTitle=1~150&usage_type=default&display_rank=1

Teruya, J. (2021). Red blood cell transfusion in infants and children: Administration and complications. *UpToDate*.
https://www.uptodate.com/contents/red-blood-cell-transfusion-in-infants-and-children-administration-and-co
mplications?search=blood%20product%20administratoin&source=search_result&selectedTitle=2~150&usage_
type=default&display_rank=2

Vichinsky, E. P. (2020). Overview of the clinical manifestations of sickle cell disease. *UpToDate*. https://www.uptoda
te.com/contents/overview-of-the-clinical-manifestations-of-sickle-celldisease?search=sickle%20cell%20anemia
&source=search_result&selectedTitle=1~150&usage_type=default&display_rank=1

Williams, H., & Tanabe, P. (2017). Sickle cell disease: A review of non-pharmacological approaches for pain.
UpToDate. https://www.ncbi.nlm.nih.gov/pmc/articles/PMC4733641/

MUSCULOSKELETAL SYSTEM

DEVELOPMENTAL DYSPLASIA OF THE HIP

Overview

- *Developmental dysplasia of the hip*, or hip dysplasia, is an abnormal musculoskeletal development that involves the acetabulum, proximal femur, and hip joint.
- It can be idiopathic or teratologic.
- Risk factors are family history of childhood hip disorders and birth in the breech position.

> **COMPLICATIONS**
>
> If untreated in infancy, children may develop a limp when they begin walking or one leg may be longer than the other.

Signs and Symptoms

- Asymmetric gait
- Hip clunk sound with abduction
- Restricted hip abduction
- Shorter affected leg
- Unequal gluteal folds

Diagnosis

Labs
There are no labs specific to diagnose developmental dysplasia of the hip.

Diagnostic Testing
- Barlow test
- Hip ultrasound
- Hip x-ray
- Ortolani test

Treatment

- Pavlik harness for infants
- Surgical reduction with a spica cast

Nursing Interventions

- Assess infant's hips and extremities for abnormalities.
- Educate family about possible need for modified car seat or securement devices.
- Evaluate for complications related to spica cast.
  - Assess for signs of infection.
  - Monitor neurovascular status and perform frequent neurovascular checks.
  - Monitor skin integrity.
    - Ensure skin is clean and dry.
    - Reposition frequently.
- Optimize skin integrity with Pavlik harness use.
  - Ensure harness is not causing skin breakdown.
  - Keep skin clean and dry.

Patient and Family Education

- Pavlik harness:
  - Adhere to the harness schedule. It is most often worn for 23 hours per day and is only removed for bathing.
  - Avoid using lotions or cream under the Pavlik harness.
  - Change diapers frequently to keep skin and harness clean.
  - Do not adjust Pavlik harness.
- Spica cast:
  - Do not put anything in spica cast.
  - Help with frequent position changes.
  - Keep spica cast dry.
  - Watch for pain, swelling, or blue toes.

 ALERT!

If lower extremities are itchy, do not place anything in spica cast. Use a hair dryer on cool setting to blow air down cast to relieve itchiness.

FRACTURES

Overview

- A *fracture* is an injury to a bone from an external applied stress.
- The most common fracture in children is in the distal forearm (radius or ulna).
- Fractures are most often caused by recreational activities, a motor vehicle crash, trauma, or incidents at home or at school.
- Common types of fractures in children include:
  - *Buckle*: raised or bulging area at fracture site caused by compression
  - *Closed (simple)*: fracture without a break in the skin
  - *Complete*: bone is divided into fragments
  - *Complicated*: fracture with injury to other organs
  - *Greenstick*: incomplete fracture, with compressed side bending
  - *Oblique*: slanting or diagonal across bone
  - *Open* (compound): fracture that protrudes through an open wound
  - *Plastic deformation*: bone is bent, but not broken
  - *Spiral*: circular and twisting around bone
  - *Transverse*: perpendicular or right angle to long axis of bone

 COMPLICATIONS

Fractures can cause a painful medical emergency called compartment syndrome. Compartment syndrome can result after a fracture when edema occurs. Pressure increases within that enclosed space and compromises circulation to the muscles, blood vessels, and nerves within that space. This can lead to decreased blood flow, ischemia, infection, and deformity. Important nursing interventions include performing frequent neurovascular assessments and monitoring the 6 Ps.

Signs and Symptoms

- Decreased ROM
- Deformity
- Ecchymosis
- Edema/swelling
- Pain
- Redness

Diagnosis

Labs

There are no labs specific to diagnose fractures.

 NURSING PEARL

6 Ps of compartment syndrome:
- Pain
- Pallor
- Paresthesia
- Pulselessness
- Paralysis
- Pressure

Diagnostic Testing
- CT
- MRI
- X-ray

Treatment

- Cast
- Surgical intervention
- Traction

Nursing Interventions

- Assess neurovascular status of affected extremity and compare to the nonaffected extremity.
  - Capillary refill
  - Pulse
  - ROM
  - Sensation
  - Skin temperature
- Assess skin integrity if wearing cast, traction, pin sites, etc. Perform pin care as ordered and assess for any redness, swelling, or drainage at site.
- Assess pain levels and administer medications as ordered and necessary.
- Assist with position changes and encourage active ROM as able in fingers or toes of affected extremities and unaffected extremities.
- Consult social work if fracture is from nonaccidental trauma or if abuse is suspected; report any abuse per policy.
- Escalate concerns of compartment syndrome to healthcare provider when symptoms present.
- Identify whether child's cast prevents safe transport in car seat or vehicle.
- Obtain history of how injury occurred.
- Prepare child for cast removal procedure when fracture is healed.

Patient and Family Education

- Avoid placing any foreign objects down or in casts.
- Continue passive and active ROM exercises.
- Continue to limit weight-bearing activities of lower extremity injuries and use crutches with movement.
- Follow up with orthopedics, pediatrician, and physical therapy as indicated.
- Keep affected extremity supported by a sling or by pillows.

 NURSING PEARL

Traction can be used for fractures to maintain alignment or used instead of surgery. Types of traction include:

- Skin: applied directly to the skin surface (Bucks, Bryant)
- Skeletal: applied directly to the skeletal structure with a pin, wire, or tongs (halo, cervical, external fixator)

JUVENILE IDIOPATHIC ARTHRITIS

Overview

- *Juvenile idiopathic arthritis* is an autoimmune disease that causes chronic inflammation of the synovial joints with joint effusion.
- It is characterized by onset before the age of 16, fever, and arthritis in one or more joints for 6 weeks or longer.
- Possible complications include difficulty with activities of daily living, walking, and playing.
- Remission is possible with treatment, but many patients have recurrent flare ups.

 COMPLICATIONS

In addition to causing synovial joint problems, juvenile idiopathic arthritis can also cause inflammation of the eye, or uveitis, which can lead to vision problems, glaucoma, and cataracts.

Signs and Symptoms

- Fever
- Joint pain
- Joint stiffness in the morning or after inactivity
- Rash
- Swelling

Diagnosis

Labs

There are no labs specific to diagnose juvenile idiopathic arthritis. However, the following may be helpful when determining severity and treatment:

- CBC to monitor hemoglobin levels
- CRP to monitor for elevated levels
- ESR to monitor for elevated levels
- Ferritin to monitor for elevated levels

Diagnostic Testing

X-rays.

Treatment

- Corticosteroids (Table A.3)
- DMARDs (Table 12.1*)
  - Etanercept
  - Methotrexate
- NSAIDs for symptom relief

Nursing Interventions

- Apply heat packs to affected joints.
- Assess pain and ROM.
- Encourage ROM exercises.
- Promote rest periods instead of naps during day to prevent stiffness.

Patient and Family Education

- Perform low-impact exercises regularly to help ease joint stiffness.
- Participate in physical therapy.
- Take warm baths to help ease joint stiffness.

 POP QUIZ 12.1

A patient is having a juvenile idiopathic arthritis flareup and complains of joint stiffness. What interventions would the nurse recommend to improve the stiffness?

OSTEOGENESIS IMPERFECTA

Overview

- *Osteogenesis imperfecta* is an inherited connective tissue disorder.
- It results in bone fragility, fractures, deformities, and restricted growth.
- The disorder can be classified as mild, moderate, severe, or lethal.
- Risk factors include having a family history of osteogenesis imperfecta.

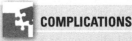 **COMPLICATIONS**

Osteogenesis imperfecta complications can include osteoporosis, hearing loss, and permanent deformities.

---

*Table 12.1 is located at the end of this chapter.

Signs and Symptoms

- Blue sclera
- Bone fractures (excess or atypical)
- Hearing loss
- Short stature
- Scoliosis
- Teeth deformities or discoloration

Diagnosis

Labs
- Bone mineral density
- Genetic testing

Diagnostic Testing
- Bone biopsy
- Dual energy x-ray absorptiometry scan
- X-ray

Treatment

- Medication: pamidronate (Table 12.1)
- Physical therapy
- Supportive treatment
- Surgical interventions: placement of rods

Nursing Interventions

- Assess skin integrity around casts, braces, and splints.
- Assist with braces, splints, and casts.
- Assist with position changes to maintain neutral alignment of extremities.
- Refer to physical therapy.

Patient and Family Education

- Adhere to physical therapy schedule and take medications as prescribed.
- Encourage use of assistive devices as necessary to prevent mobility limitations.
- Participate in low-impact exercises, such as swimming.
- Prevent fractures by avoiding activities that are high risk for falls or collisions.

OSTEOMYELITIS

Overview

- *Osteomyelitis* is an infection of the bone that causes inflammation. It can be acute or chronic.
- It typically occurs within the long bones.
  - Femur
  - Humerus
  - Metacarpals
  - Metatarsals
  - Tibia
- Onset is usually under age 5.
- Risk factors include trauma, wounds, open fractures, and foreign bodies such as implanted pins or screws.

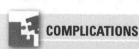

COMPLICATIONS

If osteomyelitis occurs in growth plates, it may lead to impaired growth.

Signs and Symptoms

- Fever
- Limited use of extremity
- Limping if lower extremity affected
- Pain
- Redness
- Swelling

Diagnosis

Labs

- Blood culture to screen for infection
- CBC to monitor for elevated WBCs
- CRP to monitor for elevated levels
- ESR to monitor for elevated levels

Diagnostic Testing

- Bone biopsy
- MRI
- X-ray

Treatment

- IV antibiotics
  - Cephalosporins (Table A.1)
  - Vancomycin (Table A.1)

Nursing Interventions

- Administer antibiotics as ordered.
- Assess pain and ROM.
- Monitor IV site.
- Monitor infection site for increased swelling or redness.
- Plan for placement of central access, such as PICC line, if intravenous antibiotics continue for longer than 7 days.

Patient and Family Education

- Follow up with physical therapy to help restore any lost function or ROM.
- Learn how to administer IV antibiotics at home.
- Restrict activity to tolerance.
- Take entire course of oral antibiotics.

NURSING PEARL

Vancomycin should be administered over at least an hour to prevent side effects and reactions, including vancomycin flushing syndrome, which is an itchy erythema that appears on the face and upper body and presents with tachycardia and hypotension.

POP QUIZ 12.2

A 6-year-old patient admitted for osteomyelitis of the femur has been ordered intravenous vancomycin to infuse over 30 minutes. Why should the nurse question this order prior to administering it?

SCOLIOSIS

Overview

- *Scoliosis* is a deformity characterized by a lateral curvature of the spine.
- It is more common in females and is typically diagnosed in school-age children or in early adolescence.

COMPLICATIONS

Scoliosis may lead to psychosocial issues such as having low self-esteem, feeling self-conscious about wearing a brace, and being embarrassed of poor-fitting clothing due to the brace.

Signs and Symptoms

- Asymmetry in scapula, shoulders, ribs, and hips
- Curvature of the spine

Diagnosis

Labs

There are no labs specific to diagnose scoliosis.

Diagnostic Testing

- Spine assessment using Adam's forward bend test
- Possible x-ray if positive bend test
- Spinal curvature measurement with a scoliometer

Treatment

- Brace to slow progression
- Surgery including spinal fusion or rod placement

Nursing Interventions

- Complete scoliosis screenings using Adam's forward bend test.
  - Observe children with an exposed back from behind as the children bend at their waist with their arms at their side.
  - Note any asymmetry of ribs, hips, or shoulders.
- Identify and discuss body image concerns about wearing a brace.
- If surgery is offered, provide preoperative education to patient and family.
- Monitor for postoperative complications:
  - Assess for postoperative bleeding.
  - Monitor pain level and administer analgesics as needed.
  - Perform a complete neurologic exam for 48 hours post-op due to risk of delayed neurologic injury.
  - Perform frequent neurovascular checks.
  - Provide skin care and assess surgical sites for signs of infection.

Patient and Family Education

- Brace:
  - Do not get brace wet. Remove it when swimming or bathing.
  - Wear brace as scheduled.
    - It is usually ordered for 13 to 18 hours per day.
    - Continue to use when playing non-water sports.
- Surgery:
  - Attend all orthopedic follow-up appointments.
  - Limit activity for 6 to 12 months or until spine has fused.

NURSING PEARL

Improperly fitting clothing in school-age children and adolescents can be indicative of scoliosis.

POP QUIZ 12.3

An 11-year-old girl complains that her shoulders appear uneven. What screening test is appropriate, and how is it performed?

Table 12.1 Medications for Musculoskeletal System

Indications	Mechanism of Action	Contraindications, Precautions, and Adverse Effects
Antineoplastic agent (methotrexate)		
• Reduce inflammation • Used to manage juvenile idiopathic arthritis	• Interfere with DNA synthesis, repair, and cellular replication	• Adverse effects include Stevens–Johnson syndrome, GI toxicity, bone marrow suppression, hepatotoxicity, and opportunistic infections. • Monitor liver function and albumin levels as well as monitor for neutropenia.
Bisphosphonate (pamidronate)		
• Decrease amount of calcium released from bones	• Inhibit bone resorption	• Adverse effects include hyperkalemia. • Monitor for dehydration and electrolyte imbalances.
Immunosuppressant (etanercept)		
• Used to manage juvenile idiopathic arthritis	• Bind to tumor necrosis factor and block interaction with cell receptors	• Adverse effects include inflammatory bowel disease in those with juvenile idiopathic arthritis. • Medication may increase risk of infection and malignancy.

RESOURCES

Arthritis Foundation. (n.d.). *Juvenile idiopathic arthritis*. https://www.arthritis.org/diseases/juvenile-idiopathic-arthritis

Beary, J., III. (2021). Osteogenesis imperfecta. *UpToDate*. https://www.uptodate.com/contents/osteogenesis-imperfecta-an-overview?search=osteogenesis%20imperfecta%20children&source=search_result&selectedTitle=1~76&usage_type=default&display_rank=1

Beutler, A. (2021). General principles of fracture management. *UpToDate*. https://www.uptodate.com/contents/general-principles-of-fracture-management-bone-healing-and-fracture-description?sectionName=Orientation:%20Transverse,%20oblique,%20and%20spiral&search=fractures%20in%20children&topicRef=6536&anchor=H6&source=see_link#H6

Centers for Disease Control and Prevention. (2020, July 27). *Childhood arthritis*. U.S. Department of Health and Human Services, Centers for Disease Control and Prevention. https://www.cdc.gov/arthritis/basics/childhood.htm

Children's Hospital of Philadelphia. (2018, November). *Osteomyelitis in children*. https://www.chop.edu/conditions-diseases/osteomyelitis-children

International Hip Dysplasia Institute. (n.d.). *Spica cast maintenance*. https://hipdysplasia.org/spica-cast-maintenance/

Lexicomp. (n.d.[a]). Entanercept: Pediatric drug information [Drug Information]. *UpToDate*. https://www.uptodate.com/contents/etanercept-including-biosimilars-of-etanercept-pediatric-drug-information?search=etanercept&source=panel_search_result&selectedTitle=2~148&usage_type=panel&kp_tab=drug_pediatric&display_rank=1

Lexicomp. (n.d.[b]). *Methotrexate: Pediatric drug information [Drug Information]*. *UpToDate*. https://www.uptodate.com/contents/methotrexate-pediatric-drug-information?search=methotrexate&source=panel_search_result&selectedTitle=2~148&usage_type=panel&kp_tab=drug_pediatric&display_rank=1

Lexicomp. (n.d.[c]). Pamidronate: Pediatric drug information [Drug Information]. *UpToDate*. https://www.uptodate.com/contents/pamidronate-pediatric-drug-information?search=pamidronate&source=panel_search_result&selectedTitle=2~71&usage_type=panel&kp_tab=drug_pediatric&display_rank=1

Lexicomp. (n.d.[d]). Prednisone: Pediatric drug information [Drug Information]. *UpToDate*. https://www.uptodate
.com/contents/prednisone-pediatric-drug-information?search=prednisone&source=panel_search_result&select
edTitle=2~148&usage_type=panel&kp_tab=drug_pediatric&display_rank=1

Lexicomp. (n.d.[e]). Vancomycin: Pediatric drug information [Drug Information]. *UpToDate*. https://www.uptodate
.com/contents/vancomycin-pediatric-drug-information?search=vancomycin&source=panel_search_result&sele
ctedTitle=2~148&usage_type=panel&kp_tab=drug_pediatric&display_rank=1

McGraw Hill Medical. (n.d). Vancomycin [Drug Information]. *Davis's Drug Guide for Rehabilitation Professionals*.
https://fadavispt.mhmedical.com/content.aspx?bookid=1873&sectionid=139029768

OrthoInfo. (2018). *Developmental dislocation (dysplasia) of the hip*. https://orthoinfo.aaos.org/en/diseases--conditio
ns/developmental-dislocation-dysplasia-of-the-hip-ddh/

Pediatric Infectious Disease Society. (2021, April). *Pediatric Infectious Disease Society endorses new terminology:
Vancomycin flushing syndrome*. https://pids.org/wp-content/uploads/2021/04/PIDS-Endorses-New-Terminology
_Vanc-Flushing-Syn_Final_4.27.21-1.pdf

Scherl, S. (2021). Adolescent idiopathic scoliosis. *UpToDate*. https://www.uptodate.com/contents/adolescent-idiopat
hic-scoliosis-management-and-prognosis?search=scoliosis%20treatment&source=search_result&selectedTitle=
1~150&usage_type=default&display_rank=1#H6

The Spinal Program at Boston's Children's Hospital. (n.d). School nurse's guide to scoliosis. *Boston Children's
Hospital*. https://www.childrenshospital.org/-/media/Centers-and-Services/Programs/O_Z/Spine-Division/Scoli
osisEBook.ashx?la=en&hash=F14737FD524A6751BBC1448C51667CE52B84AC1B

13

INTEGUMENTARY SYSTEM

BURNS

Overview

- *Burns* can be caused by heat, cold, chemicals, electricity, or radiation.
- The severity of a burn is based on the percentage of TBSA.
  - Minor: less than 10% of TBSA
  - Moderate: 10% to 20% of TBSA
  - Major: greater than 20% of TBSA

Signs and Symptoms

Burns can be classified as follows:
- First-degree: superficial
  - Affects the epidermal layer
  - Erythema
  - Pain
- Second-degree: partial thickness
  - Affects the epidermal and dermal layer
  - Blistering, moist, and red in appearance
  - Pain
- Third-degree: full thickness
  - Affects the epidermal layer, dermal layer, and subcutaneous tissue
  - Discoloration: red, tan, waxy white, brown, black
  - Dry, leathery appearance
  - Nerve endings and hair follicles destroyed
- Fourth degree
  - Damage to muscle, fascia, and tendons
  - Possible exposure of ligaments and bones

Diagnosis

Labs
- ABG for patients with inhalation injuries
- BMP for kidney function and fluid shifts
- Carboxyhemoglobin for carbon monoxide
- CBC for low hemoglobin, hematocrit, and platelet count
- Urinalysis for myoglobin level

COMPLICATIONS

Burn shock is a complication of severe burns due to fluid loss, inadequate circulation, and airway compromise. Patients should be monitored for changes in vital signs, urine output, respiratory status, gas exchange, and neurologic status.

ALERT!

The Lund–Browder diagram (Figure 13.1) is more accurate than the rule of nines for estimating the TBSA of burns in children due to infants and young children having larger heads and smaller lower extremities than adults.

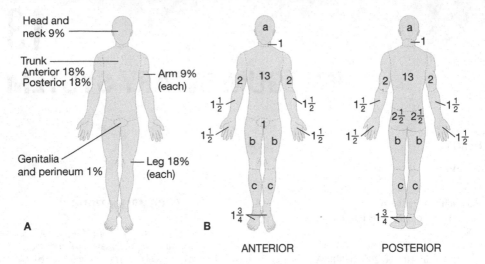

Relative percentage of body surface areas (% BSA) affected by growth

	0 yr	1 yr	5 yr	10 yr	15 yr
a - $\frac{1}{2}$ of head	$9\frac{1}{2}$	$8\frac{1}{2}$	$6\frac{1}{2}$	$5\frac{1}{2}$	$4\frac{1}{2}$
b - $\frac{1}{2}$ of 1 thigh	$2\frac{3}{4}$	$3\frac{1}{4}$	4	$4\frac{1}{4}$	$4\frac{1}{2}$
c - $\frac{1}{2}$ of 1 lower leg	$2\frac{1}{2}$	$2\frac{1}{2}$	$2\frac{3}{4}$	3	$3\frac{1}{4}$

(A) Rule of "nines"

(B) Lund–Browder diagram for estimating extent of burns

Figure 13.1 Lund–Browder diagram for estimating extent of burns in children.

Source: U.S. Department of Health and Human Services: Radiation Emergency Medical Management. Adapted from Artz, C. P., & Moncrief, J. A. (1969). *The Treatment of Burns* (2nd ed.), WB Saunders Company. https://remm.hhs.gov/burns.htm

Diagnostic Testing
- Chest x-ray for smoke injury

Treatment

- Analgesics
- Debridement for partial-thickness burns
- Fluid replacement with lactated Ringer's solution
  - Parkland formula used for burns greater than 10% of TBSA
  - Formula: 3 mL/kg/%TBSA to be given over 24 hours
  - Administration:
    - First half of the total amount over the first 8 hours
    - Second half of the total amount over the next 16 hours
- Skin coverings:
  - Allograft
  - Synthetic skin covering
  - Xenograft

- Surgical excision and grafting for full-thickness burns:
  - Mesh graft
  - Sheet graft
- Topical antimicrobial agents:
  - Bismuth-impregnated petroleum gauze: for small superficial or partial-thickness burns
  - Chlorhexidine: for superficial or partial-thickness burns
- Topical antimicrobial ointments (Table 13.1*):
  - Bacitracin
  - Neomycin
  - Polymyxin B

Nursing Interventions

- Administer tetanus vaccine (or immunoglobulin) if not up to date.
- Assess pain and administer analgesics as ordered.
- Assess skin integrity and monitor burns and dressings.
- Change dressings as ordered and as tolerated.
- Encourage a high-protein, high-calorie diet to promote healing.
- Manage vascular access, including if located on burned skin.
- Monitor vital signs, urine output, neurologic status, and neurovascular checks.
- Place NG or ND tube for feeding to promote nutrition.
- Promote comfort, rest, and psychosocial support.
- Report nonaccidental burns or suspected abuse as appropriate.

Patient and Family Education

- Recognize the importance of preventing burns.
  - Cover electrical outlets.
  - Install smoke detectors on each floor of the home.
  - Keep the following out of the reach of children:
    - Burning candles
    - Chemicals
    - Electrical cords
    - Hot liquids
    - Lighters or matches
  - Teach fire safety, including stop, drop, and roll and an escape route from home.
  - Test bath water or any heated liquid or food before giving it to a child and keep hot water heater set to 120 °F (48.8 °C) or less.
- Encourage recovery following a burn.
  - Attend all follow-up medical appointments.
  - Perform ROM exercises and activities as tolerated.
  - Perform dressing changes as instructed.
  - Remain adequately hydrated and continue a high-protein, high-calorie diet for healing.
  - Wear pressure garments to prevent scarring if ordered.
  - Remain up to date on immunizations, specifically DTaP and Tdap.

 POP QUIZ 13.1

A 35 lb, or 15.9 kg, 5-year-old has suffered major burns from a house fire on their back and the back of their legs, equaling 25% TBSA. Using the Parkland formula, how much total lactated Ringer's solution should the nurse plan to administer to provide fluid replacement for this child? What is the rate per hour for the first 8 hours of replacement?

---

* Table 13.1 is located at the end of this chapter.

IMPETIGO

Overview

- *Impetigo* is a bacterial skin infection caused by group A *streptococcus* and *Staphylococcus aureus* organisms that start as a red macule and become vesicular.
- It is a contagious infection around the mouth, nose, arms, or legs.
- Toddlers and preschoolers are the most common age groups to be affected.

> **COMPLICATIONS**
>
> Although rare, *poststreptococcal glomerulonephritis* can occur after having impetigo caused by group A *streptococcus*.

Signs and Symptoms

- Dry, honey-colored crusts
- Pruritus
- Red sores around mouth, nose, arms, or legs

Diagnosis

Labs
Culture of exudate

Diagnostic Testing
There are no diagnostic tests specific to diagnose impetigo.

Treatment

Antibiotics:
- Topical ointment: mupirocin (Table 13.1)
- Oral antibiotics for severe cases

Nursing Interventions

- Prevent the spread of infection with hand hygiene.
- Prevent the spread of infection for hospitalized patients by initiating contact precautions per facility guidelines.
- Recommend follow-up with a healthcare provider if new sores appear after initiating treatment.

Patient and Family Education

- Avoid sharing towels while infected with impetigo.
- Avoid swimming while the infection is active.
- Clean sores with mild soap and water.
- Cover draining sores with a bandage to prevent touching and spreading infection.
- Perform hand hygiene for prevention.
- Return to school is possible 24 hours after starting oral antibiotics and covering sores.
- Wash clothing, bedding, and towels each day.

PEDICULOSIS (LICE)

Overview

- Lice, or *pediculosis capitis*, is a parasitic infection of the scalp and head common among school-age children.
- The infection is spread by direct contact with infected persons or objects such as bedding, clothing, hairbrushes, and hats.
- The parasites are found on the hair and survive by feeding on human blood.

Signs and Symptoms

- Itching head and hair
- Observable white nits in the hair

Treatment

- Pediculicides (Table 13.1): permethrin shampoo
- Removal of nits

Nursing Interventions

- Inspect head and scalp.
- Monitor for secondary skin infections.
- Reassure the family that anyone can get lice.
- Utilize distraction techniques to prevent scratching.

Patient and Family Education

- Avoid sharing hats, hairbrushes, combs, and hair accessories.
- While infected, comb hair daily with a metal comb to remove nits.
- Have all household members checked for lice and treated if active infections are found.
- Place nonwashable items in a sealed bag for 14 days.
- Repeat treatment with permethrin shampoo on day 9.
- Review shampoo application instructions and expected course of nit treatment.
- Soak hairbrushes, combs, and hair accessories in boiling water.
- Wash bedding, clothing, and towels in 130 °F (54.4 °C) hot water and dry in a hot dryer.

COMPLICATIONS

Infestations of *pediculus humanus corporis*, or body lice, cause infected skin areas to be thick and dark due to the many bites. Body lice are also known to carry diseases such as typhus and relapsing fever. *Pthirus pubis*, or pubic lice, are usually found on pubic hair and if found on children may be a sign of sexual exposure or abuse.

PRESSURE INJURY RISK

Overview

- A *pressure injury* is localized skin damage, most commonly over a bony prominence, the sacrum, ears, or occiput, and may include various levels of tissue involvement.
- Risk factors include:
  - Chronic illness
  - Cognitive impairment
  - Impaired perfusion
  - Limited mobility
  - Long hospitalizations
  - Loss of sensation

COMPLICATIONS

Deep tissue injuries can occur from prolonged pressure and present with nonblanchable discoloration of intact or nonintact skin that can be red, maroon, or purple. Common presenting symptoms are pain and elevated temperature at the injury site.

Overview *(continued)*

- Medical device use:
  - ○ NIPPV interfaces
  - ○ Pulse ox probes
  - ○ Tracheostomies
- Nutritional deficiency

Signs and Symptoms

- Stage 1 pressure ulcer:
  - Intact skin
  - Nonblanchable erythema
- Stage 2 pressure ulcer:
  - Open ulcer with red or pink wound bed or serosanguineous filled blister
  - Partial-thickness skin loss with exposed dermis
- Stage 3 pressure ulcer:
  - Full-thickness tissue loss
  - Possible undermining and tunneling
  - Visible subcutaneous fat
- Stage 4 pressure ulcer:
  - Exposed muscle, tendon, or bone
  - Full-thickness tissue loss
  - Possible slough or eschar tissue
  - Undermining and tunneling often present
- Unstageable:
  - Obscured full-thickness tissue loss
  - Slough or eschar cover base of an ulcer

Treatment

- Topical antimicrobial dressings
- Wound care for open wounds

Nursing Interventions

- Apply preventative protection, such as foam dressings.
- Assess skin after procedures and surgeries.
- Assess skin frequently under devices, casts, splints, and tracheostomy collars.
- Change dressings according to policy.
- Complete Braden Q risk assessment.
- Consult wound care nurse for any skin breakdown; early recognition and treatment prevent further damage.
- Keep dressings clean, dry, and intact.
- Monitor nutrition status.
- Protect moist skin with a barrier cream.
- Turn or reposition patients who have impaired mobility at least every 2 hours.

 NURSING PEARL

The Braden Q scale is used for predicting pediatric pressure ulcer risk based on categories of mobility, activity, sensory perception, moisture, friction/shear, nutrition, tissue perfusion, and oxygenation. The lower the score, the higher the risk for injury.

Patient and Family Education

- Maintain activity, changing position, and movement as able.
- Ensure proper nutrition and hydration.
- Keep the area of injury clean.
- Observe skin for any changes, tears, or blisters.
- Review positioning needed to prevent pressure injury.

POP QUIZ 13.2

A 13-year-old nonambulatory patient with a history of obstructive sleep apnea and feeding intolerances requiring a GT has had a prolonged hospital stay trying to manage a feeding schedule. What risk factors for pressure injury should the nurse recognize?

TINEA INFECTIONS (RINGWORM)

Overview

- A *tinea infection* is a superficial fungal infection on the skin, scalp, or nails.
- *Tinea capitis* is ringworm of the scalp.
- *Tinea corporis* is a ringworm of the body.
- *Tinea pedis* is commonly known as athlete's foot and is usually found between the toes or plantar surface of feet.

COMPLICATIONS

Untreated athlete's foot or scratching *tinea corporis* can lead to a fungal infection of the nail, *tinea unguium*, or a bacterial infection.

Signs and Symptoms

- Tinea capitis
  - Alopecia
  - Pruritic
  - Scaly lesion
- Tinea corporis
  - Annular, ring-shaped plaque
  - Circular or oval
  - Erythematous scaly plaque
  - Spreads centrifugally with a raised border and clears centrally
- Tinea pedis
  - Lesions between toes
  - Patches on the plantar surface of feet
  - Pruritic, erythematous scales

Diagnosis

Labs

- Fungal cultures
- KOH preparation: uses potassium hydroxide solution to diagnose fungal infections

Diagnostic Testing

There are no diagnostic tests specific to diagnose tinea infections.

Treatment

Antifungals (Table 13.1)
- Griseofulvin
- Terbinafine
- Topical cream, ointment, or powder: nystatin

Nursing Interventions

Encourage good hygiene habits to prevent infection.

Patient and Family Education

- Avoid sharing clothing, socks, hats, and towels with affected children.
- Avoid touching the affected area to prevent spreading.
- Examine household pets for symptoms, as it can spread from animal to human.
- Keep feet dry after showering, swimming, or sweating.
- Practice proper hygiene after doing activities on gymnasium mats.

POP QUIZ 13.3

A high-school student presents with a red circular-shaped plaque on the forearm that is clear in the center and asks how they can make it go away. What education should the nurse give for treatment and prevention?

WOUND CARE

Overview

- Assessment of wounds includes the following:
  - Color, drainage, edges, and odor
  - Location on body
  - Size, length, width, and depth
  - Skin and tissue involvement: Staging pressure injuries
  - Wound bed
    - Granulation tissue
    - Necrotic tissue
    - Tunneling
- Common pediatric wounds include:
  - Abrasions
  - Diaper dermatitis
  - Lacerations
  - Moisture associated skin damage:
    - Incontinence-associated dermatitis
    - Intertriginous dermatitis
    - Periwound moisture-associated dermatitis
    - Peristomal-associated dermatitis
  - Pressure injuries
  - Skin tears
  - Surgical incisions
- Complications of wound healing include:
  - Further damage to the skin, blood vessels, or tissue
  - Infections
- Expected wound healing includes:
  - Inflammation around the injury
  - Scab formation as the skin heals and new tissue forms
  - Scarring at the site

COMPLICATIONS

Surgical wound dehiscence is a post-op emergency where the incision separates, commonly due to too much stress applied too soon after surgery. It can lead to evisceration when internal organs protrude through. The nurse should manage these complications by staying with the patient to monitor for shock, calling for help, notifying the provider, and placing a sterile soaked dressing over the incision opening.

Signs and Symptoms

- Color
  - Ecchymosis
  - Erythema
  - Pallor

- Edges
  - Approximated
  - Defined
  - Diffuse
  - Edematous
- Exudate
  - Purulent
  - Sanguineous
  - Serosanguineous
  - Serous
- Tissue
  - Granulation: beefy red, shiny
  - Necrotic: soft gray slough and hard leathery eschar

Treatment

- Antimicrobial agents:
  - Medical honey for environmental moisture and bacteria dehydration
  - Silver containing dressings for short-term use
- Debridement for necrotic tissue:
  - *Autolytic debridement*: dressings that support moisture retention
  - *Enzymatic debridement*: topical agent that liquefies necrotic tissue with enzymes
  - *Surgical debridement*: sterile procedure for removing decaying tissue
- Negative pressure wound therapy, known as *wound vac*, for tissue edema, perfusion increase, exudate removal, and granulation tissue formation
- Vacuum-assisted closure, or wound vac, to help wounds heal by using a device to decrease air pressure on the wound by removing fluid, reducing inflammation, and bringing edges together
- Wet-to-dry dressings: sterile solution and gauze over the wound; changed when dry or indicated by provider's order
- Wound cleansing: normal saline or sterile water

Nursing Interventions

- Assess for signs of active or uncontrolled bleeding.
- Assess pain level and notify healthcare provider of any increasing pain.
- Cleanse wounds as ordered.
- Measure wounds and document characteristics.
- Monitor for signs of infection, including erythema, edema, exudate, odors, and temperature.
- Monitor for skin injury around medical devices, interfaces, GTs, and any stomas.
- Premedicate for dressing changes with analgesics if needed.
- Prevent pressure, friction, and shear.
- Provide home care instructions for minor wounds.
- Remove previous dressing to assess the wound.
- Review tetanus immunization status for lacerations, punctures, and other wounds.
- Use protective barrier cream when changing diapers.
- Use hydrocolloid dressings for skin injury prevention.

Patient and Family Education

- Apply barrier cream or products with zinc oxide for diaper dermatitis.
- Avoid picking at or touching the wound.
- Dry wounds gently with a clean towel.
- Follow up with healthcare provider if wounds, lacerations, or minor skin injuries are not healing with home treatment.

(continued)

Patient and Family Education *(continued)*

- Keep wounds clean, moist, and covered.
- Protect healing and resolved wounds from the sun, as new tissue is susceptible to sunburn.
- Treat minor cuts, scrapes, and lacerations at home with bandages and OTC products.
- Wash hands and apply and change the dressing as prescribed.
- Watch for redness, streaking, warmth, swelling, pus, or new drainage.

Table 13.1 Skin Medication

Indications	Mechanism of Action	Contraindications, and Precautions and Adverse Effects
Antibacterial: topical (mupirocin)		
• Treat skin infections	• Inhibit bacterial protein and RNA synthesis	• Adverse effects include headache, localized burning, and rash. • Medication is contraindicated for use on infants less than 3 months old and also contraindicated to use on burns. • Use caution with prolonged use because of the overgrowth of resistant organisms.
Antifungal: systemic (griseofulvin)		
• Treat tinea infections	• Disrupt the mitotic spindle structure of the fungal cell	• Adverse reactions include serious rashes and Stevens–Johnson syndrome. • Medication is contraindicated in those with hepatic disease. • Use caution in patients with systemic lupus erythematosus and with sunlight exposure while taking medication.
Antifungal: topical (nystatin)		
• Treat candidiasis (cutaneous candidiasis and candidal diaper dermatitis)	• Bind to sterols in the cell membrane of fungal cells	• Adverse reactions include Stevens–Johnson syndrome, eczema, bronchospasm, and angioedema. • Use caution in patients with paraben hypersensitivity and diabetes mellitus.
Antifungal: topical (terbinafine)		
• Treat tinea infections	• Interfere with fungal biosynthesis by inhibiting enzyme activity	• Adverse reactions include depression, suicidal ideation, anxiety, insomnia, serious rashes, and Stevens–Johnson syndrome. • Medication is contraindicated in those with liver disease or renal impairment. • Use caution in children under 4 years old.

(continued)

Table 13.1 Skin Medication *(continued)*

Indications	Mechanism of Action	Contraindications, and Precautions and Adverse Effects
Pediculicide (permethrin)		
• Treat and kill lice and mites	• Disrupt the sodium channel current of the nerve cell membrane • Result in delayed repolarization and paralysis/death of parasites such as lice, ticks, fleas, and mites	• Adverse effects include skin irritation. • Medication is contraindicated for children less than 2 months old. • Medication is contraindicated for patients with chrysanthemum allergy.
Topical aminoglycosides (bacitracin/neomycin/polymyxin B)		
• Neomycin and polymyxin B: effective against gram-negative, aerobic bacteria • Bacitracin: effective against gram-positive bacteria • Used for wound management, skin abrasions, and minor burns	• Bacitracin: inhibit bacterial cell wall synthesis • Neomycin: prevent formation of functional proteins and inhibit DNA polymerase • Polymyxin B: bind to phospholipids on cell membranes of gram-negative bacteria	• Adverse reactions include hypersensitivity reactions, diarrhea, hearing loss, and pruritus. • Medication is contraindicated for use against viral or fungal infections. • Medication is contraindicated in children under 2 years old. • Use caution in systemic exposure, especially in children with renal failure.

RESOURCES

Berlowitz, D. (2020). Epidemiology, pathogenesis, and risk assessment of pressure-induced skin and soft tissue injury. *UpToDate.* https://www.uptodate.com/contents/epidemiology-pathogenesis-and-risk-assessment-of-pres sure-induced-skin-and-soft-tissue-injury?search=braden%20scale&source=search_result&selectedTitle=1~4&u sage_type=default&display_rank=1#H3711283010

Centers for Disease Control and Prevention. (2019, September 11). *Parasites: Lice.* U.S. Department of Health and Human Services, Centers for Disease Control and Prevention. https://www.cdc.gov/parasites/lice/index.html

Centers for Disease Control and Prevention. (2020, September 17). *Parasites: Pubic "crab" lice.* U.S. Department of Health and Human Services, Centers for Disease Control and Prevention. https://www.cdc.gov/parasites/lice/ pubic/gen_info/faqs.html

Centers for Disease Control and Prevention. (2021a, July 8). *Body lice.* U.S. Department of Health and Human Services, Centers for Disease Control and Prevention. https://www.cdc.gov/parasites/lice/body/disease.html

Centers for Disease Control and Prevention. (2021b, July 15). *Impetigo: All you need to know.* U.S. Department of Health and Human Services, Centers for Disease Control and Prevention. https://www.cdc.gov/groupastrep/dis eases-public/impetigo.html

Cox, J. (2019). Wound care 101. *Nursing, 49*(10), 32–39. https://doi.org/10.1097/01.NURSE.0000580632.58318.08

Freundlich, K. (2017). Pressure injuries in medically complex children: A review. *Children, 4*(4). https://doi.org/10 .3390/children4040025

Goldstein, A., & Boldstein, B. (2021). Dermatophyte (tinea) infections. *UpToDate.* https:// www.uptodate.com/contents/dermatophyte-tinea-infections?search=tinea%20 corporis&source=search_result&selectedTitle=1~77&usage_type=default&display_rank=1#H300483

Hockenberry, M., Wilson, D., & Rodgers, C. (2017). *Wong's essentials of pediatric nursing.* Elsevier.

King, A., Stellar, J., Blevins, A., & Shah, K. (2014). Dressings and products in pediatric wound care. *Advances in Wound Care, 3*(4), 324–334. https://doi.org/10.1089/wound.2013.0477

Lexicomp. (n.d.[a]). Elimite: Pediatric drug information [Drug Information]. *UpToDate.* https://www.uptodate .com/contents/permethrin-pediatric-drug-information?search=%20Elimite&source=panel_search_ result&selectedTitle=2~148&usage_type=panel&kp_tab=drug_pediatric&display_rank=1

Lexicomp. (n.d.[b]). Griseofulvin: Pediatric drug information [Drug Information]. *UpToDate.* https://www.uptodate .com/contents/griseofulvin-pediatric-drug-information?search=Griseofulvin&source=panel_search_result&se lectedTitle=2~33&usage_type=panel&kp_tab=drug_pediatric&display_rank=1

Lexicomp. (n.d.[c]). Lamisil: Pediatric drug information [Drug Information]. *UpToDate*. https://www.uptodate.com/contents/terbinafine-systemic-pediatric-drug-information?search=Lamisil&source=panel_search_result&selectedTitle=2~39&usage_type=panel&display_rank=2

Lexicomp. (n.d.[d]). Mupirocin: Pediatric drug information [Drug Information]. *UpToDate*. https://www.uptodate.com/contents/mupirocin-pediatric-drug-information?search=Mupirocin&source=panel_search_result&selectedTitle=2~69&usage_type=panel&kp_tab=drug_pediatric&display_rank=1

Lexicomp. (n.d.[e]). Neosporin: Pediatric drug information [Drug Information]. *UpToDate*. https://www.uptodate.com/contents/bacitracin-neomycin-and-polymyxin-b-topical-patient-drug-information?search=Neosporin&source=search_result&selectedTitle=1~23&usage_type=default&display_rank=1

Lexicomp. (n.d.[f]). Nystatin: Pediatric drug information [Drug Information]. *UpToDate*. https://www.uptodate.com/contents/nystatin-topical-pediatric-drug-information?search=Nystatin&source=panel_search_result&selectedTitle=2~45&usage_type=panel&display_rank=2

Lexicomp. (n.d.[g]). Silvadene: Pediatric drug information [Drug Information]. *UpToDate*. https://www.uptodate.com/contents/silver-sulfadiazine-pediatric-drug-information?search=Silvadene&source=panel_search_result&selectedTitle=2~33&usage_type=panel&kp_tab=drug_pediatric&display_rank=1

Rice, P., & Orgill, D. (2021). Assessment and classification of burn injury. *UpToDate*. https://www.uptodate.com/contents/assessment-and-classification-of-burn-injury?sectionName=CLASSIFICATION%20BY%20DEPTH&search=pediatric%20burn%20treatment&topicRef=6567&anchor=H10&source=see_link#H2361857401

Schmitt, B. D. (2012). *Pediatric telephone protocols: Office version* (14th ed.). American Academy of Pediatrics.

Tenehaus, M., & Rennekampff, H. (2020). Topical agents and dressings for local burn wound care. *UpToDate*. https://www.uptodate.com/contents/topical-agents-and-dressings-for-local-burn-wound-care#H2130890734

14

INFECTIOUS DISEASES

INFECTIOUS DISEASE

Overview

- *Infectious*, or *communicable*, *diseases* are caused by bacteria, viruses, parasites, or fungi.
- They are spread directly or indirectly from one person to another through airborne transmission, droplets of nasal or oral secretions, or direct contact with an infected person or their bodily fluids.
- Some diseases and infections are discussed within their respective body systems in the following chapters:
  - Epiglottitis, RSV (bronchiolitis), pertussis (Chapter 7)
  - Impetigo (Chapter 13)
  - Infectious mononucleosis (Chapter 5)
  - Infectious diarrhea (Gastroenteritis in Chapter 8)

FIFTH DISEASE (ERYTHEMA INFECTIOSUM)

Overview

- *Fifth disease*, or *erythema infectiosum*, is a mild, acute viral illness caused by human parvovirus B19.
- It is transmitted through respiratory secretions and blood
- Fifth disease most commonly affects school-age children.
- Symptoms usually appear within 14 days after infection.

> **COMPLICATIONS**
>
> In children with sickle cell disease, fifth disease may cause severe anemia and vaso-occlusive crisis.

Signs and Symptoms

- Fatigue
- Fever
- Headache
- Maculopapular spots
  - First appear on upper and lower extremities
  - Then appear on soles of hands and feet
- Nasal congestion
- Slapped cheek (red cheeks) rash on face
- Sore throat

Diagnosis

Labs
There are no labs specific to diagnose fifth disease.

Diagnostic Testing
There are no diagnostic tests specific to diagnose fifth disease.

Treatment
- Antipyretics for fever
- IVIG for severe cases
- Supportive care (rest, drinking fluids)

Nursing Interventions
- Maintain standard and droplet precautions, if hospitalized.
- Monitor RBC counts for children who are immunosuppressed or have sickle cell disease.
- Prepare patient and family for blood transfusion (Chapter 11) if child experiences an aplastic crisis.

Patient and Family Education
- Child is contagious until the rash appears and then can return to school or day care.
- Learn symptoms that require contacting provider or seeking medical evaluation:
  - Worsened fever or symptoms
  - Initially recovering, then developing difficulty breathing
  - Sores that appear infected, red, inflamed, or have drainage
- Pregnant caregivers should follow up with provider, if exposed.
- Perform proper and frequent hand hygiene.

HAND, FOOT, AND MOUTH DISEASE

Overview
- *Hand, foot, and mouth disease* is a viral illness commonly caused by coxsackie A16, an enterovirus.
- It is transmitted through direct contact with saliva, mucus, feces, or drainage from sores, respiratory droplets, and contaminated surfaces.
- The most commonly affected age group is children under the age of 5.

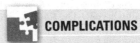 **COMPLICATIONS**

Children may become dehydrated from not eating and drinking due to mouth sores. Other possible complications include fingernail and toenail loss and viral meningitis.

Signs and Symptoms
- Decreased oral intake
- Drooling
- Fever
- Mouth sores: small red ulcers in the back of the mouth that become painful and blister
- Skin rash primarily on palms of hands and soles of feet, but can appear on knees, elbows, and genitals
- Skin rash appears as flat red macules, or papules that can become vesicles
- Sore throat

Diagnosis

Labs
There are no labs specific to diagnose hand, foot, and mouth disease.

Diagnostic Testing
There are no diagnostic tests specific to diagnose hand, foot, and mouth disease.

Treatment

- Fluids to prevent dehydration
- OTC analgesics

Nursing Interventions

- Advise families that most children will recover in 7 to 10 days without any treatment.
- Monitor skin integrity and oral intake.

Patient and Family Education

- Encourage fluid intake to prevent dehydration.
- Notify healthcare provider for signs of dehydration or fever greater than 105 °F (40.6 °C).
- Offer cold fluids and use cup or syringe to feed infants.
- Prevent the spread of infection with good hand hygiene. Young children may need help to wash hands.
- Hydration is the priority, and the child may not want solid foods until the mouth is no longer painful.
- Review signs and symptoms of dehydration and when to follow up with healthcare provider.
- Wash and disinfect frequently touched surfaces and toys that the infected child has touched.

 POP QUIZ 14.1

Parents of a toddler call the clinic, saying there is an outbreak of hand, foot, and mouth disease at their child's day care. Their toddler is refusing to eat and drink and has spots in their mouth. They want to know if there is an antibiotic to help. What answer should be given to educate the parent?

HEPATITIS

Overview

- *Hepatitis* is a viral illness that causes inflammation of the liver.
- *Hepatitis A* is a short-term foodborne illness transmitted through the fecal-oral route, unwashed food, and contaminated water.
- Hepatitis B and C are chronic illnesses and are transmitted through direct contact with infected body fluids. Both can be transmitted from infected mother to baby at birth.
- *Hepatitis D* is a liver infection that can be short-term or become chronic. It only occurs in those who are already infected with hepatitis B.
- *Hepatitis E* is an acute liver illness transmitted through the fecal-oral route. Many children infected do not show symptoms.

 NURSING PEARL

To remember hepatitis transmission routes, remember vowels are bowels. Hepatitis A and E are transmitted via the fecal-oral route.

COMPLICATIONS

Complications of hepatitis are cirrhosis and liver failure.

Signs and Symptoms

- Abdominal pain
- Dark-colored urine
- Fatigue
- Fever
- Jaundice
- Joint pain
- Light, clay-colored stools
- Loss of appetite
- Nausea
- Vomiting

Diagnosis

Labs
- Hepatitis viral panel
- LFTs

Diagnostic Testing
- Liver biopsy
- Liver ultrasound

Treatment

- Hepatitis A: supportive measures
- Hepatitis B: antiviral medications (see Table 14.2*)
- Hepatitis C:
  - Antiviral medications (see Table 14.2)
    - DAA
    - Ribavirin with pegylated interferon
  - Immune globulin helpful right after exposure

Nursing Interventions

- Recommend Hepatitis A and B vaccines.
- For Hepatitis A, monitor for dehydration and replace fluid loss with IVF.

Patient and Family Education

- Hepatitis A
  - Administer hepatitis A vaccine between 12 and 23 months old.
  - Wash hands after using the bathroom or changing a diaper and before eating.
  - Wash fruits and vegetables before eating.
- Hepatitis B and C:
  - Administer the hepatitis B vaccine at birth, at 2 to 4 months, and at 6 to 18 months.
  - There is no vaccination to prevent hepatitis C at this time.
  - Hepatitis C is transmitted via blood and body fluids:
    - During birth from an infected mother to baby
    - Sharing or reusing needles with an infected person
    - Sharing personal items such as toothbrushes with an infected person
    - During unprotected sex with an infected person
  - Adolescents should learn the dangers of IV drug use.
  - Adolescents should learn and follow safe sex practices and use condoms.

INFLUENZA

Overview

- *Influenza*, commonly known as *the flu*, is caused by viruses, most commonly flu A and flu B.
- Influenza affects the respiratory system and is transmitted through respiratory droplets.
- Children at higher risk for the flu are those under 5 years old, especially children under 2 years old, and children with asthma.
- Symptoms have an abrupt onset.

 COMPLICATIONS

Most flu infections resolve within a few days to a few weeks, but can lead to pneumonia, dehydration, and respiratory distress. Rarely, some severe cases can lead to death.

---

* Table 14.2 is located at the end of this chapter.

Signs and Symptoms

- Aches
- Chills
- Cough
- Diarrhea
- Fatigue
- Fever
- Headache
- Muscle pain
- Nasal congestion
- Photophobia
- Vomiting

Diagnosis

Labs
- Rapid influenza detection test
- RT-PCR
- Viral culture from nasopharyngeal swab or aspirate for both COVID-19 and influenza

Diagnostic Testing
There are no diagnostic tests specific to diagnose influenza.

 ALERT!

Pediatric patients presenting with flu-like symptoms should be assessed for COVID-19, which is caused by the SARS-CoV-2 virus. COVID-19 in pediatrics generally presents as asymptomatic or with mild symptoms and requires basic supportive care. However, they are still at risk for developing complications, such as multisystem inflammatory syndrome. Children at risk for severe illness from COVID usually have preexisting health conditions such as metabolic diseases (genetic, endocrine, obesity), neurological diseases, cardiac diseases, lung diseases, or conditions that cause immunosuppression, such as cancer. Care parameters are continually evolving. For current information on caring for patients with COVID-19, consult the National Institute of Health and the CDC.

Treatment

- Acetaminophen for fever
- Antivirals (see Table 14.2):
  - Oseltamivir
  - Zanamivir
  - Peramivir
  - Baloxavir
- Fluids for dehydration
- Supplemental oxygen

Nursing Interventions

- Administer IV fluids for severe dehydration.
- Administer supplemental oxygen for worsening respiratory status.
- Educate patients on the difference between the flu and the common cold (Table 14.1).
- Monitor and assess respiratory status.
- Recommend the flu vaccine for prevention each year.
- Suction nares as needed in infants and young children.

Patient and Family Education

- Children with influenza or flu-like illness should stay home from school or day care until 24 hours after fever has resolved.
- Clean and disinfect toys and surfaces that an infected child touched.
- Oseltamivir can help shorten duration of illness if started within the first 48 hours of flu-symptom onset.
- Encourage fluid intake to avoid dehydration.
- Understand expected course of illness and recommend follow-up with healthcare provider if symptoms continue beyond expected course:
  - Fever up to 3 days
  - Runny nose up to 10 days
  - Cough up to 3 weeks

(continued)

Table 14.1 Distinguishing Symptoms for Influenza, COVID-19, and the Common Cold

Symptoms	Influenza	COVID-19	Common Cold
Onset	Abrupt	Gradual	Gradual
Aches	Common	Common	Sometimes milder
Chills	Common	Common	Uncommon
Cough	Common	Common	Common
Fatigue	Common	Common	Sometimes
Fever	Common	Common	Uncommon
Headache	Common	Common	Uncommon
Nasal congestion	Uncommon	Common	Common
Loss of Taste and/or Smell	Uncommon	Common	Occasional

Patient and Family Education *(continued)*

- Notify healthcare provider or go to the ED for difficulty breathing.
- The flu vaccine is recommended for everyone 6 months and older, including caregivers of infants less than 6 months old, yearly by the end of October.
- Two types of vaccines are available:
  - Injectable influenza vaccine for children 6 months and older
  - Live inactivated influenza vaccine (nasal spray) for children 2 years and older
- Cover cough and sneezes and use proper hand hygiene to avoid spreading to others.
- Use saline nose drops or humidifier and suction nares with bulb suction to alleviate blocked nares.

 POP QUIZ 14.2

A 14-year-old child developed a 102 °F (38.9 °C) fever, aches, chills, and cough suddenly yesterday. Through a subjective history, the nurse is told that the patient's peers on their sports team have been diagnosed with the flu. What should the nurse anticipate being ordered for this child?

MEASLES

Overview

- *Measles* is an acute, highly contagious viral respiratory illness.
- It is transmitted by direct contact, respiratory droplets, or contaminated air from coughing and sneezing.
- Symptoms appear 7 to 14 days after viral infection, and rash appears 3 to 5 days after the first symptoms appear.

 COMPLICATIONS

Complications are more likely to occur in children under 5 years old. The most common complications are ear infections and diarrhea, but more severe complications are pneumonia and encephalitis.

Signs and Symptoms

- Conjunctivitis
- Cough
- Fatigue
- Fever

- Koplik spots in mouth: small, bluish-white spot with a red background on the inside of the cheek
- Maculopapular rash
  - Starts as flat red spots on face
  - Spreads to neck and down the body to trunk, arms, legs, and feet
  - Small, raised bumps may appear over red spots
- Nasal congestion
- Sore throat

Diagnosis

Labs
- Measles antibody (IgM)
- Measles RNA RT-PCR

Diagnostic Testing
There are no diagnostic tests specific to diagnose measles.

Treatment

- Management includes:
  - Antipyretics (Table A.2)
  - Clean skin and eyes
  - Fluids
  - Rest
- Vitamin A in severe cases

Nursing Interventions

- Maintain standard and airborne precautions.
- Recommend the MMR vaccine for prevention.
- Prepare child for immunoglobulin IM or IV administration, if exposed and unable to vaccinate (i.e., immunocompromised).

Patient and Family Education

- A child with measles is considered contagious from 4 days prior to rash appearing until 4 days after.
- Stay home from school or day care until no longer contagious to avoid spreading to others.
- The measles virus can live up to 2 hours in the air after an infected person has been in the area.
- Prevent measles with the MMR vaccine.
- Cover mouth when coughing and sneezing and use proper hand hygiene.

MUMPS

Overview

- *Mumps* is a contagious viral illness caused by a paramyxovirus that affects the parotid and salivary glands.
- It is transmitted through direct contact and saliva or respiratory droplets.
- Symptoms appear 16 to 18 days after becoming infected.

 COMPLICATIONS

Complications include inflammations of organs such as brain, testicles, ovaries, and pancreas; meningitis; and deafness.

Signs and Symptoms

- Earaches
- Fatigue
- Fever
- Headache
- Muscle aches
- Parotitis (swollen parotid glands)
- Swollen cheeks and jaw

Diagnosis

Labs
- Mumps IgM antibody
- RT-PCR and viral buccal or oral swab

Diagnostic Testing
There are no diagnostic tests specific to diagnose mumps.

Treatment

Supportive management:
- Analgesics for pain (Table A.2)
- Fluids
- Hot and cold compresses for neck and swelling discomfort
- Rest

Nursing Interventions

- Maintain standard contact and droplet precautions.
- Monitor airway patency.
- Recommend MMR vaccine for prevention.

Patient and Family Education

- A child with mumps is contagious a few days prior to salivary gland swelling and up to 5 days after swelling starts.
- Stay home from school or day care until no longer contagious to avoid spreading to others.
- Infected children should cover mouth and nose when coughing or sneezing and use proper hand hygiene.
- Prevent mumps infection with MMR immunization.

TUBERCULOSIS

Overview

- *TB* is a lung infection caused by *Mycobacterium tuberculosis.*
- It is categorized as either latent TB infection or active TB disease.
  - Only patients with active TB can infect others.
  - Patients with latent TB do not present with respiratory symptoms.
- Risk factors include:
  - Being a child born outside of the United States
  - Having a compromised immune system

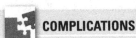

COMPLICATIONS

Tuberculosis meningitis is caused by *Mycobacterium tuberculosis* and results from bacteria spreading to the brain and spinal cord from the lungs. Symptoms include headache, fever, stiff neck, vomiting, irritability, and confusion.

- Having close contact with infected individuals
- Homelessness
- Living in a correctional facility
- Using IV drugs

Signs and Symptoms

- Chest pain
- Chronic cough
- Fever
- Hemoptysis
- Malaise
- Productive cough
- Weight loss

Diagnosis
Labs

- QuantiFERON gold (IGRA) for TB
- Sputum culture for TB infection
- Tuberculin skin test
  - Positive if greater than 10 mm in children less than 4 years old
  - Positive if greater than 15 mm in those with no risk factors

Diagnostic Testing
Chest x-ray to confirm lung consolidation consistent with TB.

Treatment

- Isoniazid (Table 14.2)
- Rifampin (Table 14.2)

Nursing Interventions

- Administer supplemental oxygen.
- Assess for any barriers to care or adherence to the treatment regimen.
  - Access to care or providers
  - Financial concerns
  - Language barriers
  - Side effects of medications
- Assess the size of induration of tuberculin skin test.
- Encourage drinking fluids to prevent dehydration.
- Ensure hospitalized patients are placed on airborne precautions and a negative air pressure room.
- Monitor for complications or evidence of pneumonia:
  - Coughing up blood
  - Decrease in pulse oximetry
  - Increased work of breathing
  - Worsening cough
- Refer to the local public health department to report TB.

Patient and Family Education

- Avoid others with respiratory illness and perform hand hygiene.
- Encourage family members, including children, to be screened for TB; an adult typically infects children.
- Utilize support services, such as social workers, social or community resources, if necessary for financial concerns, homelessness, or substance use and abuse.

(continued)

Patient and Family Education *(continued)*

- Prevent dehydration by drinking fluids.
- Remain up to date on immunizations.
- Take medications as prescribed. Following the treatment regimen prevents relapsing symptoms, decreases the risk of clinical deterioration, and prevents bacteria from developing resistance to medications.

VARICELLA

Overview

- *Varicella* is caused by the varicella-zoster virus and is commonly known as *chicken pox*.
- It is transmitted through direct contact, airborne droplets, and contaminated objects.
- It is communicable 1 to 2 days before lesions appear until 6 days after lesions form crusts.

COMPLICATIONS

Infants, adolescents, and those who are immunocompromised are at higher risk for complications such as bacterial skin infections or encephalitis.

Signs and Symptoms

- Fatigue
- Fever
- Headache
- Malaise
- Pruritic rash
  - Initially presents as macules (raised, red bumps)
  - Progresses to vesicles
  - Lesions crust or scab over

Diagnosis

Labs

Varicella-zoster virus skin lesion

Diagnostic Testing

There are no diagnostic tests specific to diagnose varicella.

Treatment

- Acetaminophen for fever (Table A.2)
- Acyclovir (Table 14.2)
- Supportive therapies, such as calamine lotion or oatmeal baths, to relieve itching
- Varicella-zoster immune globulin

Nursing Interventions

- Maintain standard contact and airborne precautions.
- Monitor rash and inform healthcare provider if any lesions appear infected or lesions continue after the sixth day.
- Recommend the varicella vaccine.
- Provide distractions to help children avoid scratching.

Patient and Family Education

- A child with chicken pox is considered contagious from 1 to 2 days before rash appears until all the lesions have crusted over.
- Call healthcare facility prior to entering so clinic or hospital can initiate precautions to prevent exposure before the child enters the building.
- Children will need to stay home from school or day care until lesions are all crusted over and they are no longer contagious to avoid spreading to others.
- Never give aspirin to children with chicken pox due to the association with Reye's syndrome.
- Lesions will appear daily until the fifth day of illness.
- Prevent varicella infections with immunization.
- Use calamine lotion or a cool bath with baking soda or oatmeal to relieve itching.
- Trim fingernails short and avoid scratching blisters to prevent skin infections and to prevent spreading disease to others. Family may apply mittens to help prevent young children from scratching.
- Wash hands with soap and water after scratching any lesions or blisters.

 POP QUIZ 14.3

A patient is admitted with suspected chicken pox. Their lesions have not crusted over yet. What precautions and PPE should be implemented?

Table 14.2 Infectious Disease Medications		
Indications	**Mechanism of Action**	**Contraindications, Precautions, and Adverse Effects**
Antibiotic (rifampin)		
• Antituberculosis agent	• Inhibit bacterial and mycobacterial RNA synthesis	• Administer 1 hour before or 2 hours after meals and with a glass of water. • Adverse effects include discoloration of teeth, urine, sweat, tears, and sputum.
Antituberculosis agent (isoniazid)		
• Antimycobacterial agent	• Inhibit the synthesis of mycolic acid, a component of the bacterial cell wall	• Monitor for hepatotoxicity. • Medication may increase metabolism and hepatotoxic effects of acetaminophen.
Antiviral (acyclovir)		
• Antiviral therapy for varicella-zoster virus	• Inhibit DNA synthesis and viral replication	• Begin within 24 hours of appearance of rash for maximum benefit. • Adverse effects include acute kidney injury and neurotoxicity; administer over 1 hour or longer to reduce adverse effects.
Antiviral (interferon)		
• Treatment of hepatitis B and hepatitis C	• Inhibit viral replication	• Adverse effects include inhibition of growth. • Adverse effects include fatigue, headache, insomnia, alopecia, weakness, and nausea. • Monitor for bone marrow suppression and neuropsychiatric disorders. • Caution that it may aggravate autoimmune, infectious, and ischemic disorders.

(continued)

Table 14.2 Infectious Disease Medications *(continued)*

Indications	Mechanism of Action	Contraindications, Precautions, and Adverse Effects
Antiviral (ribavirin)		
• Treatment of chronic hepatitis C when used with interferon	• Act as RNA virus mutagen	• Medication is contraindicated as monotherapy. • Monitor for hepatic decompensation and toxicity. • Use with caution in patients with anemia or cardiac disease. • Adverse effects include growth inhibition and suicidal ideation. • Medication is contraindicated in children less than 3 years old.
Antivirals (oseltamivir, zanamivir, peramivir, baloxavir)		
• Treatment and prevention of infections due to Influenza A and Influenza B	• Inhibit action of viral neuraminidase to prevent the spread of viral illness in respiratory tract	• Medication is most effective if started within 48 hours of symptom onset or exposure. • Monitor for drug toxicity with intermittent blood work. • Adverse effects include nausea, vomiting, and headaches.
DAA		
• Reduce rates of chronic hepatitis C in children	• Inhibit viral replication	• Medication is contraindicated in children less than 3 years old. • Medication is contraindicated in children who also have Hepatitis B infection.

RESOURCES

Centers for Disease Control and Prevention. (2021a, April 28). *Chickenpox.* U.S. Department of Health and Human Services, Centers for Disease Control and Prevention. https://www.cdc.gov/chickenpox/index.html

Centers for Disease Control and Prevention. (2021b, June 21). *Cold versus flu.* U.S. Department of Health and Human Services, Centers for Disease Control and Prevention. https://www.cdc.gov/flu/symptoms/coldflu.htm

Centers for Disease Control and Prevention. (2021c, February 2). *Complications of hand, foot, and mouth disease.* U.S. Department of Health and Human Services, Centers for Disease Control and Prevention. https://www.cdc.gov/hand-foot-mouth/about/complications.html

Centers for Disease Control and Prevention. (n.d.[a]). *Coronavirus Disease 2019 (COVID-19) treatment guidelines.* U.S. Department of Health and Human Services, Centers for Disease Control and Prevention. https://www.covid19treatmentguidelines.nih.gov

Centers for Disease Control and Prevention. (n.d.[b]). *COVID data tracker: Pediatric data.* U.S. Department of Health and Human Services, Centers for Disease Control and Prevention. (n.d.[b])https://covid.cdc.gov/covid-data-tracker/#pediatric-data

Centers for Disease Control and Prevention. (2020a, December 30). *Information for pediatric health care providers: COVID-19.* U.S. Department of Health and Human Services, Centers for Disease Control and Prevention. https://www.cdc.gov/coronavirus/2019-ncov/hcp/pediatric-hcp.html

Centers for Disease Control and Prevention. (2020b, November 5). *Measles (rubeola).* U.S. Department of Health and Human Services, Centers for Disease Control and Prevention. https://www.cdc.gov/measles/index.html

Centers for Disease Control and Prevention. (2020c, July 28). *What is viral hepatitis?* U.S. Department of Health and Human Services, Centers for Disease Control and Prevention. https://www.cdc.gov/hepatitis/abc/index.htm

Centers for Disease Control and Prevention. (2021a, June 21). *Flu & young children.* U.S. Department of Health and Human Services, Centers for Disease Control and Prevention. https://www.cdc.gov/flu/highrisk/children.htm

Centers for Disease Control and Prevention. (2021b, March 31). *Healthcare workers: Information on COVID-19.* U.S. Department of Health and Human Services, Centers for Disease Control and Prevention. https://www.cdc.gov/coronavirus/2019-ncov/hcp/

Centers for Disease Control and Prevention. (2021c, March 8). *Mumps*. U.S. Department of Health and Human Services, Centers for Disease Control and Prevention. https://www.cdc.gov/mumps/index.html

Centers for Disease Control and Prevention. (2021d, June 1). *What you should know about flu antiviral drugs*. U.S. Department of Health and Human Services, Centers for Disease Control and Prevention. https://www.cdc.gov/flu/treatment/whatyoushould.htm

Hockenberry, M., Wilson, D., & Rodgers, C. (2017). *Wong's essentials of pediatric nursing*. Elsevier.

Jhaveri, R. (2021). Hepatitis C virus infection in children. *UpToDate*. https://www.uptodate.com/contents/hepatitis -c-virus-infection-in-children?search=hepatitis%20c%20daa&source=search_result&selectedTitle=1~150&usage _type=default&display_rank=1#H2151009193

Jordan, J. (2021). Clinical manifestations and diagnosis of parvovirus B19 infection. *UpToDate*. https://www. uptodate.com/contents/clinical-manifestations-and-diagnosis-of-parvovirus-b19-infection?search=fifth%20 disease%20children&source=search_result&selectedTitle=1~64&usage_type=default&display_rank= 1#H525137743

Lexicomp. (2021a). Acyclovir [Drug Information]. *UpToDate*. https://www.uptodate.com/contents/acyclovir-system ic-pediatric-drug-information?search=acyclovir%20&source=panel_search_result&selectedTitle=2~142&usage _type=panel&display_rank=2#F54964689

Lexicomp. (2021b). Ioniazid [Drug Information]. *UpToDate*. https://www.uptodate.com/contents/isoniazid-pediatri c-drug-information?search=isoniazid&source=panel_search_result&selectedTitle=2~148&usage_type=panel& kp_tab=drug_pediatric&display_rank=1

Lexicomp. (2021c). Oseltamivir [Drug Information]. *UpToDate*. https://www.uptodate.com/contents/oseltamivir-pe diatric-drug-information?search=Oseltamivir&source=panel_search_result&selectedTitle=2~46&usage_type= panel&kp_tab=drug_pediatric&display_rank=1

Lexicomp. (2021d). Rebetol [Drug Information]. *UpToDate*. https://www.uptodate.com/contents/ribavirin-systemic -pediatric-drug-information?search=rebetol&source=panel_search_result&selectedTitle=2~142&usage_type= panel&display_rank=2&showDrugLabel=true

Lexicomp. (2021f). Rifampin [Drug Information]. *UpToDate*. https://www.uptodate.com/ contents/rifampin-rifampicin-pediatric-drug-information?search=rifampin&source=pa nel_search_result&selectedTitle=2~148&usage_type=panel&kp_tab=drug_pediatric&display_rank=1

National Institutes of Health. (2021). *COVID-19 treatment guidelines*. U.S. Department of Health and Human Services, National Institutes of Health. https://www.covid19treatmentguidelines.nih.gov/about-the-guidelines/ whats-new/

Sick-Samuels, A. C. (2021, July 8). *MIS-C and COVID-19: Rare inflammatory syndrome in kids and teen*. John Hopkins Medicine. https://www.hopkinsmedicine.org/health/conditions-and-diseases/coronavirus/misc-and -covid19-rare-inflammatory-syndrome-in-kids-and-teens

Williams, N., Radia, T., Harman, K., Agrawal, P., Cook, J., & Gupta, A. (2020). COVID-19 Severe acute respiratory syndrome coronavirus 2 (SARS-CoV-2) infection in children and adolescents: A systematic review of critically unwell children and the association with underlying comorbidities. *European Journal of Pediatrics*, *180*, 689–697. https://doi.org/10.1007/s00431-020-03801-6. https://link.springer.com/article/10.1007/s00431-020-03801-6

BEHAVIORAL AND MENTAL HEALTH

ANXIETY

Overview

- *Anxiety* is characterized by persistent thoughts of worry and fear and can also cause physical symptoms such as increased heart rate and sweating.
- Anxiety can be associated with educational underachievement and risks for depression, substance abuse, and suicide.
- Types of childhood anxiety disorders include:
  - *Agoraphobia*: fear of public transportation, open spaces, enclosed spaces
  - *GAD*: constant dread or worry
  - *OCD*: reoccurring obsessions (thoughts, sensations) that drive repetitive behaviors (compulsions)
  - *Panic disorder*: recurrent unexpected panic attacks
  - *PTSD*: develops after a traumatic or catastrophic event, such as witnessing or experiencing a serious injury, abuse, an accident, or a natural disaster
  - *Social anxiety*: fear of social situations, interactions, or performing in front of others
  - *Specific phobia*: fear of heights, flying, animals, injections

> **COMPLICATIONS**
>
> Anxiety interferes with daily activities. Children may start avoiding everyday activities such as going to school.

Signs and Symptoms

- Anxiety
  - Chest pain or racing heartbeat
  - Difficulty concentrating
  - Dizziness or lightheadedness
  - Fatigue
  - Fear
  - Muscle tension
  - Nausea and abdominal discomfort
  - Restlessness or irritability
  - Sleep disturbances
  - Sweating
  - Trembling or shaking
- PTSD
  - Avoidance of anything that may remind the patient of traumatic event (feelings, places, thoughts)
  - Feelings of numbness, denial, or detachment
  - Depression, phobias, anxiety, conversion reactions, flashbacks, obsessions
  - Intrusive thoughts: displaying repetitive actions, desire to play out the situation

(continued)

Signs and Symptoms *(continued)*

- Irritability, angry outbursts, physical aggression
- Nightmares
- Uncontrolled thoughts, dreams, or flashbacks about traumatic event
- OCD
  - Repeated, unwanted, or aggressive thoughts
  - Fear of germs or contamination
  - Repetitive and compulsive behaviors:
    - Placing objects in specific, precise order (symmetry)
    - Excessive compulsions (handwashing, cleaning, counting)
    - Repeated checking on things (e.g., locks)
    - Rituals

Diagnosis

Labs
There are no labs specific to diagnose anxiety.

Diagnostic Testing
Children experiencing anxiety should be assessed by a trained pediatric psychotherapist.

Treatment

- Cognitive behavioral therapy
- Medications:
  - Benzodiazepine (Table A.2)
  - SSRIs (Table 15.1*)
  - Tricyclic antidepressants (Table 15.1)

Nursing Interventions

- Encourage seeing a mental health counselor/professional, psychologist, or psychiatrist.
- Screen for anxiety symptoms and disorders as well as symptoms of depression.
- Encourage the patient to discuss their feelings, generally or about a specific event.
- Suggest a specialist or psychologist with any change in behavior that can be traced to a traumatic event.
- Use screening tools to identify symptoms of anxiety, PTSD, and OCD.

Patient and Family Education

- Continue to take prescribed medications and follow the treatment plan, even if feeling better.
- Family should allow children to express their feelings.
- Learn that it may take up to 4 weeks to see a therapeutic effect with SSRI medication.
- Maintain routines that are reassuring for children.
- Manage symptoms by maintaining a healthy lifestyle with diet, exercise, and proper sleep.
- Practice mindfulness or relaxation techniques.
- Prevent traumatic events from occurring, such as maltreatment, violence, and bullying.
- Prevent big changes or events from being traumatic by preparing child as much as possible.

---

*Table 15.1 is located at the end of this chapter.

BULLYING AND SOCIAL MEDIA USE

Overview

- *Bullying* is unwanted aggressive behavior that involves a real or perceived imbalance of power.
  - Physical bullying includes hurting a person or their possessions, such as hitting, kicking, spitting, pushing, tripping, or breaking possessions.
  - Social bullying includes hurting someone's reputation or relationships.
    - Cyberbullying, insulting texts, or embarrassing on social media
    - Telling peers not to be friends with someone, rumors, embarrassing on purpose
  - Verbal bullying includes saying mean things about another person. Examples include teasing, name-calling, taunting, threatening, or making inappropriate sexual comments.
- Social media are web and mobile platforms that promote virtual social interaction, communication, networking, and entertainment.
  - Examples include Facebook, Snapchat, Instagram, email, Twitter, and TikTok.
  - Risks include cyberbullying, sexting, depression, suicide, and self-esteem issues.

 COMPLICATIONS

Children who are bullied are more likely to have low self-esteem, depression, suicidal thoughts, headaches, stomachaches, tired and anxious feelings, and poor performance/frequent absences in school.

Signs and Symptoms

- Changes in eating habits, coming home from school hungry
- Destroyed or lost clothing, books, or other possessions
- Difficulty sleeping
- Loss of self-esteem
- Not wanting to go to school
- Unexplainable injuries

Nursing Interventions

- Advise families to talk to children about social media use and bullying.
- Ask child privately about bullying or abuse (Chapter 16) for unexplainable injuries.
- Evaluate for access to firearms and promote firearm safety.
- Evaluate screen time and recommend less than 2 hours per day.

Patient and Family Education

- Discuss bullying and how to recognize it.
- Learn internet safety. Families should check privacy settings on children's online profiles and devices.
- Learn ways to respond to bullies, such as walking away and getting help.
- Talk to a trusted adult when bullying occurs.
- Use established screen time limits per day.

 POP QUIZ 15.1

A school-aged girl states she is not being bullied but does not like to go to school because other girls send mean texts about her to her classmates. How can the nurse educate and inform this patient?

DEPRESSION

Overview

- *Depression* causes feelings of profound sadness, often accompanied by hopelessness and/or a loss of interest in activities.
- It interferes with the abilities to perform well in school and to develop and maintain relationships.
- Risk factors include a history of depression in a parent or sibling, exposure to adversity, gender dysphoria, and chronic medical illness.

Signs and Symptoms

- Changes in appetite
- Crying
- Decreased energy
- Difficulty concentrating
- Sad, hopeless, or worthless feelings
- Loss of interest or pleasure in activities
- Tendency to be alone or poor social engagement
- Trouble sleeping or sleeping too much

Diagnosis

Labs
There are no labs specific to diagnose depression.

Diagnostic Testing
Depression screening.

Treatment

- Cognitive behavioral therapy
- Medications:
  - SSRIs (Table 15.1)
  - Tricyclic antidepressants (Table 15.1)

Nursing Interventions

- Screen for depression and suicidal thoughts.
- Encourage talking or expressing feelings and positive coping mechanisms.
- Ensure a safe environment if a suicidal risk is identified.
- Monitor for self-harm.

Patient and Family Education

- Continue to take prescribed medications, even if feeling better.
- Keep in mind that antidepressants may take 2 to 4 weeks to show effect.
- Family and caregivers:
  - Be aware of signs of suicidal ideation.
  - Establish a safety plan, including calling healthcare providers, going to the local ED, or calling the National Suicide Prevention Lifeline.

COMPLICATIONS

Depression can lead to thoughts of suicide, but antidepressants can also cause children and adolescents to have suicidal thoughts. Patients should be monitored for suicidal thoughts especially when starting antidepressant medication.

NURSING PEARL

Depression Symptoms Mnemonic: A SAD FACES

A: Appetite change

S: Sleep change

A: Anhedonia (loss of interest or pleasure)

D: Dysphoria (feeling uneasy or unhappy)

F: Fatigue

A: Agitation changes

C: Concentration difficulty

E: Esteem: low

S: Suicidal ideation

POP QUIZ 15.2

A mother states that her teenage daughter has not been sleeping through the night and is too tired for school. She is not interested in playing sports anymore, appears moody, and has not eaten as much as usual. She is wondering if this is normal teenage behavior or if something is wrong. How should the nurse respond?

EATING DISORDERS

Overview

- *Eating disorders* are disturbances in eating behaviors and related thoughts.
- Eating disorders are characterized by preoccupation with food, body weight, and body shape.
- Common eating disorders include anorexia nervosa, bulimia nervosa, and binge-eating disorder.

Signs and Symptoms

- Anorexia
  - Anemia
  - Bradycardia
  - Brittle nails
  - Distorted body image
  - Emaciation
  - Fear of gaining weight
  - Hair loss
  - Restricted eating
- Binge eating
  - Eating alone or in secret
  - Eating fast and when not hungry
  - Eating unusually large amounts of food in a short amount of time
  - Feeling ashamed or guilty about eating
  - May be overweight
- Bulimia
  - Binge-eating followed by vomiting, laxative use, fasting, or excessive exercise
  - Chronic sore throat
  - Decaying teeth
  - Dehydration
  - Electrolyte imbalance

COMPLICATIONS

Hypotension, bradycardia, and hypothermia can be associated with extremely low weight. For extremely low weight and severe malnutrition, it is important to avoid rapid weight gain due to refeeding syndrome, which leads to cardiovascular, neurologic, and hematologic complications.

ALERT!

Be aware of the physical side effects of eating disorders, such as urinary tract problems from limiting fluids, orthostatic hypotension, bradycardia, and hypothermia. Rapid weight gain can lead to refeeding syndrome, which causes metabolic abnormalities.

Diagnosis

Labs
There are no labs specific to diagnose eating disorders.

Diagnostic Testing
There are no diagnostic tests specific to diagnose eating disorders.

Treatment

- Medications: antidepressants
- Nutrition therapy
- Psychotherapies

Nursing Interventions

- Establish healthy eating patterns.
- Help identify emotions attached to food.

(continued)

Nursing Interventions *(continued)*

- Monitor daily weight.
- Monitor heart rate for bradycardia.
- Monitor meals/snacks and document intake.
- Place NG tube for supplemental nutrition.
- Promote a positive body image.
- Recommend speaking with a dietician or mental health professional about concerns for disordered eating habits.

Patient and Family Education

- Establish regular eating patterns.
- Prepare nutritional meals and snacks.
- Seek treatment for disordered eating that cannot be managed at home.
- Watch for behavior changes that may indicate depression or suicidal thoughts.
- Educate caregivers to supervise meals.

POP QUIZ 15.3

A parent of a 12-year-old female patient expresses concerns of their child's eating patterns. The parent states the child never complains of abdominal or GI issues but does complain of a sore throat often. Which eating disorder is this a symptom of, and what causes it?

GENDER IDENTITY AND SEXUAL ORIENTATION

Overview

- *Gender* refers to cultural roles, behaviors, activities, and attributes expected of people based on their sex.
- *Sex* is an individual's biologic status as male, female, or something else. Sex is assigned at birth and associated with physical attributes, anatomy, and chromosomes.
- *Sexual orientation* is a person's sexual and emotional attraction to another person and behavior. Examples include bisexual, heterosexual, gay, lesbian, and others.
- *Gender identity* is an individual's sense of themself as a man, woman, transgender, and so on.
  - *Cisgender* refers to individuals whose current gender identity is the same as the sex assigned at birth.
  - *Nonbinary* refers to individuals who do not identify their gender as male or female.
  - *Transgender* refers to individuals whose current gender identity differs from the sex assigned at birth.

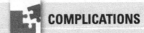

COMPLICATIONS

Adolescents and teens who identify as a sexual minority are at a greater risk for suicidal behaviors than their heterosexual peers.

Clinical Presentation

- Childhood: Children may prefer clothing, activities, toys, and role models that are typically associated with the opposite sex.
- Adolescence: Puberty and the development of secondary sex characteristics can cause gender dysphoria and cause adolescents to feel uncomfortable in their own body.

ALERT!

LGBTQ+ children and adolescents may fear family/peer rejection and social isolation and be at risk for psychosocial issues.

Nursing Interventions

- Ask adolescents their first name and which pronouns they prefer staff to use.
- Encourage children and adolescents planning to come out to have a support and safety plan.
- Screen for suicidal thoughts or history of suicide attempts.
- Use nonjudgmental communication.

NURSING PEARL

Asking and correctly using someone's pronouns is one way to respect their gender identity.

Patient and Family Education

- Avoid using alcohol or drugs to relieve depression or low self-esteem.
- Tell a supportive adult of bullying or violence.
- Get involved in gay/straight alliances or organizations at school.
- For families:
  - Access LGBTQ+ organizations for resources on how to support child.
  - Use honest and open communication.

NEONATAL ABSTINENCE SYNDROME

Overview

- An infant born to a mother with a substance use disorder is at risk for withdrawal.
- *NAS* is a withdrawal syndrome in newborns exposed to opioids, nicotine, benzodiazepines, and SSRIs during the prenatal period.

Signs and Symptoms

- Excessive sucking
- Feeding difficulty
- Fever
- Frequent yawning
- High-pitched cry
- Hypertonicity
- Irritability
- Jitteriness
- Loose stools
- Mottling
- Nasal stuffiness/sneezing
- Short sleep cycles
- Sweating
- Tachypnea
- Tremors
- Vomiting

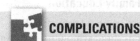

COMPLICATIONS

NAS has been attributed to low birth weights, poor feeding, and irritability. It can lead to prolonged hospitalizations after birth and the need for higher calorie formula.

Diagnosis

Labs
- Maternal blood or urine drug screen
- Meconium analysis
- Urine drug screen

Diagnostic Testing
There are no diagnostic tests specific to diagnose neonatal abstinence syndrome.

Treatment

- Methadone (Table A.2)
- Morphine (Table A.2)

Nursing Interventions

- Cluster care to decrease waking infant during rest.
- Promote comfort by providing a low-stimulation environment.
- Involve social workers for discharge planning.
- Monitor symptoms and NAS scoring to determine medication-weaning protocol.
- Offer a pacifier for excessive sucking or overactive sucking reflex.
- Provide frequent small feedings, typically with higher calorie formula, to allow rest periods and to help with any feeding or swallowing issues.
- Swaddle the infant to promote warmth to maintain body temperature and reduce tremors.
- Use barrier creams with diaper changes to protect skin from excoriation.

Patient and Family Education

Most patient education is for the family:
- Ask questions about symptoms, monitoring, and feeding difficulties.
- Breastfeeding is allowed for methadone-maintained mothers.
- Learn how to help the infant eat, sleep, and console.
- Follow up with therapies to help child with academic, behavioral, and interpersonal skill development.
- Use a breast pump and milk dumping for mothers who are rehabilitating from other illicit substances and plan to breastfeed.

 POP QUIZ 15.4

A new parent of a baby weaning off morphine for NAS states that their newborn sneezes and yawns frequently. How can the nurse use this moment to educate the new parent?

RISK BEHAVIORS

Overview

- Self-harm:
  - *Self-directed violence* is intentional self-injury.
  - Examples include cutting, scratching, burning, or attempted suicide.
  - Risk factors include a history of suicide attempts, family history of suicide, depression, stressful life events, alcohol abuse, and drug abuse.

 COMPLICATIONS

HIV is a contagious, bloodborne pathogen that can start with flu-like symptoms and progress to AIDS. Patients with AIDS are prone to frequent opportunistic infections due to a damaged immune system.

- Substance abuse:
  - *Substance abuse* is the recurrent use of alcohol or drugs that causes impairment, health problems, and failure to meet responsibilities.
    - There is a high incidence of substance use for adolescents with mental health disorders.
    - Examples include the use of alcohol, misuse of prescription drugs, use of illicit drugs, and injection drugs.
    - Alcohol, marijuana, and tobacco are the substances most commonly used by adolescents.
    - Substance abuse is likely to occur with other risky behaviors, such as unprotected sex and dangerous driving.
  - *Addiction* is psychologic dependence, compulsive use, or continued use, even after harmful consequences, including growth- and brain-development abnormalities.
- Unprotected sex
  - Unprotected sex occurs when individuals do not use prophylactic measures such as condoms and birth control.
  - Common STIs are HPV, HSV, chlamydia, gonorrhea, and HIV.
  - Risks of unprotected sex are pregnancy and STIs.

Signs and Symptoms

- Self-harm
  - Burns, scratches, bruises
  - Depression
  - Impulsiveness
  - Scars
  - Wearing long sleeves or pants even in hot weather
- STIs:
  - Chlamydia: presents with erythema, edema, and itching but may be asymptomatic; specific symptoms include:
    - Female: cervical exudate
    - Male: tenderness, dysuria, urethral discharge
  - HIV
    - Chills
    - Fatigue
    - Fever
    - Mouth ulcers
    - Muscle aches
    - Sore throat
    - Swollen lymph nodes
  - Gonorrhea
    - Female: cervicitis, discharge, dysuria, vulvovaginitis
    - Male: urethritis, yellow discharge, dysuria, frequency and urgency to urinate
  - HSV
    - Small painful, itchy vesicles on genitalia, buttocks, and thighs
    - Vesicles turn to shallow, circular painful lesions
  - HPV
    - High-risk types linked to cancers
    - Warts on male or female genitalia
- Substance abuse:
  - Eating and sleeping pattern changes
  - Changes in peer groups
  - Self-report
  - Skipping school or getting lower grades

Diagnosis

Labs

- Blood test or cheek swab for HIV
- Genital swab for STIs
- Urine culture

Diagnostic Testing

There are no diagnostic tests specific to diagnose risk behaviors.

Treatment

- Chlamydia and gonorrhea: doxycycline (Table 15.1)
- HIV: antiretroviral therapy

Nursing Interventions

- Assess for physical injuries from self-harm.
- Assist in identifying positive coping mechanisms in place of self-harming.
- Be available for questions and discussions from both adolescents and their families.
- Educate on contraceptive options.

(continued)

Nursing Interventions *(continued)*

- Educate on STIs and treatment plans.
- Help identify positive coping strategies.
- Maintain confidentiality regarding adolescent sexual health issues.
- Refer to mental health professionals.
- Start screening and asking about substance use in children at 9 years old.

Patient and Family Education

- Self-harm:
  - Call the National Suicide Prevention Lifeline if necessary.
  - Learn the number for Crisis Text Line.
  - Refrain from texting or using devices while driving.
  - Talk to a trusted adult if having thoughts of self-harm.
- Substance use:
  - Avoid peer situations where there may be pressure to use alcohol or drugs.
  - Do not get in a car with a driver who has been drinking or using legal/illegal substances.
- Unprotected sex:
  - Abstinence is the most reliable way to prevent pregnancy and avoid sexually transmitted diseases.
  - Abstain from sexual intercourse for 7 days after treatment for chlamydia and gonorrhea.
  - Condoms must be used correctly and every time to be effective.
  - The HPV vaccine is recommended at ages 11 to 12.
  - Use contraceptives to prevent pregnancy.
  - Families are encouraged to present sex education to school-age children regarding growth, development, and puberty.
  - Families should provide accurate information to adolescents about anatomy, pregnancy, contraceptives, and STIs.

NURSING PEARL

The CRAFFT screening is a tool to identify substance use and risk in adolescents. Two or more positive answers identify a positive screen.

C: Have you ever ridden in a **car** driven by someone (including yourself) who was high, drunk, or had been using drugs?

R: Have you ever used drugs or alcohol to **relax**?

A: Do you ever use substances **alone**?

F: Do you ever **forget** things that you did while using?

F: Do family or **friends** tell you to cut down?

T: Have you ever gotten into **trouble** when using?

SUICIDE

Overview

- *Suicide* is the act of self-injury with the intent that the injury results in death.
- *Suicidal ideation* is the thought, preoccupation, or planning of committing suicide.
- *Suicide attempt* is a self-directed injury behavior that is intended to cause death.
- A previous suicide attempt indicates a risk for a future suicide attempt.

COMPLICATIONS

Suicide is the second leading cause of death for adolescents ages 15 to 19 years old.

Signs and Symptoms

- Changes in behavior: sleep patterns, appetite, school performance
- Depression, loss of energy and interests, flat affect, feeling worthless
- Giving away possessions
- Preoccupation with death and dying
- Reckless behavior
- Withdrawal from friends

Diagnosis

Labs
There are no labs specific to diagnose suicide.

Diagnostic Testing
Suicidal screening.

Treatment

Depression treatment plan.

Nursing Interventions

- Patients with suicidal thoughts or plans should not be left alone; they should be in a safe, protective environment free of firearms, medications, sharp objects, shoelaces, and belts.
- Monitor or supervise adolescents that have expressed suicidal feelings or plans.
- Screen for suicide using SLAP:
  - Specificity: Ask if they feel suicidal and if they have a specific plan.
  - Lethality: Determine the lethality (gun, hanging, medications) of the plan.
  - Accessibility: Determine the availability of the planned method.
  - Proximity: Determine when they plan to commit suicide.
- Threats of suicide should always be taken seriously.

Patient and Family Education

- Family members should listen to child and provide support.
- Learn the information for the National Suicide Prevention Lifeline.
- Learn positive coping mechanisms and problem-solving skills.
- Reach out to an adult for help if a friend is considering suicide.

 ALERT!

In 2021, the American Academy of Pediatrics, the American Academy of Child and Adolescent Psychiatry, and the Children's Hospital Association declared a National Emergency in Child and Adolescent Health. In a statement, the organizations note that mental health concerns have been rising steadily for several years. The CDC reports that pediatric mental health emergencies have risen some 20% to 30%, with suicide attempts in girls approaching a 50% increase. Pediatric nurses should evaluate their patients' mental health, especially in communities with extended lockdowns or school disruptions.

 NURSING PEARL

Warning signs of suicide include giving away cherished possessions and sudden cheerfulness after a period of deep depression.

 POP QUIZ 15.5

When educating a caregiver of an adolescent with depression and history of suicidal ideations, what warning signs should the caregiver be aware of that the child may be preparing for suicide?

Table 15.1 Behavioral and Mental Health Medications

Indications	Mechanism of Action	Contraindications, Precautions, and Adverse Effects
Antibiotic (doxycycline)		
• Antibiotic treatment for chlamydia and gonorrhea	• Inhibit protein synthesis in bacterial cells	• While treating STI, medication may mask symptoms of other STIs. The patient should be tested for other STIs. • It is advised to have the partner treated to avoid reinfection. • Adverse effects include diarrhea. • Use caution for tissue hyperpigmentation and only use in children less than 8 years old in severe or life-threatening cases.

(continued)

Table 15.1 Behavioral and Mental Health Medications *(continued)*

Indications	Mechanism of Action	Contraindications, Precautions, and Adverse Effects
SSRI (citalopram, duloxitine, escitalopram, fluoxitine)		
• First-line antidepressant • Treat depression and anxiety symptoms	• Inhibit reuptake of serotonin	• Use caution with some SSRIs (citalopram) in children due to suicidal ideation and growth inhibition. Some SSRIs are not recommended or approved for children under 8 years old. • Medication is contraindicated with MAO inhibitors. • Adverse reactions include weight changes, overdose, and serotonin syndrome.
Tricyclic antidepressants (imipramine, amitriptyline)		
• Second-line antidepressant • Treat depression and anxiety symptoms	• Inhibit reuptake of both serotonin and norepinephrine, increasing the amount of neurotransmitter in the synaptic cleft	• Use with caution in children less than 12 years old. • Medication is contraindicated with MAO inhibitors. • Adverse effects include overdose, seizures, bone fractures, and anticholinergic effects.

RESOURCES

American Academy of Pediatrics (2021, October 19). *AAP-AACAP-CHA declaration of a national emergency in child and adolescent mental health*. https://www.aap.org/en/advocacy/child-and-adolescent-healthy-mental-development/aap-aacap-cha-declaration-of-a-national-emergency-in-child-and-adolescent-mental-health/

American Academy of Pediatrics. (2018, July 2). *Health concerns for gay and lesbian teens*. https://www.healthychildren.org/English/ages-stages/teen/dating-sex/Pages/Health-Concerns-for-Gay-and-Lesbian-Teens.aspx

American Academy of Pediatrics News. *AAP, AACAP, CHA declare national emergency in children's mental health*. https://www.aappublications.org/news/2021/10/19/children-mental-health-national-emergency-101921

American Psychiatric Association. (2020, October). *What is depression?* https://www.psychiatry.org/patients-families/depression/what-is-depression

Bonin, L. (2021). Patient education: Depression in children and adolescents. *UpToDate*. https://www.uptodate.com/contents/depression-in-children-and-adolescents-beyond-the-basics?search=depression%20treatment%20adolescent&topicRef=1231&source=see_link

Buckstein, O. (2021). Substance use disorder in adolescents: Epidemiology, pathogenesis, clinical manifestations and consequences, course, assessment, and diagnosis. *UpToDate*. https://www.uptodate.com/contents/substance-use-disorder-in-adolescents-epidemiology-pathogenesis-clinical-manifestations-and-consequences-course-assessment-and-diagnosis?search=CRAFFT%20screening%20substance%20use&source=search_result&selectedTitle=2~150&usage_type=default&display_rank=2#H2808800888

Centers for Disease Control and Prevention. (2019a, September 17). *Self-directed violence and other forms of self-injury*. U.S. Department of Health and Human Services, Centers for Disease Control and Prevention. https://www.cdc.gov/ncbddd/disabilityandsafety/self-injury.html

Centers for Disease Control and Prevention. (2019b, December 18). *Terminology. Adolescent and school health*. U.S. Department of Health and Human Services, Centers for Disease Control and Prevention. https://www.cdc.gov/healthyyouth/terminology/sexual-and-gender-identity-terms.htm

Centers for Disease Control and Prevention. (2020a, December 9). *LGBT youth resources*. U.S. Department of Health and Human Services, Centers for Disease Control and Prevention. https://www.cdc.gov/lgbthealth/youth-resources.htm

Centers for Disease Control and Prevention. (2020b, June 25). *People with disabilities and chronic diseases: Information about bullying*. U.S. Department of Health and Human Services, Centers for Disease Control and Prevention. https://www.cdc.gov/ncbddd/disabilityandsafety/bullying.html

Centers for Disease Control and Prevention. (2020c, March 25). *What is autism spectrum disorder?* U.S. Department of Health and Human Services, Centers for Disease Control and Prevention. https://www.cdc.gov/ncbddd/autis m/facts.html

Centers for Disease Control and Prevention. (2021, February 15). *Mental health conditions: Depression and anxiety.* U.S. Department of Health and Human Services, Centers for Disease Control and Prevention. https://www.cdc. gov/tobacco/campaign/tips/diseases/depression-anxiety.html

CrisisTextLine. (n.d). *How to deal with self-harm.* https://www.crisistextline.org/topics/self-harm/#what-is-self -harm-1

Forcier, M., & Olson-Kennedy, J. (2020). Gender development and clinical presentation of gender diversity in children and adolescents. *UpToDate.* https://www.uptodate.com/contents/gender-development-and-clinical-presentation- of-gender-diversity-in-children-and-adolescents?csi=85785c94-c2a1-4f1a-94832d46a8fc9464&source=contentShar e#H182326331

Hirsch, M., & Birnbaum, R. SSRI: Pharmacology, administration and side effects. (2022, April 11). *UpToDate.* https://www.uptodate.com/contents/selective-serotonin-reuptake-inhibitors-pharmacology-administration- and-side-effects?search=ssri&source=search_result&selectedTitle=2~145&usage_type=default&display_rank= 1#H367753

HIV.gov. (2020). *Symptoms of HIV.* https://www.hiv.gov/hiv-basics/overview/about-hiv-and-aids/symptoms-of-hiv

Hockenberry, M., Wilson, D., & Rodgers, C. (2017). *Wong's essentials of pediatric nursing.* Elsevier.

Jansson, L. (2021). Neonatal abstinence syndrome. *UpToDate.* https://www.uptodate.com/contents/neonatal-abstine nce-syndrome?search=NAS&source=search_result&selectedTitle=1~44&usage_type=default&display_rank=1 #H1521818068

Knight, J. R. (2020). *Craft+N questionnaire.* Center for Adolescent Behavioral Health Research, Boston Children's Hospital. https://crafft.org/wp-content/uploads/2021/07/CRAFFT_2.1N-HONC_Self-administered_2021-07-0 3.pdf

Lexicomp. (2021a). Alprazolam: Pediatric drug information [Drug Information]. *UpToDate.* https://www.uptodate .com/contents/alprazolam-pediatric-drug-information?search=alprazolam&source=panel_search_result&selected Title=2~120&usage_type=panel&kp_tab=drug_pediatric&display_rank=1#F132003

Lexicomp. (2021b). Citalopram: Pediatric drug information [Drug Information]. *UpToDate.* https://www.uptodate .com/contents/citalopram-pediatric-drug-information?search=celexa&source=panel_search_result&selected Title=2~103&usage_type=panel&kp_tab=drug_pediatric&display_rank=1

Lexicomp. (2021c). Doxycycline: Pediatric drug information [Drug Information]. *UpToDate.* https://www.uptodate .com/contents/doxycycline-pediatric-drug-information?search=doxycycline&source=panel_search_result&sel ectedTitle=2~148&usage_type=panel&kp_tab=drug_pediatric&display_rank=1#F163310

Lexicomp. (2021d). Methadone: Pediatric drug information [Drug Information]. *UpToDate.* https://www.uptodate .com/contents/methadone-pediatric-drug-information?search=methadone&source=panel_search_result&select edTitle=2~148&usage_type=panel&kp_tab=drug_pediatric&display_rank=1#F193961

Lexicomp. (2021e). Morphine: Pediatric drug information [Drug Information]. *UpToDate.* https://www.uptodate .com/contents/morphine-pediatric-drug-information?search=morphine&source=panel_search_result&selected Title=2~148&usage_type=panel&kp_tab=drug_pediatric&display_rank=1#F8776704

McLaughlin, K. (2019, July 8). Posttraumatic stress disorder in children and adolescents: Epidemiology, pathogenesis, clinical manifestations, course, assessment, and diagnosis. *UpToDate.* https://www.uptodate .com/contents/posttraumatic-stress-disorder-in-children-and-adolescents-epidemiology-pathogenesis-clinical -manifestations-course-assessment-and-diagnosis?search=ptsd%20children&source=search_result&selectedTi tle=2~150&usage_type=default&display_rank=2#H3276263985

Medial Mnemonics. (2021). *Symptoms of depression.* https://knowmedge.com/blog/medical-mnemonics-depressio n-sad-faces/

National Institute of Mental Health. (2016, February). *Eating disorders.* U.S. Department of Health and Human Services, National Institute of Mental Health. https://www.nimh.nih.gov/health/topics/eating-disorders/

National Suicide Prevention Lifeline. (n.d). *Youth.* https://suicidepreventionlifeline.org/help-yourself/youth/

O'Keefe, G. S., & Clarke-Pearson, K. (2011). The impact of social media on children, adolescents, and families. *Pediatrics, 127*(4), 800–804. https://doi.org/10.1542/peds.2011-0054. https://pediatrics.aappublications.org/con tent/127/4/800

Sege, R. (2021, July 5). Peer violence and violence prevention. *UpToDate.* https://www.uptodate.com/contents/peer -violence-and-violence-prevention?search=bullying&source=search_result&selectedTitle=1~46&usage_type=d efault&display_rank=1

Territo, H., & Burstein, G. (2021). CDC updates guidelines on treatments of sexually transmitted infections. *AAP News.* https://www.aappublications.org/news/2021/07/23/cdcstdguidelines072321

DE-ESCALATION STRATEGIES

Overview

- Most studies concerning de-escalation techniques apply to adults, but the techniques have been proven to work well with children.
- De-escalation strategies involve the following steps:
  - Identify the behavior as escalating as early as possible.
  - Recognize that even if verbally agitated, emotion coaching is possible.
  - Identify that the behavior may result in harm.
  - Plan for appropriate interventions.
  - Remember that the goal is to prevent injury and relieve agitation.

Signs and Symptoms

- Anger
- Crying
- Frustration
- Physical threats (to self or others)
- Physical violence: hitting or fighting behaviors
- Self-harm
- Swearing
- Throwing things
- Verbal threats or exclamations

Treatment

- Prevention: escalation of verbal aggression
- Ten domains of de-escalation

Nursing Interventions

- Assess and apply the appropriate restraint according to facility protocol.
- Keep voice calm.
- Try to find out what is bothering the child.
- Verify the child is not in pain.
- Be patient.
- Provide emotional support if needed.
- Listen and try to understand why the child is acting out.
- Avoid overreacting.

 ALERT!

Possible triggers in children, especially in a medical environment, can include:

- Unpredictability
- Sensory overload
- Feeling vulnerable or frustrated
- Feeling attacked or confronted

 NURSING PEARL

Emotion coaching is a de-escalation strategy that helps identify feelings, address the behavior, and problem-solve. Preventing injury to the patient and staff is the primary goal of emotion coaching.

 NURSING PEARL

The 10 Domains of De-Escalation

- Respect personal space.
- Do not be provocative.
- Establish verbal contact.
- Be concise; use short phrases to explain what needs to happen.
- Identify wants and feelings.
- Listen closely to the patient.
- Agree, or agree to disagree.
- Set clear limits.
- Offer choices and be optimistic.
- Debrief patient and staff when de-escalation has taken place.

(continued)

Nursing Interventions *(continued)*

- Try to be nonjudgmental and do not escalate the situation.
- Use emotion coaching to prevent escalation.
- Follow the 10 domains of de-escalation.
- Identify when de-escalating strategies fail.

Patient and Family Education

- Consult a child life therapist to assist with age-appropriate communication techniques, distractions, and things to do.
- Develop an age-appropriate plan of self-care.
- Family can learn de-escalation techniques.
- Family should reassure child that safety is the primary concern.
- Family should remember that child's thoughts and feelings are important.
- Find help in the community (support groups, or other parenting resources).
- Follow up with mental health specialists and other interdisciplinary support as indicated.
- Identify triggers.
- Implement routines at home to prevent anxiety.
- Journaling, drawing, or role-play (age appropriate) may help express emotions in a nonthreatening way.

 POP QUIZ 16.1

The nurse is preparing to assess a 16-year-old male patient after they have just received distressing news about their test results from the provider. This patient has a history of verbal and physical aggression, and the nurse recognizes his frustration as a possible trigger for violence. What can the nurse do to keep themselves and the patient safe for the remainder of the shift?

ENVIRONMENTAL SAFETY

Overview

- Pollutants and physical hazards are safety hazards for children in the environment.
  - Air pollutants, smoking, carbon monoxide, poor sanitation, unsafe agriculture, and lead poisoning (Chapter 5) can all create unsafe environments for children.
    - Because of their low body weight, children may be exposed to more toxins per mass.
    - Children may also have more time ahead of them to develop the long-term effects of early exposure.
  - Children are more vulnerable to environmental hazards because they are curious and explore without the benefit of knowledge of dangers and the health implications or solutions to hazards.
  - Many schools and neighborhoods are not environmentally safe. This may include the lack of sidewalks or the presence of mold.
  - Physical risks include stairs, construction sites, busy roads, and unsafe playground equipment.
- Unintentional injuries can include the following:
  - Accidents (bicycles, scooters, cars)
  - Burns (fires)
  - Drowning
  - Falls
  - Toxins
- Communicable diseases are also safety hazards to children.
  - Because of lower immunity levels, children may be more susceptible to communicable diseases present in their environments. However, building immunity is a necessary step for improved health. Making sure children get their immunizations and stressing their importance is part of the pediatric nurse's family education.
  - Some behaviors of small children, such as crawling, putting things in their mouth, and playing in the dirt, put them at a higher risk for safety hazards.

Signs and Symptoms

- Chronic respiratory illness from air pollutants
  - Aggravation of seasonal allergies
  - Asthma
- Common infectious diseases among children (Chapter 14)

Treatment

Treat injuries and illnesses as needed.

Nursing Interventions

- Care for the illness or injury.
- Educate family on caring for the child at home.
- Educate family on safety in the home and outside.
- Provide information on safe environments.

Patient and Family Education

- Family members who smoke should consider smoking cessation therapy or smoke outside the home.
- Implement home safety measures, including fire drills, and research neighborhood safety initiatives.
- Older children who may be experimenting with tobacco or vaping should educate themselves on the subject.
- Review good hygiene practices to keep the whole family healthier.

FACTITIOUS DISORDER IN ANOTHER/MUNCHAUSEN BY PROXY

Overview

- *FDIA*, also known as *Munchausen by proxy*, is a form of abuse where a caregiver makes up or causes an illness or injury in a person under their care, such as a child.
- The perpetrator can be anyone. Many times it is the mother, and the victim (child) can be any age.
- The caregiver invents, creates, or causes injury to the child, seemingly as a means of receiving attention from medical personnel.
- FDIA is diagnosed through a review of the patient's medical history, family history, and mother's history.
- They often seek care in multiple different hospitals.

Signs and Symptoms

- Disagreement between reported symptoms and diagnostic tests
- Presence of chemicals or substances (or nonneeded medications) in blood, stool, or urine
- Objective symptoms dependent on action inflicted by caregiver
  - Possibly including seizures, nausea and vomiting, diarrhea, and altered mental status
  - Possible poor weight gain
  - Symptoms (or worsening symptoms) usually witnessed only by the perpetrator
- Subjective symptoms include:
  - Condition improves in hospital
  - Evasive history
  - Exacerbation of illness just before discharge
  - Exaggeration or fabrication of symptoms by caregiver
  - Few visitors
  - Many hospitalizations or office visits for the child
  - Patient appearing more comfortable than they should
  - Perpetrator desires to be friends with medical staff

Signs and Symptoms *(continued)*

- Perpetrator opposed to psychiatry
- Perpetrator overly friendly, cooperative with healthcare workers, and extremely knowledgeable about the patient's alleged condition
- Perpetrator remaining at bedside and over-involved in care

Diagnosis

Labs
There are no labs specific to diagnose FDIA, but labs may be done depending on health concerns.

Diagnostic Testing
There are no diagnostic tests specific to diagnose FDIA, but diagnostic tests may be done depending on health concerns.

Treatment

Team of specialists involved in treatment including social workers, foster care, and law enforcement.

Nursing Interventions

- Assess and ensure the safety of the child.
- Contact proper authorities; use the same process of reporting as other forms of child abuse.
- Compare family's story to the physical findings.
- Identify and stop any nursing care intended for a fictional illness.
- Refer family to community resources, including counseling.
- Treat the victim's injuries.
- Visitation of the perpetrator may need to be curtailed to determine if the child gets better away from the caregiver. This should be done cautiously and only when certain an FDIA situation is evident.

Patient and Family Education

- Foster care (or family member deemed safe instead of foster care) if utilized: learn about the patient's condition, including physical and emotional trauma.
- Utilize counseling resources if age appropriate. The caregiver can also utilize counseling resources.
- Utilize support groups available for foster parents.

 POP QUIZ 16.2

A mother brings her 5-year-old daughter into the ED reporting fever and vomiting for several days. The daughter is small for her age and has been to the ED many times before with various concerns. Each time, the ED providers were unable to find a specific cause for the concern and released the patient with minimal treatment. On assessment, the patient is afebrile with unremarkable lab results. The nurse offers a snack, which the child eats with no signs of nausea or vomiting and appears happy and comfortable. The mother is friendly, but she will not leave the room and insists that her daughter still feels sick and should have further evaluation and testing done.

What should the nurse suspect, and how should the nurse handle the situation?

MALTREATMENT AND NEGLECT

Overview

- There are several types of abuse.
  - *Emotional*: behaviors that reduce a child's self-worth or well-being
  - *Neglect*: failure to meet a child's basic needs (physical and emotional) and keep them safe; this is the most common form of abuse
  - Physical:
    - *Physical abuse* is the intentional use of force that can cause physical injury.
    - Fractures that often come from abuse include rib fractures, parietal and linear skull fractures, spiral fractures, various fractures in different stages of healing, and long bone fractures in a nonambulatory child. *Shaken Baby Syndrome* is another form of abuse seen in infants and young children.

- *Sexual*: A child is sexually abused when they are involved in any type of sexual activity that they do not developmentally understand or consent to.
- There are several risk factors for abuse.
  - Children are at higher risk for abuse of all types if they have:
    - ADHD
    - Chronic illness
    - Congenital anomalies
    - Difficulty being consoled (infants)
    - Disabilities (physical, emotional, or intellectual)
    - Failed to attach or bonding with parent
    - Sibling(s) or a multiple birth challenging parents' ability to attend to all children
  - An environment at high risk for abuse includes:
    - Chronic stressors, loss of job, divorce, illness
    - Criminal or violent activities
    - Discrimination against the family
    - Disrespect within the family
    - Insufficient housing
    - Lead or toxins
    - Poverty
    - Social isolation
    - Violence in the home
  - Caregivers are more likely to abuse if the following are present:
    - Alcohol or substance abuse
    - Caregiver was abused
    - Low education level
    - Low level of child development knowledge
    - Negative perception of normal child behaviors
    - Psychiatric illness
    - Socially isolated
    - Unfamiliar with developmentally appropriate behaviors
    - Unplanned pregnancy of child
    - Unrealistic expectations of child
    - Use of physical punishment
    - Young age

Signs and Symptoms

- Anxiety
- Attempts to leave family (runaway)
- Bleeding, discharge from genitals/anal area
- Fractures/broken bones sometimes in various stages of healing
- Emotional/psychologic trauma
- Impaired socio-emotional skills
- Lack of attachment to parent
- Lack of cleanliness
- Lack of friends
- Learning, attention, and memory problems
- Nonage-appropriate sexual knowledge or curiosity, STIs
- Physical injuries
- PTSD
- Retinal detachment
- Shaken baby syndrome
- Brain hemorrhage
- Substance abuse
- Suicidal ideation

Diagnosis

Labs

- Depends on the nature of the abuse/neglect.
  - Calcium, alkaline phosphatase, albumin (malnutrition, bone mineralization disorders)
  - CBC including platelets, coagulation times (to rule out other causes for bruising or bleeding)
  - Toxicology screen (overdose or poisoning)

Diagnostic Testing

Depends on type of abuse:

- CT scan
- MRI
- Skeletal survey

Treatment

- First: ensure child's safety
- Employment services, adequate housing, healthcare, and social services; federal, state, and local agency referrals
- Safe environment for the child, including child services and foster care if needed
- Outpatient services as indicated
  - Continued counseling to help child through trauma
  - Type of therapy or psychologic counseling based on the child's injuries: physical, mental, or both
- Treatment for the abuse:
  - Physical: care of physical injuries, with possible hospital care for malnourishment
  - Sexual: medical care for physical injuries
  - Emotional: conversation, professional counseling as needed
  - Neglect:
    - ○ Talk with the child separately from the family if possible to ascertain what daily life is like for them.
    - ○ Link the family with community programs to help with basic needs, and refer to social services and/or family therapy as indicated.

Nursing Interventions

- Assess and record any physical or behavioral signs suspecting or confirming abuse.
- Assess for signs of malnutrition.
- Assess whether the child is meeting normal developmental milestones.
- Assist with investigations by law enforcement and child protective services.
- Encourage the child to express themselves in words or draw pictures. Utilize plush animals or dolls for role-play as needed. Involve a pediatric child life therapist.
- Interview child with open-ended questions.
- Monitor normal growth and development patterns.
- Observe and document any concerning interactions between parent and child.

Patient and Family Education

- Family should obtain information on community services.
- Family should understand the importance of the child's healthcare and the prevention of further abuse.
- Utilize emotional support and healthy communication.

 NURSING PEARL

Nurses are considered mandated reporters, which means that they must report suspected cases of abuse to law enforcement. Every state writes regulations for mandated reporters, including the standards for the report, the confidentiality of the reporter, and the responsibility of the reporter's institution. Abuse should be reported to the local child and youth services agency.

Most states require the following as mandatory reporters:

- Child care workers
- Clergy
- Counselors, therapists
- Law enforcement officers
- Physicians, nurses, other healthcare workers
- Social workers
- Teachers, principals, other school personnel

RESTRAINTS

Overview

- Restraints are used mostly in critical care units for children where their own safety is of paramount concern.
- Restraints are used when a patient shows agitated behavior that could compromise their safety, the safety of others, or to ensure the safe use of medical devices such as invasive lines and when intubated.
- Seclusion is a form of restraint.
- All four bed rails raised is a form of restraint.
- A new order is required upon initiation and daily for a child in restraints.
- When the child is calm, there should be an assessment for possible causes of the agitation:
  - Abnormal vital signs
  - Altered mental status
  - Hypoglycemia
  - Hypoxia
  - Neurologic deficits
  - Pain and discomfort
- Restraints (and medication used as a restraint) can be seen negatively by children and can be physically harmful and psychologically traumatic. Restraints should be the last option when dealing with children.
- The types of restraints used in pediatrics are physical (nonviolent or violent) and pharmacologic.
- Physical restraints restrict a person's free body movement.
  - Nonviolent physical restraints:
    - Bed/chair alarm
    - No-nos, arm immobilizers
    - Video, mechanical, or acoustical surveillance
  - Violent physical restraints
    - Restraints used when the patient's behavior is escalating and verbal de-escalation techniques are not effective
    - Sedation medications possible if the patient is still violent after placing restraints
- Pharmaceutical restraints are used to control a patient's behavior or restrict freedom of movement (when not needed to treat a medical condition).

Signs and Symptoms

- Indicated in one or both of the following:
  - Unsuccessful de-escalation strategies; patient cannot be redirected by verbal cues or distraction
  - Safety concerns where patient:
    - Causes harm to him/herself, other patients, staff, or family
    - Pulls at medical devices such as IVs, Foleys, NGs, or drains
    - Pulls at surgical dressings or sites

 ALERT!

There is potential harm in using restraints, including:

- Falling
- Incontinence
- Malnutrition
- Pressure injuries
- Psychologic harm
- Physical harm

 ALERT!

The Joint Commission regulates the use of restraints.

- The Joint Commission regulates the initiation and evaluation of preventative measures that, if used, will avoid the use of restraints. A primary focus is that the least restrictive restraint is to be used for the least possible period of time. It should be removed when it is no longer needed.
- The Joint Commission states that policies in facilities must describe:
  - The care required for patients who are restrained
  - The standards of monitoring the patient during the use of restraints
  - That there must be a physician order, either verbal or written, that is time-limited and must be obtained for each use
  - Hospital policy addresses the periodic observation of a patient for whom restraints or seclusion is used

Nursing Interventions

- Assess and determine the need for restraints; promote patient safety.
- Check for a written order for the restraints. If a verbal order was given, document the verbal order and obtain a written order as soon as possible, depending on the institution's policy.
- Assess the patient's anxiety level.
- Ensure elimination needs are met.
- Evaluate for adequate hydration.
- Periodic assessments must include:
  - Assessing skin integrity
  - Checking that the restraints are correctly applied
  - Neurovascular checks
  - Whether the restraints accomplish their purpose
- Monitor circulation status frequently.
- Provide range of motion exercise for restrained extremities.
- Reassure patient with every assessment.

 POP QUIZ 16.3

A nurse is called to the room of a 14-year-old patient by the family because the patient is yelling at their mother. The nurse keeps their distance, remains calm, and attempts to calm the patient. The patient refuses to respond to the nurse, who continues to attempt to engage the patient in normal conversation. Instead, the patient continues to yell at their entire family, picks up several objects in the room, and throws the objects at the family. What should the nurse's next steps be?

Patient and Family Education

- Be assured that the least amount of restraint will be used.
- Understand the need for restraints and that restraints will be removed when it is safe to do so.

SLEEP PRACTICES

Overview

- It is recommended that babies sleep on their backs to reduce the risk of SIDS (Chapter 2).
- A safe sleep environment includes a flat, firm surface with a tight-fitting sheet. Avoid placing any extra blankets, pillows, crib bumpers, stuffed animals, or toys in crib. Avoid co-sleeping.

Diagnosis

Labs
There are no labs specific to sleep practices.

Diagnostic Testing
There are no diagnostic tests specific to sleep practices.

Treatment

There is no treatment specific to sleep practices.

Nursing Interventions

- Model safe practices in the hospital.
- Swaddle babies if using blankets.

Patient and Family Education

Sleep practices patient education is directed toward the family.

 ALERT!

SIDS is defined as the sudden death of an infant under 1 year old which, after investigation, remains unexplained. Investigation includes an autopsy, review of clinical history, and death scene exploration.

Risk factors include:

- Young mother
- Maternal smoking or drinking alcohol during pregnancy
- Little or no prenatal care
- Preterm baby, low birth weight
- Sleeping prone
- Sleeping on fluffy blankets and linens
- Sleeping with accessories or toys
- Sleeping in parent's bed
- Putting a lot of clothing on the child
- Brief, resolved unexplained event or an acute life-threatening event
  - Not a diagnosis; an unexplained event involving breathing, appearance, or behavior
  - Challenging clinical question: which patient needs further testing?
  - Can include:
    - Cyanosis, pallor
    - Absent, decreased, or irregular breathing
    - Marked change in tone
    - Altered level of responsiveness

- Learn SIDS prevention techniques:
  - Sleep on back on firm surface, such as a breathable mattress.
  - Breastfeeding is associated with less incidence of SIDS.
  - Do not put blankets, bumpers, or pillows in crib.
  - The use of a pacifier at bedtime is permissible.
  - Dress the baby in few layers so as not to overheat.
- If nursing, mother should not drink alcohol or use illicit drugs.
- Engage in supervised tummy time to strengthen the baby's neck and development of the baby's head.
- Consider alternatives to blankets in bed, such as wearable blankets (sleep sacks).
- Understand the reasons for safety precautions.
- If any safety measures present challenges for the family, brainstorm possible solutions.

> **ALERT!**
>
> The AAP recommends that babies wait until they are at least 12 months old before sleeping with a blanket. It is also recommended that infants may sleep in the same room with parents but not the same bed.

RESOURCES

Arpey, N. C., Gaglioti, A. H., & Rosenbaum, M. E. (2017). How socioeconomic status affects patient perceptions of health care: A qualitative study. *Journal of Primary Care & Community Health*, 169–175. https://doi .org/10.1177/2150131917697439.

Blum, N. J., & Pipan, M. E. (2018). *Developmental and behavioral pediatrics* (2nd ed.). American Academy of Pediatrics.

Butchart, A., Kahane, T., Furniss, T., Mian, M., & Phinney, A. (2006). *Preventing child maltreatment: A guide to taking action and generating evidence.* https://apps.who.int/iris/rest/bitstreams/51614/retrieve

Centers for Disease Control and Prevention. (n.d.). *Preventing child abuse and neglect.* U.S. Department of Health and Human Services, Centers for Disease Control and Prevention. https://www.cdc.gov/violenceprevention/chil dabuseandneglect/prevention.html

Centers for Disease Control and Prevention. (2018, January 9). *Safe sleep for babies: eliminating hazards.* U.S. Department of Health and Human Services, Centers for Disease Control and Prevention. https://www.cdc.gov/ vitalsigns/safesleep/index.html

Dimsdale, J. E. (2020, October). Factitious disorder imposed on another. *Merck Manual Professional Version.* https:// www.merckmanuals.com/professional/psychiatric-disorders/somatic-symptom-and-related-disorders/factitious -disorder-imposed-on-another?query=Factitious%20Disorder%20Imposed%20on%20Another

Eunice Kennedy Shriver National Institute of Child Health and Human Development. (n.d.). *Known risk factors for SIDS and other sleep-related causes of infant death.* U.S. Department of Health and Human Services, Eunice Kennedy Shriver National Institute of Child Health and Human Development. https://safetosleep.nichd.nih.gov /safesleepbasics/risk/factors

Montovani, C. (2017, February 24). Using de-escalation techniques to prevent violent behavior in pediatric psychiatric emergencies: It is possible. *Pediatric Dimensions*, 2(1), 1–2. https://doi.org/10.15761/PD.1000138. https://www.researchgate.net/publication/314514229_Using_de-escalation_techniques_to_prevent_violent_behavi or_in_pediatric_psychiatric_emergencies_It_is_possible

National Alliance on Mental Illness. (2016). *Mental health crisis planning for children.* https://namimn.org/wp-conte nt/uploads/sites/188/2018/03/NAMI-MHCrisisPlanforChildrenFeb2016.pdf

Schmidt, M. (2021). *Attachment-informed de-escalation techniques. Adoptalk 1.* https://www.nacac.org/resource/atta chment-informed-de-escalation-techniques/

U.S. Department of Health & Human Services. (2019). *Child maltreatment 2019.* https://www.acf.hhs.gov/sites/defa ult/files/documents/cb/cm2019.pdf

Winter, H. (2021). Gastroesophageal reflux in infants. *UpToDate.* https://www.uptodate.com/contents/ gastroesophageal-reflux-in-infants?csi=4ce9d2b9-7ace-43a9-9318-225620c34402&source=contentShare

World Health Organization. (2021). *The environment and health for children and their mothers.* https://www.who.int/ ceh/publications/factsheets/fs284/en/

PROFESSIONAL RESPONSIBILITIES

Overview

- *Assent* is the agreement of someone under 18 years of age after they have been informed.
  - Children as young as 7 may give their assent, usually for research only.
  - Assent is in addition to, not a replacement for, a legal guardian's consent.
- *Consent* is the legal agreement of someone 18 and over.
  - Children's parents or legal guardians must give consent prior to any procedure, surgery, or medical treatment.
  - Legal guardians are not required to be parents and are often grandparents or other family members. Legal guardians can give consent.
  - Foster parents can legally give consent for treatment.
  - Adolescents may consent without their family's knowledge to treatment for medically emancipated conditions including STIs, mental health, and alcohol and drug treatment, pregnancy, and contraceptives.
- An *emancipated minor* is a child under 18 who is legally able to care and make decisions for themselves. Reasons can vary by state, but typically can occur after pregnancy, marriage, graduation from high school, or military service. Emancipated minors can give consent for themselves.
- *Informed consent* is when the patient, parent, or legal guardian is given information about a procedure, surgery, or treatment, including the potential risks and benefits, so that they can make their own intelligent voluntary decision regarding their healthcare.
- An informed decision is needed for both assent and consent.
- If, at any time, the family or child wishes to withdraw their consent and/or assent, they have the right to do so.

Assessment

- Identify cultural and spiritual influences that impact child and family healthcare decisions and practices:
  - Religion impacts many medical decisions including diet, medications, blood product use, modesty, and preference of gender of their caretakers.
  - Many religions reject part or all mainstream healthcare.
- Assess understanding of language or need for an interpreter.
  - Language barriers can be detrimental to giving and receiving nursing and medical care.
  - Consent should be discussed in the patient's or legal guardian's preferred language.
- Assess child and family's understanding of health/disease process.
- Assess the patient and/or caregiver's ability to understand relevant medical information and their ability to make an independent, voluntary decision.
- Assess child and family's reactions to acute stressors (e.g., hospitalization, new diagnosis, upcoming surgical procedure). Assess if the patient and family can identify positive coping strategies.

(continued)

Nursing Considerations *(continued)*

- Assess if patient and family can identify a support system. There are several normal reactions in response to crisis:
  - Avoidance
  - Broad distress (symptoms from every category)
  - Dissociation
  - Hyper-arousal symptoms
  - Reexperiencing
- The child/family should react appropriately to chronic stress.
  - Caregivers need to take care of themselves as well.
  - Chronic illnesses can be overwhelming for caregivers and families.
  - Identify educational needs of child and family:
  - Assess whether the family needs time for the following:
    - Grieve new diagnosis
    - Consider new plan of care
    - Evaluate priorities
    - Participate in discharge planning

Nursing Considerations

- Address educational needs of the child and family.
- Advocate for the child and family in managing care.
- Ensure a signed consent form is completed prior to starting procedure or treatment.
  - If provider obtains verbal consent over the phone, the nurse's role may be to witness.
  - The nurse will verify the person who is giving consent and document the consent as witness.
- Identify and address ethical and legal concerns related to pediatric practice (e.g., assent, mandatory reporting, privacy and confidentiality, custody, refusal of care).
- Incorporate cultural and spiritual needs into the plan of care.
- Implement communication strategies appropriate to child and family's developmental capabilities.
- Implement use of an interpreter (in person, over the phone, or tablet device) or translated materials in the patient's preferred language.
- Provide developmentally appropriate preparation and support for procedures.
- Understand and address refusal of treatment.
  - Parents can deny treatment for their child in certain circumstances.
  - An emancipated minor may also refuse treatment.
  - The state may take over medical decisions for a minor if all the following conditions are met:
    - The medical community is in agreement about the course of treatment for the child.
    - The expected outcome for the child would be a good quality of life.
    - The child would die without the treatment.
    - The parent is refusing to grant permission.
    - Children do not have the legal ability to say no to treatment.
  - For information on refusal for blood transfusion, see Chapter 12.

Patient and Family Education

- Ask all questions prior to giving or signing consent for procedures and treatments.
- Request translated information and materials in their preferred language or request an interpreter.
- Care must be taken to assure that a minor is developmentally capable to perform what is requested and understand what is expected of them.

 POP QUIZ 17.1

A 16-year-old patient is seeking medical treatment for an expected STI diagnosis. The patient is concerned about their parents finding out and asks the nurse if their parents will need to be informed. How should the nurse respond?

DIVERSITY

Overview

- Family dynamics
  - There are various types of family structures or households: traditional, blended, extended, single parent, nuclear and binuclear, communal, and LGBTQ+ families.
- Culture
  - *Culture* is characterized by values, beliefs, and practices learned or shared within a particular group across generations.
  - *Ethnicity* is a group of people who share cultural heritage.
  - To provide the best care, healthcare providers must understand how a patient's culture affects their healthcare. Determine what is important to patients and families regarding:
    - Clothing
    - Food
    - Gender roles
    - Language
    - Medicine
    - Rituals or practices
    - Spiritual beliefs
- Religion
  - Their families, communities, and culture often influence children's religious beliefs and spirituality. It is a source of strength and moral purpose for many people.
  - Children may want to incorporate praying or religious rituals into their daily care.
  - Religious beliefs can be central to a patient's life, but may also cause barriers to healthcare. Some religious beliefs reject part or all of mainstream healthcare.
  - Religion impacts many medical decisions regarding diet, medications, blood product use, modesty, and preference of gender of their caretakers.
- Socioeconomic status
  - Social class is the patient and family's economic and education level.
  - Families of lower socioeconomic status may have access to fewer resources.
  - Poverty can lead to lack of resources such as adequate clothing and housing or nutritious and affordable food, leading to poor nutrition.
  - Poverty can directly affect healthcare because of access to insurance, providers who will take Medicaid or uninsured patients, and the ability to pay for prescriptions.

 ALERT!

Practices such as coining and cupping in Vietnamese and Asian cultures can leave lesions or bruises on the skin but are done with the belief of treating illness or getting rid of disease.

 ALERT!

Jehovah's Witnesses have a religious belief that they should not accept blood and will commonly refuse a blood transfusion (Chapter 11).

 ALERT!

Dietary restrictions vary according to different religions. Some cultures and religions have dietary restrictions that will affect medical treatment, but be aware that some adherents are more strictly observant than others. In general:

- Hinduism: no beef, no "foods that stimulate the senses"
- Buddhism: vegetarian; some eat fish, some eat no meat
- Sikhism: no alcohol
- Mormons: no smoking, alcohol, or caffeine
- 7th Day Adventist: strict lacto-ovo vegetarian: no meat, fish, or poultry, and no alcohol, smoking, or caffeine
- Jewish: kosher, no pork or shellfish, additional restrictions on religious holidays
- Islam: no pork: can affect medication choice as heparin and some vaccinations contain pork derivatives

Assessment

- Assess family dynamics by determining legal guardian and primary caregiver, family structure, and if patient has any siblings.
- Assess if the patient or family identifies with a specific religion or culture and if there are any beliefs or rituals they would like the nurses or providers to be aware of.
- Assess patient and family or learner's education level and preferred learning style prior to teaching about a disease process or discharge education.
- Assess patient and family for their preferred language and any need for an interpreter.
- Gender roles within relationships and cultures need to be acknowledged by the healthcare team.

Nursing Considerations

- Family-centered care is an approach to patient care that involves the patient and family in partnership with the nurse and medical team in the planning, delivery, and evaluation of the patient's healthcare.
- Family-centered care is a collaborative effort between families and healthcare teams in decision-making.
- Culture: Assess for any cultural beliefs or restrictions, or dietary requirements patients and families want the nurse or provider to be aware of.
- Religion
  - Respect the patient and family beliefs and practices.
  - Incorporate care around religious rituals or daily prayer.
  - Offer chaplain services for hospitalized patients and advocate for spiritual practices prior to surgeries or at end-of-life care.
  - Seek to gain knowledge about religions of the patient population in the area.
- Socioeconomic status
  - Assess for barriers to care including transportation issues, medication payment issues, and access to providers or pharmacies.
  - Assess home environment for safety, including safe sleep surfaces, smoke detectors, carbon monoxide detectors, and car seats.
  - Coordinate care with social work or case management as needed for supplies or resources.
- Common considerations for various religions:
  - Hinduism
    - Personal hygiene of great importance
    - Death rituals, including:
      - Preference to die at home
      - Cremation on the day of death
      - Family washes body after death, priest may pour water in mouth
    - Right hand is used for eating and the left for toileting
  - Buddhism
    - Death must be peaceful and calm.
    - Family will pray and chant.
    - No mind-altering drugs permitted.
    - Often vegetarians
  - Sikhism
    - In death, the body bathed, dressed, and cremated
    - Floor covered with white sheets; no shoes worn
    - Hair on body not to be cut
  - Mormon
    - No alcohol, caffeine, or tobacco
    - Last rites for death
    - Baptism for infant
  - 7th Day Adventists
    - Many vegetarians
    - Practice fasting

- ○ Believe the dead are only unconscious
- ○ Diet is important for healing
- Judaism
  - ○ Circumcision by rabbi on 8th day of life
  - ○ Food must be kosher, separating milk and meat
  - ○ Celebrate the shiva at death
  - ○ May request the rabbi's opinion on medical matters
  - ○ Amputated limbs buried in consecrated ground
  - ○ Burial must take place as soon as possible.
  - ○ Family stays with deceased until taken away
- Islam
  - ○ Women care for the sick and dying
  - ○ After death, body wrapped in white cloth and positioned to face Mecca
  - ○ No pork or alcohol
  - ○ Handwashing rituals
  - ○ Fasting

HIPAA COMPLIANCE

Overview

- *HIPAA* is a 1996 federal law that protects patient health information from being shared without the patient's knowledge or consent.
- HIPAA is in place to protect patient privacy and confidentiality.
- HIPAA allows the parent of a minor child to have access to their child's health records in most situations, with exceptions being:
  - When the child is an emancipated minor or treated for medically emancipated conditions
  - When the child is under the care of the court and a court-appointed individual
  - When the parent agrees that the child and healthcare provider may have a confidential relationship
- Areas of concern regarding confidentiality for adolescents are:
  - Sexual health, activity, pregnancy
  - Use of recreational drugs

Nursing Considerations

- Maintain professional boundaries in therapeutic relationships (appropriate use of social media, gifting).
  - Nurses cannot accept gifts from patients or families. Gifts may be given to the unit.
  - Use of social media or social networking sites must be professional and not violate the relationship that exists with patients.
    - ○ Avoid using patient information on social networking sites.
    - ○ Maintain professional boundaries with patients and families.
    - ○ Remember that coworkers, patients, and employers may see social media postings.
    - ○ Use privacy settings for personal social media accounts.
    - ○ Report social media postings that violate HIPAA.
  - Positive uses of social media:
    - ○ Professional networking
    - ○ Professional education
    - ○ Organizational promotion
    - ○ Patient care portals
    - ○ Patient education
    - ○ Public health programs

(continued)

Nursing Considerations *(continued)*

- Negative uses of social media:
  - Breaching patient privacy
  - Creating damage to professional image
  - Disseminating poor quality health information
  - Venting about work problems
  - Violation of patient-healthcare worker boundaries
- Educate family about the HIPAA provisions and have them sign the form that states they understand.
- Explain privacy requirements to caregivers and patient and what must be done to negate this policy.
- Only the legal guardians may call and get information on the patient's condition via the telephone. Generally, there is a password that only the guardians and nurse will know.

 POP QUIZ 17.2

Explain how the HIPAA Act of 1996 affects patients today.

PALLIATIVE AND END-OF-LIFE CARE

Overview

- Palliative care supports a patient living with a debilitating chronic illness and their family.
  - Focus on improving quality of life and supportive care for symptoms.
  - Patient can receive palliative care as well as curative treatment for their illness.
  - Palliative care teams are made up of many different professionals such as providers, nurses, nutritionists, and chaplains that can help with physical, psychologic, and social distress.
  - A palliative care patient can progress to hospice if less than 6 months to live.
- Hospice care is available for patients with expected 6 months or less to live.
  - Hospice care is for patients with an illness too severe to treat, or for a patient choosing to not continue treatment for their illness.
  - Focus on pain control, comfort, dignity, and quality of life of a patient who is dying.
  - Focus on physical, psychosocial, and spiritual needs.
  - Hospice is responsible for symptom management, coordination of care, communication and decision-making, clarification of goals of care, and quality of life.
  - Hospice improves the quality of life for the patient as well as the family and provides support for siblings.
  - The hospice caregiver will prepare the family for end-of-life care.
- End-of-life care is available.
  - Infants and toddlers have no to limited understanding of death.
  - Preschoolers can believe that their thoughts or actions can cause death or think that death is temporary.
  - School-age children can begin to understand the concept of death and dying. They can start to ask questions about a disease process or fear death and dying. They realize death is irreversible.
  - Adolescents have a concrete understanding of death and dying. They may feel isolated from peers and focus on physical symptoms of their illness rather than of death.

Assessment

- Signs and symptoms of clinical deterioration leading to death:
  - Agonal, noisy breathing
  - Changes in breathing
  - Confusion
  - Decreased appetite and thirst
  - Difficulty swallowing
  - Loss of bowel, urine control
  - Loss of senses

- Mental confusion
- Physical disfigurement
- Skin color changes
- End-of-life documents:
  - Advance directives
    - A *living will* is a legal document for anyone 18 years of age and over that states a person's wishes regarding their medical treatment in a situation where they are unable to give consent. Directives can be made on behalf of a minor by a parent, spouse, or guardian.
    - A *healthcare proxy* is a legal document in which an individual designates another person to make healthcare decisions if they are incapable of making them.
    - A *durable power of attorney* is a legal document that allows another person to make bank transactions, sign social security checks, apply for disability, or pay bills for another who is medically incapacitated.
  - DNR orders
    - Providers write DNR orders.
    - The DNR order instructs healthcare workers not to do CPR if the patient's breathing stops or if their heart stops beating.
    - The patient can change their mind but must have the provider change the order.
  - Physician orders for life-sustaining treatment
    - The physician, in consultation with guardians, writes what is to be done and not done regarding life-saving interventions.
    - This is typically done for a complex patient.
  - Do not escalate orders
    - Do not escalate orders set limits on different interventions (e.g., medication amounts).
    - Families can decide and communicate with the provider what they want to withhold (e.g., medications only, or no CPR but all other medical treatments). It is easier for a family to set a limit rather than withhold all treatment.

Nursing Considerations

- Beliefs on death and dying are different for different cultures. If the healthcare team is aware of these beliefs, dying can be handled in a way that the patient and family consider correct.
  - Provide guidance for anticipated progression of condition and treatment options.
  - Provide palliative care for the child and family to promote quality of life (e.g., massage therapy for chronic condition, spiritual care for family).
  - Manage care and needs throughout the dying process (e.g., symptom management, interdisciplinary resources, support for family).
  - Discuss the possibility of organ donation and what that would entail.
  - Support end-of-life decision-making (e.g., DNR status, family presence, hospice).
  - Provide psychosocial support for the child and family dealing with grief and loss.
- Give honest, clear, and accurate information about illness, nursing care, and known prognosis.
- Involve children in decision-making processes and discuss how much information they want to know.
- Involve child life therapists to help explain death and dying to patients and siblings.
- Support the family.
  - Advocate for the patient and family and help them navigate the healthcare system.
  - Encourage families to spend time with patient.
  - Help to manage any cultural or language differences.
  - Support families with ethical concerns regarding different aspects of the healthcare process (e.g., blood administration).
  - Encourage the family to attend to their own needs as well as assist the patient.

 POP QUIZ 17.3

A patient has a chronic lung condition that limits their activity. They attend school on a limited basis but are able to complete some of their work online. The patient lives with their mother and little brother. The mother has two jobs to support both children. The patient is able to understand their medication and treatment routine if they are feeling well, but sometimes forgets. What type of care team would this patient and their family benefit from?

Patient and Family Education

- Discuss how families would like to inform child and siblings of illness or prognosis.
- Discuss options for family support from social worker, psychology professional, or child life specialist.
- Offer resources for information on hospice care, palliative care, and end-of-life care and documents.

THERAPEUTIC COMMUNICATION

Overview

- *Therapeutic communication* is a process where the nurse consciously influences the patient or helps them to better understand through verbal and nonverbal means.
- The nurse implements communication strategies appropriate to the child's and the family's developmental capabilities.
- Therapeutic communication provides mutual acceptance and respect and improves outcomes by:
  - Using understanding language
  - Active listening
  - Maintaining a low-authority profile
  - Showing empathy
  - Using open-ended questions

Assessment

- Assess child and family's understanding of health/disease process.
- Assess child and family's reactions to acute stressors (e.g., family crisis, hospitalization, violence).
- Assess coping mechanisms of child, siblings, and caregivers.
- Assess verbal and nonverbal communication needs.

Nursing Considerations

- Allow time without distractions for communication.
- Encourage the patient to express feelings.
- Introduce self to patient and family.
- Communicate at patient or family eye level; for example, sit down if they are sitting.
- Meet patient and family at their education level when communicating health information.
- Speak clearly and confidently with simple sentences.
- Use open-ended questions when gathering further information from patients and families.
- Clarify the patient's message or statement by paraphrasing or restating to ensure understanding.
- Consider the age of the child when communicating.
  - Infant
    - Use nonverbal behaviors.
    - Maintain calm, soft touch, and soft voice.
  - Toddler/preschooler
    - Be honest.
    - Use simple, direct language.
    - Give choices when available.
  - School age
    - Allow patient to discuss feelings and fears.
    - Use their hobbies and interests to reduce anxiety.
    - Explain reasoning for nursing care and treatments.
  - Adolescent
    - Maintain privacy and confidentiality.
    - Give attention and listen.

- Avoid using medical jargon.
- Education for patients and families should be appropriate for age level. If adolescent or adult, materials should be at a 6th-grade level.
- Integrate psychosocial assessment in the plan of care in collaboration with the child and family.

RESOURCES

American Nurses Association. (n.d.). *Social media.* https://www.nursingworld.org/social/

Amoah, V. M. K., Anokye, R., Boakye, D. S., Acheampong, E., Budu-Ainooson, A., Okyere, E., Kumi-Boateng, G., Yeboah, C., & Afriyie, J. O. (2019). A qualitative assessment of perceived barriers to effective therapeutic communication among nurses and patients. *BMC Nurse, 18*(4). https://doi.org/10.1186/s12912-019-0328-0

Campbell, Y., Machan, M., & Fisher, M. (2016). The Jehovah's Witness population: Considerations for preoperative optimization of hemoglobin. *AANA Journal, 84*(3), 173–178. https://www.aana.com/docs/default-source/aana -journal-web-documents-1/jehovahs-witness-0616-pp173-178.pdf?sfvrsn=d1d348b1_6

Centers for Disease Control and Prevention. (2018). *Health insurance portability and accountability act of 1996 (HIPAA). Centers for Disease Control and Prevention.* U.S. Department of Health and Human Services, Centers for Disease Control and Prevention. https://www.cdc.gov/phlp/publications/topic/hipaa.html

Bruijn, W., Daams de., G. J., van Hunnik F., Arends, A. J., Boelens, A. M., Bosnak, E. M., Meerveld, J., Roelands, B., van Munster, B. C., Verwey, B., Figee, M., de Rooij, S. E., & Mocking, R. (2020). Physical and pharmacological restraints in hospital care: Protocol for a systematic review. *Frontiers in Psychiatry, 10,* 921. https://www.ncbi .nlm.nih.gov/pmc/articles/PMC7058582/

Myers-Wallis, J. A. (2020, May 23). Family life education for families facing acute stress: Best practices and recommendations. *Family Relations Interdisciplinary Journal of Applied Family Science, 69*(3), 662–676. https:// onlinelibrary.wiley.com/doi/abs/10.1111/fare.12452

National Cancer Institute. (2020). *Children's assent.* U.S. Department of Health and Human Services, National Cancer Institute. https://www.cancer.gov/about-cancer/treatment/clinical-trials/patient-safety/childrens-assent

Psychology Today. (2021). *Understanding family dynamics.* https://www.psychologytoday.com/us/basics/family -dynamics

RegisteredNursing.org. (2021, August 9). *Therapeutic communication: NCLEX RN.* https://www.registerednursing. org/nclex/therapeutic-communication/

Rumum, A. J. (2014, April). Influence of religious beliefs on healthcare practice. *International Journal of Education and Research, 2*(4), 37–48. https://www.ijern.com/journal/April-2014/05.pdf

18

ANSWERS

CHAPTER 2

POP QUIZ 2.1

3 months

POP QUIZ 2.2

Educate these parents that toddlers must stay in rear-facing car seats until age 3 or until they meet the maximum weight and height requirements for rear-facing car seats. When toddlers outgrow the rear-facing car seat, they can use a forward-facing car seat until at least age 5, and then ultimately graduate to a booster seat when they are the appropriate height and weight.

POP QUIZ 2.3

Trust versus mistrust, because infants develop trust through their primary caregiver, providing stability, consistency, loving care, and meeting their basic needs.

POP QUIZ 2.4

A patient who just turned 4 should be able to combine three to four words to form complex sentences, stand on one foot, pedal a tricycle, and be able to dress themselves. The child may start to be able to communicate using four- to five-word sentences and be able to skip, hop, throw a ball overhead, and catch a ball.

POP QUIZ 2.5

Side effects are mild fever and injection site soreness. Fever can be managed with a cool bath or nonaspirin pain reliever, such as acetaminophen. Patient is too young for ibuprofen. Injection site soreness can be managed by placing a cool, damp cloth on the site.

CHAPTER 3

POP QUIZ 3.1

The nurse should explain that the medication needs to be administered separately in order to ensure the infant receives all the medication. If the infant does not finish the bottle, the infant may not receive the entire dose of medication.

POP QUIZ 3.2

The nurse should check the six rights of medications: right patient, right drug, right dose, right route, right time, right documentation. The nurse should calculate the safe dose range. The nurse should check patency and confirm placement of NG tube.

POP QUIZ 3.3

The nurse should ask open-ended questions such as:
- What natural supplements, herbs, or vitamins are you taking?
- What OTC products are you taking?
- What is the dose or how often do you take them?

CHAPTER 4

POP QUIZ 4.1

Assess for abnormal eye contact, delays or impairment with communication milestones, and unusual repetitive behavior. Assess and rule out any other diagnosis, such as performing a hearing screen.

POP QUIZ 4.2

The child can have the cheeseburger and the broccoli. The bun, french fries, and ice cream are not permitted on a ketogenic diet.

POP QUIZ 4.3

The patient is most likely suffering from a malfunctioning shunt. High ICP would cause the symptoms that the child is suffering. A head CT or shunt series in x-ray should be done to assess the shunt. If it is not draining, the patient needs surgery to have it replaced.

POP QUIZ 4.4

The nurse should prepare the mother that blood tests for genetic disorders might be indicated. If the blood test/chromosomal analysis is ordered by the provider and confirms trisomy 21, then the infant should be referred to a cardiologist, an ophthalmologist, and an audiologist. The nurse should enlist the help of social workers, chaplains, or community support as appropriate to support the family.

CHAPTER 5

POP QUIZ 5.1

The eye patch is worn over the stronger eye, not over the affected eye. Using the patch will help the child to use their left eye (lazy eye) more and stimulate it without the right eye compensating.

POP QUIZ 5.2

This patient's assessment and past medical history are concerning for sensorineural hearing loss because an 8-month-old should be vocalizing, and gentamicin is an ototoxic medication.

POP QUIZ 5.3

To avoid pollen and prevent allergic rhinitis symptoms, the patient can stay indoors or keep windows closed on high pollen days. They should also change clothes after being outside on high pollen days or take a shower after coming inside.

POP QUIZ 5.4

The child may return to school after being afebrile or taking antibiotics for at least 24 hours.

POP QUIZ 5.5

Tachycardia, pallor, frequent swallowing, and vomiting bright red blood could indicate hemorrhage. Respiratory distress, stridor, and drooling post-op would indicate airway obstruction.

CHAPTER 6

POP QUIZ 6.1

The neonate may have poor lower extremity pulses, be pale in color, have a heart murmur, and have a blood pressure discrepancy between the upper and lower extremities. Diagnostic testing will be done to determine the severity of the coarctation. Family should be informed of the needed interventions as soon as possible.

POP QUIZ 6.2

These are signs and symptoms of TOF. First, the nurse should try to calm the toddler down and put them on oxygen. The nurse should anticipate an order for an opioid, such as morphine, and propranolol.

POP QUIZ 6.3

The nurse should advise the parents that their child will be monitored with both blood and urine tests. To evaluate the patient's heart, an echocardiogram will be done. Since they have been sick less than 10 days, they will most likely be given IVIG and aspirin. The patient's temperature will be monitored closely, and the nurses will administer IV fluids to keep them hydrated.

CHAPTER 7

POP QUIZ 7.1

Follow asthma care plan, avoid triggers as much as possible, and take controller medication as prescribed, even when not having symptoms. Rescue, or quick relief, inhalers are used only for asthma attacks and should not be used on a daily basis. Monitor for trouble breathing or wheezing.

POP QUIZ 7.2

These conditions are indicative of cystic fibrosis, and the provider will likely order a sweat chloride test.

POP QUIZ 7.3

No longer having a seal-like barky cough, stridor, increased restlessness, drooling, hypoxia, and tripod positioning.

CHAPTER 8

POP QUIZ 8.1

Abdominal distention, inability to swallow due to injury or abnormality, need for more calories than patient can take in orally, heart conditions, IBD, and other GI issues

POP QUIZ 8.2

- Mucus and pus from anus
- Bloody stools
- No fistulas or anal fissures; no upper GI symptoms

POP QUIZ 8.3

Patient is very irritable, demands to be fed despite recently vomiting, and has a palpable small mass in the RUQ.

CHAPTER 9

POP QUIZ 9.1

The nurse should anticipate orders for a urinalysis to look for proteinuria and hematuria and a BMP to measure BUN, creatinine, and electrolyte changes.

POP QUIZ 9.2

The female urethra is shorter than in males and is closer to the rectum, allowing *Escherichia coli* to enter the urethra more easily. Teach girls to wipe front to back after going to the bathroom to avoid introducing *E. coli* into the urethra.

POP QUIZ 9.3

Education on preventing UTIs includes the following: avoid tight-fitting clothing, empty bladder completely and frequently to avoid holding urine, perform proper perineal hygiene, and stay adequately hydrated.

CHAPTER 10

POP QUIZ 10.1

Patient questions: Have you had any trouble seeing? Have you had a bad taste in your mouth?

Caregiver questions: How much is she sleeping daily? How much has she been drinking daily? How often is she urinating? How is her appetite?

POP QUIZ 10.2

The nurse could recommend point-of-care testing because the results are received sooner, and therefore treatment can begin promptly. It has also been shown to shorten hospital stays, reduce complications, and increase adherence. Patients feel better sooner and can get back to a normal routine faster.

POP QUIZ 10.3

The patient needs to take medicine on an empty stomach and at the same time every day. No other medications or supplements should be taken with the medication.

CHAPTER 11

POP QUIZ 11.1

Educate on starting iron supplementation (ferrous sulfate) now that the baby is 4 months old. Anticipate introducing iron-fortified cereals after the infant turns 6 months old.

POP QUIZ 11.2

First, turn off the infusion. Stay with the patient to monitor for anaphylaxis. Ask a coworker to notify the provider. Provide any treatment that is ordered, such as starting oxygen or 0.9% sodium chloride infusion. Give the patient and the family emotional support.

POP QUIZ 11.3

The provider will order oxygen via nasal cannula for shortness of breath and opioids and warm compresses for pain relief.

CHAPTER 12

POP QUIZ 12.1

The nurse should recommend low-impact exercises such as walking and stretching, active ROM exercises, and heat therapy.

POP QUIZ 12.2

Vancomycin should be infused over at least 1 hour to prevent adverse effects of extravasation, phlebitis, and vancomycin flushing syndrome.

POP QUIZ 12.3

The Adam's forward bend test is recommended to screen for scoliosis. It is performed by observing children with an exposed back from behind as they bend forward with their arms at their side.

CHAPTER 13

POP QUIZ 13.1

The total amount of lactated Ringer's solution to provide fluid replacement for this child is 1,192.5 mL.
Explanation: 3 mL × 15.9 kg × 25% TBSA = 1,192 mL.
    The rate for the first 8 hours is 74.5 mL.
    Explanation: Half of 1,192.5 mL = 596.25 mL.
    Administering 596.25 mL over 8 hours = 74.5 mL/hr.

POP QUIZ 13.2

This patient's immobility, nutritional deficiency, chronic conditions, extended hospital stay, and NIPPV medical devices for obstructive sleep apnea and GT for feeding are risk factors for pressure injury.

POP QUIZ 13.3

Use antifungal treatment on the arm as prescribed, perform proper hygiene after activities, avoid sharing clothing and towels with peers, and have any pets examined for tinea.

CHAPTER 14

POP QUIZ 14.1

Hand, foot, and mouth disease is a viral illness that will resolve in about a week. Antibiotics are not effective against viruses. Analgesics like acetaminophen can help with any fever or pain. They should encourage the child to sip fluids or eat ice pops to prevent dehydration.

POP QUIZ 14.2

Rapid flu detection test and oseltamivir, if the test is positive, because it is within 48 hours of flu or flu-like symptoms starting.

POP QUIZ 14.3

Standard contact and airborne precautions should be practiced for this patient.

CHAPTER 15

POP QUIZ 15.1

Inform the patient that even though the classmates are not physically hurting her, they are still engaging in social bullying or cyberbullying. Encourage her to talk to her family about it. Suggest she find a trusted teacher at school and inform them about what is going on.

POP QUIZ 15.2

The nurse should discuss with the mother the rationale for screening for mental health issues such as anxiety, depression, and suicide, since the teenager shows signs of anhedonia, behavior changes, appetite changes, and changes in normal sleep cycle.

POP QUIZ 15.3

Chronic sore throat is a symptom of bulimia due to repetitive irritation from vomiting.

POP QUIZ 15.4

Always educate in a nonjudgmental manner. Teach the parent that sneezing, nasal congestion, and yawning multiple times in a row are symptoms of autonomic dysfunction due to withdrawal, along with sleep-wake cycle disturbances, alterations in tone such as hypertonicity and tremors, GI disturbances, and sensitivity to stimulation.

POP QUIZ 15.5

Warning signs of suicide include sudden cheerfulness after a period of depression and the child giving away their favorite or cherished possessions.

CHAPTER 16

POP QUIZ 16.1

The nurse can recognize the need for de-escalation techniques and remain vigilant for escalation in behavior. The nurse can provide and respect the patient's space after receiving bad news and establish a verbal contract for the remainder of the day's nursing care, setting clear expectations, and offering choices.

POP QUIZ 16.2

The nurse should suspect FDIA and inform the providers. The nurse should also report to social workers and follow policy for reporting abuse while ensuring the patient's safety.

POP QUIZ 16.3

The nurse should first ask the family to leave the patient's room. If all the nurse's de-escalation strategies have failed, the nurse should notify the attending physician and apply appropriate restraints, assuring the patient that safety is the primary concern. The nurse should then make sure an order for restraints is placed. Afterwards, the nurse can work with the patient and family to identify triggers and assist the family by teaching them de-escalation techniques. The nurse will also need to do restraint and extremity checks for proper skin integrity, to ensure that the restraints are correctly applied, and perform neurovascular checks.

APPENDIX A:
COMMON MEDICATIONS
FOR PEDIATRICS

Table A.1 Common Antibiotics and Antifungals for Pediatrics

General Indications	General Mechanism of Action	General Contraindications, Precautions, and Adverse Effects
Aminopenicillins (amoxicillin)		
• Treat otitis media and streptococcal pharyngitis • Used for UTI prophylaxis	• Inhibit bacterial cell wall synthesis by binding to penicillin-binding proteins	• Medication is contraindicated in patients with a penicillin allergy. • Adverse effects include diarrhea, abdominal pain, vomiting, and headache. • Avoid use in patients with infectious mononucleosis due to erythematous rash. • Avoid prolonged use due to development of superinfections or *Clostridium difficile* associated diarrhea.
Cephalosporins (cephalexin)		
• Treat bacterial infections • Used for treatment of UTIs • Used for treatment of osteomyelitis • Used for treatment of otitis media, pneumonia, and skin and soft tissue infection	• Inhibit bacterial cell wall synthesis by binding to penicillin-binding proteins	• Use with caution in children with a history of penicillin allergy and with patients with seizure disorders. • Adverse effects include pruritus, diarrhea, abdominal pain, nausea, and headache. • Avoid prolonged use due to development of superinfections or *C. difficile* associated diarrhea.

(continued)

Table A.1 Common Antibiotics and Antifungals for Pediatrics *(continued)*

General Indications	General Mechanism of Action	General Contraindications, Precautions, and Adverse Effects
Cephalosporin (ceftriaxone)		
• Treat epiglottitis caused by haemophilus influenza • Treat gonococcal infections, meningitis, acute otitis media, UTI, and skin and soft tissue infections	• Inhibit cell wall synthesis by binding to penicillin-binding proteins	• Adverse effects include rash, nausea, vomiting, and diarrhea. • Medication is contraindicated in patients with cephalosporin or penicillin hypersensitivity and in premature infants. • Use with caution in patients with inflammatory bowel disease, liver disease, vitamin K deficiency, or urinary tract obstructions.
Glycopeptide antibiotic (vancomycin)		
• Treat bacterial infections • Treat gram positive osteomyelitis bacterial infections • Treat blood stream infections, pneumonia, meningitis, and skin and soft tissue infections	• Bind to bacterial cell wall inhibiting synthesis.	• Adverse effects include vancomycin flushing syndrome, chest pain, chills, and dizziness; medication can have ototoxic effects. • Adverse effects may include pruritus, Stevens–Johnson syndrome, leukopenia, thrombocytopenia, myalgia, vertigo, malaise, dyspnea, wheezing, and fever. • Adverse effects include ototoxicity, renal toxicity, extravasation, and phlebitis. • Administer over at least 60 minutes and monitor for adverse effects including redness in face, neck, torso, and upper extremities (vancomycin flushing syndrome, formerly known as red man/neck syndrome), and hypotension.
Macrolide antibiotic (erythromycin)		
• Treat pertussis • Treat impetigo and pneumonia • Used as prophylaxis for patients with sickle cell disease • Used as a GI motility agent	• Inhibit RNA-dependent protein synthesis	• Adverse effects include nausea, vomiting, diarrhea, and skin rashes. • Adverse effects seen in infants include hypertrophic pyloric stenosis. • Use with caution in patients with liver or inflammatory bowel disease, seizure disorders, and myasthenia gravis.

(continued)

Table A.1 Common Antibiotics and Antifungals for Pediatrics *(continued)*

General Indications	General Mechanism of Action	General Contraindications, Precautions, and Adverse Effects
Topical aminoglycosides (bacitracin/neomycin/polymyxin B)		
• Neomycin and polymyxin B: effective against gram-negative, aerobic bacteria • Bacitracin: effective against gram-positive bacteria • Used for wound management, skin abrasions, and minor burns	• Bacitracin: inhibit bacterial cell wall synthesis • Neomycin: prevent formation of functional proteins and inhibit DNA polymerase • Polymyxin B: bind to phospholipids on cell membranes of gram-negative bacteria	• Adverse reactions include hypersensitivity reactions, diarrhea, hearing loss, and pruritus. • Medication is contraindicated for use against viral or fungal infections. • Medication is contraindicated in children under 2 years old. • Precaution for systemic exposure, especially in children with renal failure.

Note: All agents are contraindicated in the presence of hypersensitivity to the medication or one of its components.

RESOURCES

Lexicomp. (2021a). Budesonide (oral inhalation): Pediatric drug information [Drug information]. *UpToDate*. https://www.uptodate.com/contents/budesonide-oral-inhalation-drug-information?search=budesonide&source=panel_search_result&selectedTitle=1~140&usage_type=panel&display_rank=1

Lexicomp. (2021b). Dexamethasone: Pediatric drug information [Drug information]. *UpToDate*. https://www.uptodate.com/contents/dexamethasone-systemic-pediatric-drug-information?search=dexamethasone&source=panel_search_result&selectedTitle=2~145&usage_type=panel&display_rank=2#F8015706

Lexicomp. (n.d.[a]). Methylprednisone: Pediatric drug information [Drug Information]. *UpToDate*. https://www.uptodate.com/contents/methylprednisolone-pediatric-drug-information?search=methylprednisolone&source=panel_search_result&selectedTitle=2~148&usage_type=panel&kp_tab=drug_pediatric&display_rank=1#F195345

Lexicomp. (n.d.[b]). Prednisone: Pediatric drug information [Drug Infromation]. *UpToDate*. https://www.uptodate.com/contents/prednisone-pediatric-drug-information?search=prednisone&source=panel_search_result&selectedTitle=2~148&usage_type=panel&kp_tab=drug_pediatric&display_rank=1

Table A.2 Common Pain and Sedation Medications for Pediatrics

General Indications	General Mechanism of Action	General Contraindications, Precautions, and Adverse Effects
Analgesics with antipyretic activity: acetaminophen		
• Reduce fever temporarily • Manage mild to moderate pain	• Activate descending serotonergic inhibitory pathways • Inhibit the hypothalamic heat-regulating center	• Adverse effects include nausea, vomiting, hearing loss, and erythema of the skin. • Contraindications include severe liver disease. • Use cautiously while taking other OTC drugs that may contain acetaminophen.

(continued)

Table A.2 Common Pain and Sedation Medications for Pediatrics *(continued)*

General Indications	General Mechanism of Action	General Contraindications, Precautions, and Adverse Effects
Benzodiazepine (diazepam)		
• Treat acute seizures, status epilepticus, and febrile seizures	• Enhance the inhibitory effect of GABA on neuronal excitability	• Contraindications include untreated open-angle glaucoma, infants younger than 6 months, severe respiratory impairment, sleep apnea, and severe hepatic impairment. • Precautions include amnesia, CNS depression, paradoxical reactions, sleep activity, and suicidal ideation. • Use caution in patients with depression, glaucoma, hepatic and renal impairment, and respiratory disease. • Use with opioids may result in coma, respiratory depression, and death. • Adverse effects include drowsiness. • Medication may be given rectally (diazepam rectal gel).
Benzodiazepine (lorazepam)		
• Used for status epilepticus, anxiety, and sedation	• Enhance the inhibitory effect of GABA on neuronal excitability	• Contraindications include narrow-angle glaucoma, severe respiratory insufficiency, sleep apnea, and premature infants. • Precautions include risk of sleep activities such as driving or cooking while asleep. • Use caution in patients with renal and hepatic impairment or respiratory disease. • Use with opioids may result in coma, respiratory depression, and death. • Adverse effects include local pain at injection site, drowsiness, and sedation.

(continued)

Table A.2 Common Pain and Sedation Medications for Pediatrics *(continued)*

General Indications	General Mechanism of Action	General Contraindications, Precautions, and Adverse Effects
Benzodiazepine (midazolam)		
• Treat acute seizures, status epilepticus, sedation, and anxiolysis	• Enhance the inhibitory effect of GABA on neuronal excitability	• Contraindications include narrow-angle glaucoma and concurrent use with protease inhibitors. • Precautions include risk for amnesia, respiratory depression, hypoxia, apnea, hypotension, paradoxical reactions, and suicidal ideation. • Use with opioids may result in coma, respiratory depression, and death. • Only use in a setting where vital signs can be monitored. • Adverse effects include respiratory depression or arrest, hypoxia, sedation, desaturation, apnea, nasal discomfort (with intranasal administration), and vomiting.
Nonsteroidal anti-inflammatory (ibuprofen)		
• Relief of minor aches and pains as analgesic • Reduce fever temporarily as an antipyretic • Used for juvenile idiopathic arthritis	• Inhibit COX 1 and 2 enzymes to decrease formation of prostaglandin precursors	• Adverse effects include acute kidney injury, increased risk of cardiovascular thrombotic events and gastrointestinal bleeding, ulceration, and inflammation. • Medication is contraindicated in infants less than 6 months old. • Use cautiously in patients with coagulation disorders, liver disease, renal impairment, and hyperkalemia.
Nonsteroidal anti-inflammatory (ketorolac)		
• Pain management	• Inhibit COX 1 and 2 enzymes decreasing formation of prostaglandin precursors	• Adverse effects include abdominal pain, nausea, dyspepsia, increased liver enzymes, and headache. • Medication is contraindicated with NSAID hypersensitivity, recent GI bleeding, and cerebrovascular bleeding. • Monitor for increased risk of acute kidney injury and bleeding.

(continued)

Table A.2 Common Pain and Sedation Medications for Pediatrics *(continued)*

General Indications	General Mechanism of Action	General Contraindications, Precautions, and Adverse Effects
Opioids (methadone)		
• Treat severe pain, opioid withdrawal and neonatal abstinence syndrome	• Bind to opiate receptors and inhibit pain pathways	• Adverse effects include respiratory depression, bradycardia, QT DEprolongation, and constipation. • Methadone may cause CNS depression, constipation, and hypotension. • Medication is contraindicated with severe respiratory depression, hypercarbia, and GI obstructions.
Opioids (morphine)		
• Treat acute and chronic moderate to severe pain • Management of chronic severe pain in patients who require daily, around-the-clock long-term opioid treatment • Dyspnea in patients with end-stage cancer or pulmonary disease • Procedural sedation	• Act at the mu receptor, causing changes in perception to pain at the spinal cord and into the CNS	• Medication is contraindicated in significant respiratory depression in unmonitored settings, acute or severe bronchial asthma (oral solutions), respiratory depression or hypoxia, upper airway obstruction, acute alcoholism or delirium tremens (rectal route), known or suspected GI obstruction or paralytic ileus, hypovolemia, circulatory shock, cardiac arrhythmia or heart failure secondary to chronic lung disease, and concurrent use with MAO inhibitor therapy. • Use caution in substance abuse, alcoholism, opioid naïve patients, CNS depression, head trauma, seizures or increased ICP, cardiac disease, adrenal insufficiency, hypothyroidism, and myxedema. • Do not abruptly discontinue, as withdrawal symptoms can occur. • Adverse effects include ileus, bradycardia, arrhythmia, increased ICP, bronchospasm, GI obstruction, laryngospasm, depression, confusion, hypoxia, edema, euphoria, delirium, dysphagia, hallucinations, psychosis, physiologic dependence, adrenocortical insufficiency, drowsiness, diarrhea, constipation, headache, fever, nausea, restlessness, and vomiting.

(continued)

Table A.2 Common Pain and Sedation Medications for Pediatrics *(continued)*

General Indications	General Mechanism of Action	General Contraindications, Precautions, and Adverse Effects
Opioid (hydromorphone, oxycodone)		
• Acute moderate or severe pain • Sedation and patient-controlled PCA	• Bind to opioid receptor in CNS and inhibit ascending pain pathways	• Adverse effects on the CNS include abnormal dreams, abnormal gait, agitation, CNS depression, fatigue, sleep disorder, and restlessness. • Monitor for CNS depression, constipation, hypotension, and respiratory depression. • Medication is contraindicated in patients with severe asthma or GI obstruction. • Prolonged use during pregnancy can cause neonatal opioid withdrawal syndrome.
Platelet aggregation inhibitors, salicylates (aspirin)		
• Used in Kawasaki Disease, rheumatic fever, MIS-C • Used to treat ischemic stroke and in children with prosthetic heart valves	• Inhibit COX 1 and 2 enzymes • Inhibit platelet aggregation • Has antipyretic, analgesic, and anti-inflammatory properties	• Adverse effects include bleeding and GI disturbances. • Medication is contraindicated in children with or recovering from viral illnesses, specifically varicella or influenza, due to association with Reye's syndrome. • Medication is contraindicated in children with asthma, rhinitis, and nasal polyps. • Use cautiously in patients with bleeding disorders, liver disease, renal impairment, and gastritis.

RESOURCES

Lexicomp. (2021a). Acetaminophen: Pediatric drug information [Drug Information]. *UpToDate.* https://www.uptod ate.com/contents/acetaminophen-paracetamol-pediatric-drug-information?search=acetaminophen&source=pa nel_search_result&selectedTitle=2~148&usage_type=panel&kp_tab=drug_pediatric&display_rank=1#F129282

Lexicomp. (2021b). Aspirin: Pediatric drug information [Drug Information]. *UpToDate.* https://www.uptodate.com /contents/aspirin-pediatric-drug-information?search=aspirin&source=panel_search_result&selectedTitle=2~14 8&usage_type=panel&kp_tab=drug_pediatric&display_rank=1

Lexicomp. (2021c). Diazepam: Pediatric drug information [Drug Information]. *UpToDate.* https://www.uptodate .com/contents/diazepam-drug-information?source=auto_suggest&selectedTitle=1~3---1~3---diaz&search=diaz epam#F158987

Lexicomp. (2021d). Hydromorphone: Pediatric drug information [Drug Information]. *UpToDate.* https://www.upto date.com/contents/hydromorphone-pediatric-drug-information?search=hydromorphone&source=panel_searc h_result&selectedTitle=2~148&usage_type=panelkp_tab=drug_pediatric&display_rank=1#F180566

Lexicomp. (2021e). Ibuprofen: Pediatric drug information [Drug Information]. *UpToDate.* https://www.uptodate .com/contents/ibuprofen-pediatric-drug-information?search=ibuprofen&source=panel_search_result&selectedTit le=2~148&usage_type=panel&kp_tab=drug_pediatric&display_rank=1

Lexicomp. (2021f). Ketorolac: Pediatric drug information. *UpToDate.* https://www.uptodate.com/contents/ketorolac -systemic-pediatric-drug-information?search=ketorolac&source=panel_search_result&selectedTitle=2~143&us age_type=panel&display_rank=2&showDrugLabel=true#F8345802

Lexicomp. (2021g). Lorazepam: Pediatric drug information. *UpToDate*. https://www.uptodate.com/contents/lorazep am-pediatric-drug-information?search=lorazepam&source=panel_search_result&selectedTitle=2~148&usage_ type=panel&kp_tab=drug_pediatric&display_rank=1#F189951

Lexicomp. (2021h). Methadone: Pediatric drug information. *UpToDate*. https://www.uptodate.com/contents/metha done-pediatric-drug-information?search=methadone&source=panel_search_result&selectedTitle=2~148&usag e_type=panel&kp_tab=drug_pediatric&display_rank=1#F193961

Lexicomp. (2021i). Midazolam: Pediatric drug information. *UpToDate*. https://www.uptodate.com/contents/midazo lam-pediatric-drug-information?search=midazolam&source=panel_search_result&selectedTitle=2~148&usage _type=panel&kp_tab=drug_pediatric&display_rank=1#F196402

Lexicomp. (2021j). Morphine: Pediatric drug information. *UpToDate*. https://www.uptodate.com/contents/morphin e-pediatric-drug-information?search=morphine&source=panel_search_result&selectedTitle=2~148&usage_ty pe=panel&kp_tab=drug_pediatric&display_rank=1

Lexicomp. (2021k). Oxycodone: Pediatric drug information. *UpToDate*. https://www.uptodate.com/contents/oxyco done-drug-information?source=auto_suggest&selectedTitle=1~4---1~4---oxyco&search=oxycodone#F204871

Table A.3 Common Steroids for Pediatrics

General Indications	General Mechanism of Action	General Contraindications, Precautions, and Adverse Effects
Corticosteroids (dexamethasone)		
• Used for moderate to severe asthma exacerbations or status asthmaticus • Used for croup and airway edema	• Reduce swelling and inflammation in airways by suppression of neutrophil migration	• Adverse effects include effects on growth, adrenal suppression, infection, and increased ocular pressure. • Use caution in immunosuppression and inhibition of bone growth; monitor for fractures.
Corticosteroids (methylprednisolone, prednisone, prednisolone)		
• Used for moderate to severe asthma exacerbations or status asthmaticus • Administration: oral (prednisolone and prednisone) or IV or IM (methylprednisolone) • Used for juvenile idiopathic arthritis, Kawasaki disease, nephrotic syndrome, and ulcerative colitis	• Suppress or decrease inflammation	• Adverse effects include GI upset, weight gain, and mood changes. • Medication is contraindicated in patients with fungal, viral, and bacterial infections. • Prednisolone is contraindicated in patients with sulfite or tartrazine hypersensitivity. • Use with caution in patients with immunosuppression, growth inhibition, adrenal suppression, and increased intracranial pressure.
Inhaled corticosteroid (budesonide, fluticasone)		
• Decrease airway inflammation and bronchoconstriction	• Reduce allergic responses associated with allergies	• Adverse effects include thrush; rinse mouth after each use. • Adverse effects include growth suppression. • Use with caution in immunocompromised patients. • Use with caution in long-term use for nasal septum perforation or ulcers. • Do not abruptly discontinue; monitor for adrenal insufficiency.

RESOURCES

Lexicomp. (2021a). Budesonide (oral inhalation): Pediatric drug information [Drug information]. *UpToDate.* https://www.uptodate.com/contents/budesonide-oral-inhalation-drug-information?search=budesonide&source=panel_search_result&selectedTitle=1~140&usage_type=panel&display_rank=1

Lexicomp. (2021b). Dexamethasone: Pediatric drug information [Drug information]. *UpToDate.* https://www.uptodate.com/contents/dexamethasone-systemic-pediatric-drug-information?search=dexamethasone&source=panel_search_result&selectedTitle=2~145&usage_type=panel&display_rank=2#F8015706

Lexicomp. (n.d.[a]). Methylprednisone: Pediatric drug information [Drug Information]. *UpToDate.* https://www.uptodate.com/contents/methylprednisolone-pediatric-drug-information?search=methylprednisolone&source=panel_search_result&selectedTitle=2~148&usage_type=panel&kp_tab=drug_pediatric&display_rank=1#F195345

Lexicomp. (n.d.[b]). Prednisone: Pediatric drug information [Drug Information]. *UpToDate.* https://www.uptodate.com/contents/prednisone-pediatric-drug-information?search=prednisone&source=panel_search_result&selectedTitle=2~148&usage_type=panel&kp_tab=drug_pediatric&display_rank=1

References

APPENDIX B:
ACRONYMS FOR PEDIATRICS

AAP	American Academy of Pediatrics
ABG	arterial blood gases
ABR	auditory brainstem response test
ACE	angiotensin-converting enzyme
ADA	Americans with Disabilities Act
ADHD	attention-deficit hyperactivity disorder
ADLs	activities of daily living
AIDS	acquired immunodeficiency syndrome
AKI	acute kidney injury
ALL	acute lymphoblastic leukemia
ALT	alanine aminotransferase
AML	acute myeloid leukemia
ANC	absolute neutrophil count
ANCC	American Nurses Credentialing Center
AP	anteroposterior
ARDS	acute respiratory distress syndrome
ASD	atrial septal defect
AST	aspartate aminotransferase
AV	atrioventricular
AVSD	atrioventricular canal defect
BAER	brainstem auditory evoked response
BBB	blood brain barrier
BiPAP	bilevel positive airway pressure
BMI	body mass index
BMP	basic metabolic panel
BP	blood pressure
BUN	blood urea nitrogen
CAUTI	catheter-associated urinary tract infection
CaEDTA	calcium ethylenediaminetetraacetate
CaNa$_2$EDTA	edetate calcium disodium
CBC	complete blood count
CDC	Centers for Disease Control and Prevention
CF	cystic fibrosis
CLABSI	central line-associated bloodstream infection
CMP	comprehensive metabolic panel
CNS	central nervous system
CO	carbon monoxide
COX	cyclooxygenase
CP	cerebral palsy
CPAP	continuous positive airway pressure
CPN	Certified Pediatric Nurse
CPR	cardiopulmonary resuscitation
CRIES	crying, requires increased oxygen administration, increased vital signs, expression, sleeplessness
CRP	C-reactive protein
CSF	cerebrospinal fluid
CT	computed tomography

CV	cardiovascular
CVC	central venous catheter
DAA	direct-acting antiviral
DI	diabetes insipidus
DIC	disseminated intravascular coagulation
DMARD	disease-modifying anti-rheumatic drug
DNR	do not resuscitate
DTaP	diphtheria and tetanus toxoids and acellular pertussis vaccine
EEG	electroencephalogram
EKG	electrocardiogram
ER	extended release
ESR	erythrocyte sedimentation rate
ETT	endotracheal tube
FACES	facial analysis comparison and elimination system
FDA	U.S. Food and Drug Administration
FDIA	factitious disorder in another
FFP	fresh frozen plasma
FLACC	faces, legs, activity, cry, consolability
FTT	failure to thrive
GABA	gamma-aminobutyric acid
GAD	generalized anxiety disorder
GAS	group A streptococcus
GCS	Glasgow Coma Scale
GER	gastroesophageal reflux
GERD	gastroesophageal reflux disease
GFR	glomerular filtration rate
GI	gastrointestinal
GT	gastrostomy tube
HbA1C	glycated hemoglobin
HDL	high-density lipoprotein
HiB	*Haemophilus influenzae* type B vaccine
HIPAA	Health Insurance Portability and Accountability Act
HIV	human immunodeficiency virus
HLHS	hypoplastic left heart syndrome
HOB	head of bed
HPV	human papillomavirus
HR	heart rate
HSV	herpes simplex virus
HVAC	heating, ventilation, and air conditioning
I/O	intake and output
IBD	inflammatory bowel disease
ICP	intracranial pressure
IgA	immunoglobulin A
IgM	immunoglobulin M
IGRA	Interferon gamma release assay
IM	intramuscular
INR	international normalized ratio
IR	interventional radiology
ITP	immune thrombocytopenic purpura
IV	intravenous
JT	jejunostomy tube
KOH	potassium hydroxide
LABA	long-acting beta agonists
LDL	low-density lipoprotein
LFT	liver function tests
LGBTQ+	lesbian, gay, bisexual, transgender, queer, other sexual identities
LOC	level of consciousness

LR	lactated Ringer's
MAO	monoamine oxidase inhibitor
MIS-C	multisystem inflammatory syndrome in children
MMR	measles, mumps, and rubella vaccine
MR	mitral regurgitation
MRI	magnetic resonance imaging
MVA	motor vehicle accident
Na$_2$EDTA	ethylenedinitrilotetraacetic acid disodium salt dihydrate
NAS	neonatal abstinence syndrome
ND	nasoduodenal
NG	nasogastric
NJ	nasojejunal
NICU	neonatal intensive care unit
NIPPV	nasal intermittent positive pressure ventilation
N-PASS	neonatal pain, agitation, and sedation scale
NPH	neutral protamine hagedorn
NPO	nothing by mouth
NS	normal saline
NSAID	non-steroidal anti-inflammatory drug
NSS	nephron-sparing surgery
OCD	obsessive-compulsive disorder
ORT	oral rehydration therapy
OTC	over the counter
PAS	pediatric appendicitis score
PCOS	polycystic ovary syndrome
PCR	polymerase chain reaction
PDA	patent ductus arteriosus
PED-BC	Pediatric Nursing Board certification
PFT	pulmonary function test
pH	potential/power of hydrogen
PICC	peripherally inserted central catheter
PICU	pediatric intensive care unit
PNCB	Pediatric Nursing Certification Board
PO	by mouth
PPI	proton pump inhibitor
PRBC	packed red blood cells
PT	prothrombin time
PTSD	posttraumatic stress disorder
PTT	partial thromboplastin time
PUCAI	pediatric ulcerative colitis activity index
RBC	red blood cell
RLQ	right lower quadrant
RN	registered nurse
ROM	range of motion
ROME	respiratory opposite, metabolic equal
RR	respiratory rate
RSV	respiratory syncytial virus
RT-PCR	reverse-transcriptase polymerase chain reaction
RUQ	right upper quandrant
SA	sinoatrial
SABA	short-acting beta-agonists
SCWOARA	spinal cord injury without radiographic abnormality
SIADH	syndrome of inappropriate antidiuretic hormone secretion
SIDS	sudden infant death syndrome
SSRI	selective serotonin reuptake inhibitor
STI	sexually transmitted infection
TB	tuberculosis

TBI	traumatic brain injury
TBSA	total body surface area
Tdap	tetanus, diphtheria, and acellular pertussis vaccine
TNF	tumor necrosis factor
TOF	tetralogy of fallot
TSH	thyroid-stimulating hormone
UA	urinalysis
UC	ulcerative colitis
URI	upper respiratory infection
UTI	urinary tract infection
VP	ventriculoperitoneal
VSD	ventricular septal defect
WAGR	Wilms' tumor, aniridia, genitourinary
WBC	white blood count
WHO	World Health Organization

INDEX

Printed in the United States
by Baker & Taylor Publisher Services